*A Manual of Central
Venous Catheterization and
Parenteral Nutrition*

A Manual of Central Venous Catheterization and Parenteral Nutrition

Edited by **J. L. Peters** FRCS

Resident Assistant Surgeon
University College Hospital
London

with a Foreword by
H. J. C. Swan MD

WRIGHT · PSG

Bristol London Boston
1983

Published by:
John Wright & Sons Ltd, 823–825 Bath Road,
Bristol BS4 5NU, England.
John Wright PSG Inc., 545 Great Road, Littleton,
Massachusetts 01460, USA.

British Library Cataloguing in Publication Data
A Manual of Central Venous Catheterization and Parenteral Nutrition.
  1. Cardiac catheterization
  I. Peters, J. L.
  616.1′20754   RC683.5.C25

ISBN 0 7236 0549 1

Library of Congress Catalog Card Number: 82–70100

Typset and printed in Great Britain by John Wright & Sons (Printing) Ltd at The Stonebridge Press, Bristol

Preface

Experience has shown that in surgery and medicine all techniques, procedures and drugs have their own particular drawbacks. Often these may not always be apparent at first sight, and even when recognized, there is a natural desire to dismiss these undesirable features of a particular technique or therapeutic advance. During the past 50 years central venous catheterization has gradually gained a place in the management of critically ill patients. The associated insertion techniques and devices have proved to be of immense benefit for those patients who require temporary haemodynamic monitoring, circulatory support, prolonged intravenous feeding or chemotherapy in order to restore their health.

During the past 30 years central venous catheterization and parenteral nutrition have been associated with hazards, many of which have been undoubtedly iatrogenic in origin, whilst others can be ascribed to technical failures in the equipment provided by manufacturers. Furthermore, junior clinical staff often learn the techniques and knowledge concerning the maintenance of such systems by a process of trial and error. Complications have become accepted almost as inherent hazards of the techniques.

Should this be the case? Is there an unwarranted attitude of complacency prevailing? What improvements in this field of patient care could be made?

The aim of this book is to help final year medical students and junior medical and nursing staff to avoid the associated pitfalls that have already been documented in the literature. An attempt has been made by the contributors to cover the clinical spectrum in which the techniques of central venous catheterization and the related devices are used. The intention is to provide a review of both the past history and the current state of the art (excluding diagnostic angiocardiographic techniques) and to provide an introduction to the essential principles of parenteral nutrition. Rather than present a multiple choice of approaches, which would only serve to confuse the beginner, the descriptions of percutaneous insertion procedures have been limited to a few techniques for each vein which are known to be safe and effective.

It is the hope of the contributors that through this book the incidence of inherent hazards may be reduced and the safety of patients ensured.

J. L. P.

Contributors

Rodney F. Armstrong FFARCS
Consultant Anaesthetist, Intensive Care Unit, University College Hospital, London

Phillip A. Belsham FRCS
Resident Surgical Officer, Brompton Hospital, London; and Surgical Registrar to University College Hospital, London

Alan C. Edwards FRACP
Staff Cardiologist, Royal North Shore Hospital, St Leonard's, Sydney, Australia.

Ian C. W. English FFARCS
Emeritus Consultant Anaesthetist to the Brompton Hospital, London

John V. Farman FFARCS
Consultant Anaesthetist to Addenbrooke's Hospital, Cambridge

Cyril Fisher MRC PATH
Consultant Pathologist, Royal Marsden Hospital, Fulham Road, London

Christopher P. O. Garrett FFARCS
Senior Registrar in Anaesthesia to The Hospital for Sick Children, Great Ormond Street, London and to University College Hospital, London

Reuben Grüneberg MD MRCPATH
Consultant Microbiologist to University College Hospital, London

Rowland B. Hopkinson FFARCS
Consultant Anaesthetist and Director of the Intensive Therapy Unit, East Birmingham Hospital, Bordesley Green East, Birmingham

Julian Jessop MB BS
Surgical Registrar to Queen Elizabeth Hospital for Children, Hackney, London and to University College Hospital, London

Andrew J. Macnab MD
Neonatologist, Department of Paediatrics, The University of British Columbia, Vancouver, Canada

John Moxham MRCP
Consultant Physician, Chest Unit, Kings College Hospital, London

Malcolm Panter-Brick DCH, MRCP
Consultant Paediatrician to Sunderland and South Shields District General Hospitals; formerly Lecturer in Paediatrics, The Children's Hospital, Ladywood, Birmingham

David L. H. Patterson MD, FRCP
Consultant Physician and Cardiologist to the Whittington Hospital and the Royal Free Hospital, London

Joseph L. Peters FRCS
Resident Assistant Surgeon and Senior Registrar to University College Hospital, London

Michael J. Rennie PHD
Wellcome Senior Lecturer, Department of Human Metabolism, The Rayne Institute, University College School of Medicine, London

J. C. St George
District Sterile Services Manager, University
College Hospital, Gower Street, London

Lynne T. Sawyer SRN, DN RNCT
Formerly Sister to the Accident and
Emergency Ward, University College Hospital,
London; and formerly Sister to the
Intensive Care Unit, Barnet General
Hospital, Barnet, Hertfordshire

Jonathan C. L. Shaw MRCP
Consultant Paediatrician, Regional Neonatal
Intensive Care Unit, University College
Hospital, London

Peter D. Wright MD, FRCS
Consultant Surgeon to the Freeman
Hospital, Newcastle upon Tyne

Acknowledgements

I should like to thank Professor Charles G. Clark, the surgeons and nursing staff of University College Hospital, London, for their support, advice, ideas and criticism during the development of this book. I am also indebted to Dr Bernard Lucas, Consultant Anaesthetist to University College Hospital and the National Heart Hospital, London, for his encouragement during the project and to Mr J. C. R. Lincoln, Consultant Cardiothoracic Surgeon to the Brompton Hospital, for providing the initial stimulus to create the manuscript. I also owe a great deal to Mr Roy Baker of John Wright and Sons Ltd for being so patient over the years and illuminating the way forward with such good humour.

A special debt of gratitude is owed by all the contributors to Mr Robert N. Lane for his excellent illustrations; to Mr V. K. Astor and Mr D. Ellis of University College Hospital Medical School for producing such fine graphs, figures and clinical photographs; and to the clinicians who have generously contributed photographs for publication. Furthermore, I am indebted to the editors of several journals for granting permission to reproduce important items and due acknowledgement has been made appropriately in the text.

Finally, this work could not have been completed without the dedication shown by my wife nor without the secretarial expertise of Miss Yvonne Bisset, Mrs Marisa Nottley and the assistants of the individual contributors.

Contents

II. CENTRAL VENOUS CATHETERS AND PARENTERAL NUTRITION

Foreword

by **H. J. C. Swan** MD, PhD, FRCP. Director of Cardiology, Cedars–Sinai Medical Center, Los Angeles, California

In the past it has been a near universally accepted truth that successful outcome of surgical procedures was largely, if not entirely, a consequence of the inherent skills, speed and sagacity of the operating surgeon. Many adhered to the belief that careful and detailed evaluation of the condition of the patient resulted only in delay in the important business at hand: completion of the surgical procedure. It is now evident that an increasing population stands in need of, and many substantively benefit from, surgical interventions. The results in these patients, however, may be dependent upon the management of disorders of multiple systems throughout the body, the severity or intensity of the primary surgical problem, and the effective participation of health care personnel other than the operating surgeon.

In this respect, the past two decades have been characterized by an enormous increase in the skills of the anaesthetist. The development of a wide variety of pharmacological agents to manipulate many aspects of biological behaviour, techniques to measure and control gas exchange, and to maintain the seriously compromised patient in a relatively optimal state, now extends the potential of surgical therapy by an order of magnitude.

This monograph addresses a vital part of these processes, namely central venous cannulation and catheterization. The importance of these techniques allows for not only optimal adjustment of circulatory parameters by haemodynamic measurements, but is frequently and in a complementary manner, a fundamental part of the nutritional management of the critically ill. The application of techniques of central venous cannulation is the particular responsibility of the modern anaesthetist. Because the broad principles of venous cannulation are relatively simple, sloppy techniques and careless application have crept into their effective implementation. Thus, complications, which are inevitable in any invasive procedure, are inversely related to experience and the development of appropriate skills. But it should not be necessary for all users to repeat all the complications with the same degree of frequency. Awareness of the potential for complications and application of strict protocols in detail will minimize the occurrence of such complications.

One of the major complications, although frequently not addressed as such, is the failure on the part of the treating physician to understand and apply in an optimal manner the data obtained by haemodynamic measurements. It has been not unknown for treating physicians to ignore completely adverse haemodynamic measurement data in an apparently stable clinical situation, only to have disaster strike within a predictably short time. Hence, it is essential for medical care personnel to be adequately trained in the application of principles of measurement, to be aware of measurement artifacts, and to be able to confirm the validity or error of measurements of vital functions. The ability to make such measurements in the surgical patient was developed initially in response to the needs of cardiac surgery. As the emphasis in primary cardiac procedures moved from younger patients with relatively healthy mycardium to patients with overt and relatively severe coronary artery disease, then the issues of perioperative management in the avoidance of myocardial infarction became vital. The application of haemodynamic measurements and monitoring then was extended to aortic surgery—in particular, the correction of aneurysm or disection in the thorax. Prostatic surgical procedures are common in the elderly patient in whom there is a significant incidence of overt or covert coronary artery disease. These patients also are subjected to massive fluid shifts during the course of the surgical procedure. Extensive multisystem disease or large scale excision for malignancy, again more common in the elderly, can only be successful if accompanied by optimal stabilization of vital organ functions.

One of the newer areas of interest is in the management of the trauma and burn patient. Relatively important alterations occur in the pulmonary circulation under these circumstances and the outcome may be decided by failure of the right ventricle, whether by reason of changes in the lungs or depression of overall myocardial function. Correction of these aspects of complex disorders may be vital for survival in such instances.

Central venous cannulation and catheterization is a vital part of all aspects of modern surgery. There is no reason to believe that it will diminish in the future. Its effective application in minimizing mortality and morbidity and maximizing the optimal recovery of the critically ill or injured patient is of vital concern to all. This monograph sets important guidelines and standards that will materially assist in these objectives.

I   General Principles of Central Venous Catheter Insertion

Chapter 1

Historical Review

J. L. Peters

The venous system has been the subject of close observation since the dawn of civilization. The ancient philosophers and natural scientists attempted to provide rational explanations for bodily functions; Alcmaeon of Crotona, in the late sixth century BC, thought that sleep arose from the retreat of blood to blood-carrying veins and that death occurred by the total retreat of blood into these vessels. Aristotle (384–322 BC), a great natural historian and the first person to illustrate a biological treatise, considered the heart to be the seat of intelligence, and he noted that 'as they advance, blood vessels become ever smaller, until at last their tubes are too fine to admit the blood'.

Praxagoras of Cos (335 BC) distinguished between arteries and veins. The first footholds in anatomical knowledge were placed by Herophilus of Chalcedon at Alexandria in the third century BC. He was also the first to count the pulse and to make an analysis of its variations using a water-clock or clepsydra. In the same period at the Alexandrian school, Eristratus of Chios, who, alongside Galen, may be considered as one of the 'fathers of physiology', thought that in life blood was present in the liver, veins and heart alone. Air was taken up by the lungs and changed into a 'pneuma' or 'spirit of life' in the left heart. The reasoning behind this concept, which misled the early philosophers, including Aristotle, was that after violent death, the liver, veins and right heart are engorged with blood. The spirit of life, according to Eristratus, was carried to all parts of the body by the arteries and in the brain this spirit changed to the second 'pneuma' or 'psychic spirit'.

Galen of Pergamum (AD 130–200) projected his views so well that they dictated medicine for more than a thousand years. He postulated the existence of three pneumata. Foodstuffs were taken as chyle from the gut to the liver and there changed to blood. The lowest pneuma, the 'spirit of growth', was located in the liver, veins and right heart. The ebb and flow of venous blood distributed this spirit to all parts of the body. He disproved the work of Eristratus concerning arteries and by experiment showed that they and the left heart contained blood. The second pneuma, the 'spirit of life', was situated in the left heart and arteries, and was formed there from the combination of air brought in from the lungs by the pulmonary vein with the blood reaching the left heart from the right side of the heart via minute pores in the interventricular septum. This pneuma was responsible for pulsatile force, anger, courage, rage and personality. The spirit of life reached the ventricles of the brain and here the third pneuma, the 'spirit of pysche', was formed. The dogma created by Galen concerning the passage of venous blood through invisible pores held up physiological progress for centuries.

Not all philosophers and natural scientists agreed with classical Galenical teaching and Ibn an-Nafis (al-Qurashi, circa 1210–1288) of Damascus postulated that blood was heated and refined in the right ventricle and passed up the artery-like vein or pulmonary trunk; a fraction of the blood was further refined by transudation through the thick walls of the vein and the least refined portion was used for nutrition of the lungs. The filtered fraction and air passed back to the heart after penetrating the walls of the pulmonary venous plexus, and further mixture with air occurred in the left ventricle in order to make the spirit of life.

Leonardo da Vinci (1452–1519) was the next man after Aristotle to recognize the scientific value of illustration. He provided a great impetus to the study of anatomy and he dissected cadavers and animals. He considered that it was impossible for air to reach the heart. He performed inflation experiments using lungs and considered that the pulmonary arteries received the 'freshness of air' from the bronchi. Whilst Galen taught that the liver was the origin of the great veins, Leonardo maintained that the heart gave rise to these vessels.

Vesalius (1514–1564) published 'De humani corporis fabrica libri septem', a work of fundamental importance to physiology, which provided a complete and accurate description of the whole human body. He later demonstrated that the pulsation of arteries depended on the heart and was not an inherent feature of these vessels. He described the presence of pericardial fluid, and he performed an important experiment in an animal in which he showed that if the lungs of an animal were collapsed with a tube situated in the trachea, the heart could be brought almost to a standstill and that successive artificial ventilations of the lungs would restore the heart's activity to normal. He noted that although the interventricular system was pitted, no pores penetrated from the right to the left ventricle.

Thus, Vesalius and Ibn an-Nafis cast doubt upon the classical Galenical dogma. Botallus (1564) thought that blood passed from the right to the left side of the heart via the foramen ovale which he had noted in dissection of calves and other animals. Andreas Caesalpius (1519–1603) of Arezzo, first used the word 'circulatio'; however, he adopted Aristotle's belief in the supremacy of the heart and did not oppose Galen's view that the blood was strained through pores in the interventricular septum. The next most important discovery concerning circulatory physiology was made by Hieronymus Fabricius (1530–1619) who, in 1574, was the first to discover 'valves' during the course of his dissections in Padua, where he succeeded Fallopius as Professor of Surgery with charge of anatomy. William Harvey (1578–1657) visited Padua shortly after leaving Caius and Gonville College, Cambridge, in 1599. He produced his first book, 'Exercitatio anatomica de motu cordis et sanguinis', in 1628. Henry Power (1623–1668) mentioned the 'circulatio harveiana inventa ab authore A.D. 1614', suggesting that people were aware of Harvey's work well before the publication of his book. In the 9 years prior to the publication of his work, Harvey had convinced and obtained the agreement of his colleagues at the College of Physicians by providing numerous demonstrations. This manuscript was indeed one of the most important medical works ever written, and a most excellent, comprehensive review is provided by Franklin (1).

THE ORIGINS OF VENOUS ACCESS

Shortly after Harvey's discovery, Sir Christopher Wren made the first attempts at providing intravenous nutrition and injecting drugs (2). In 1656, using a goose quill attached to a pig's bladder, he infused a mixture of wine, ale and opium into dogs. He was not alone in this field of inquiry, for Richard Lower (3, 4) and Major in 1662 (5) performed intravenous infusions and transfusions on animals. Robert Boyle described the work of Wren, and he performed experiments using intravenous infusion from animals to man (6, 7). Denys transfused blood from a lamb into a human being in 1667 in Paris (8) and Lower performed the first successful transfusion of animal blood into a human in the same year. These practices soon fell into disrepute, as fatal reactions occurred and a Church and Parliamentary Edict prevented further transfusions until 1818, when James Blundell, an English obstetrician, saved the lives of several patients with postpartum haemorrhage by injecting blood using a syringe (9).

In 1733 Stephen Hales conceived the idea of introducing a glass tube into the venous and arterial systems of a live mare in order to measure blood pressure. He also made the first attempts to estimate the cardiac output by bleeding the animal to death and filling its left ventricle with melted beeswax. He multiplied the volume of the solidified wax by the normal resting heart rate in order to achieve figures for the cardiac output of dogs, oxen, sheep and men (10).

Cardiac catheterization was first performed by Claude Bernard in order to determine the temperature of the blood in the right and left ventricles. Lavoisier had suggested that animal heat was produced as a result of respiratory gas exchange in the lungs (11) whilst Gustav Magnus had advanced the alternative hypothesis that 'combustion' took place in the tissues (12). In 1844 Bernard operated upon a horse and cannulated the carotid artery and left ventricle, followed by the internal jugular vein and right ventricle, using a long mercury thermometer (13). He disproved the pulmonary combustion theory, and later he went on to measure intracardiac pressures using glass tubes. Bernard also noted in an autopsy on a dog that the right ventricle had been perforated by the tube, causing intrapericardial haemorrhage, and thus he recorded the first complication of central catheterization (13).

The first systematic study, description and interpretation of intracardiac pressure recordings was made in 1861 by Chauveau and Marey after working at the School of Veterinary Medicine of Alfort near Paris (14). They developed a special double lumen catheter, and Marey wrote, 'one can be reassured of the innocuity of this method by examining the horse, who is scarcely disturbed, walks and eats as usual. In only a few instances is the pulse rate slightly increased, especially at the time of the catheter's introduction within the heart cavities'. Thus, he first noted the potential for arrhythmias to occur as a complication. He also emphasized the importance of extending the clinical examination to include the exploration of many cavities and canalicular systems with catheters; however, neither he nor Chauveau extended their investigations to man. During the following years cardiac catheterization developed rapidly as an investigation in circulatory physiology and new manometric systems were developed. Rolleston pointed out the role of friction along the tube from the exploring cannula to the manometer (15). Porter studied the canine heart using silver-plated brass tubes with a single or double lumen and an internal diameter of 3 mm, connected by a 30–40 cm length of rubber tubing with the same diameter as the manometer (16). At this time arguments surrounded the question of whether or not such catheters and manometers accurately reflected the intracardiac pressures. These questions were finally resolved by Otto Franck in 1903 when he published his classic papers (17, 18).

Controversy surrounds the earliest pioneers of central venous catheterization in man. Werner Forssmann, André Cournand and Dickinson Richards jointly shared the 1956 Nobel Prize for Medicine. The first to report the use of a catheter in man for obtaining mixed venous blood and for the measurement of right atrial pressure or cardiac output were Cournand and Ranges in 1941 (19). They mention Forssmann as the originator of central venous catheterization technique. In 1929, shortly after the publication of Forssmann's paper in which he described his self-catheterization experiment (20), an addendum was published in which Forssman referred to a communication stating

> Professor E. Unger informs me that Bleichroeder, Unger and Loeb carried out the same experiment in 1912. This was published under the title—'Intra-arterielle Therapie'. He [Unger] had passed a ureteric catheter into the arm veins up to the axilla on four human subjects, among them Dr Bleichroeder, and also from the thigh to the vena cava. To judge from the length of the catheter and a stabbing pain, he believed that in the case of Dr Bleichroeder, the catheter must reach the right heart. This latter experiment was not published.

The reference provided by Unger alluded to presentations by Bleichroeder, Unger and Loeb before the Hufeland Medical Society in Berlin (21). Bleichroeder reported in 1905 that he had passed catheters into the arteries and veins of dogs as well as of human beings. He did not believe the experiments to be of any practical value and left them unpublished. However, in 1912, with the opening of the 'chemotherapeutic era', he perceived a use for his method, as it was believed at the time that a chemotherapeutic agent should be applied as near as possible to the diseased organ. Thus, in four patients with puerperal sepsis, Bleichroeder and Unger inserted a catheter via the femoral artery up to the region of the aortic bifurcation and injected 'Collargol'. In his address, Bleichroeder did not specify the nature of his experiments in 1905, but remarked that he had used the catheter to obtain blood from the inferior vena cava close to the hepatic vein. He was interested in the morbid anatomy of cirrhosis and these investigations may have been related (22). In his paper concerning intra-arterial therapy he stated that he had passed the catheter well over a hundred times through the femoral vein and left it in place for several hours without clot formation or other ill-effects. Naturally, he was unable to verify the exact position of catheters using contrast radiology.

Werner Forssmann conceived the idea of introducing a catheter into the right heart in order to administer emergency drugs on the operating table in the most rapid and effective way during episodes of sudden cardiac failure. He was opposed to percutaneous intracardiac injections because of the risks of cardiac tamponade from either a coronary vessel laceration caused by the needle or leakage of blood from the heart itself, and of pneumothorax from pleural laceration. He first attempted the approach on cadavers using a vein in the antecubital fossa of the left arm. He chose the left arm because the catheter had to make less of a curve when it passed through the subclavian and innominate veins. He also realized that this occurred because of the relatively acute angle at which various tributaries entered the main brachial, axillary and subclavian veins, pointing always in the direction of blood flow (*Fig.* 1.1).

At the time Forssmann was working in the small town of Eberswalde, 50 miles north-east of Berlin, as assistant in the surgical department under Dr Schneider. Although a friend and mentor, Schneider denied permission for Forssmann's plans to attempt the procedure on patients or on himself. Forssmann could not be deterred, however, and he decided to carry out the experiment upon himself. A wide-bore needle was inserted into a right cubital fossa vein, through which an ureteric catheter (4 French) was passed for 35 cm without difficulty. His colleague, who performed the operation, flinched and abandoned the procedure. One week later, Forssmann anaesthetized his own left cubital fossa, advanced the catheter into his right atrium and then climbed several flights of stairs to the X-ray department and documented his achievement. This account was published on 5 November 1929. The first and only clinical application in which he used his catheter was to administer glucose, epinephrine hydrochloride and strophanthin to a woman with terminal purulent peritonitis following perforation of the appendix. After a temporary improvement, the patient relapsed and died; at autopsy the catheter was found to have passed through the right atrium and its tip was situated in the inferior vena cava.

Forssmann pointed out that such a catheter could be used for central venous blood sampling as well as for injections. He also realized that the technique he had pioneered provided many possibilities for future metabolic studies and investigations into cardiac function. Later he was the first to inject a radio-opaque substance directly into the right heart via both arm and thigh veins (on himself) using Uroselectan (23). Thus, he demonstrated that a well-known experimental technique could be applied to the study and treatment of disease in man.

His enthusiasm for this discovery did not extend to his contemporary German colleagues, and little interest was shown in his work. He spent 6 years as an army surgeon in Germany, Norway and Russia and returned weary and malnourished to civilian medical practice. He turned to urology before receiving his unexpected and belated academic reward.

A short hiatus in this field of clinical physiology occurred until the systematic physiological investigations of Cournand, Richards and others commenced in 1936. A new flexible radio-opaque catheter was designed to enable intravenous and intracardiac blood sampling to be performed together with pressure recordings

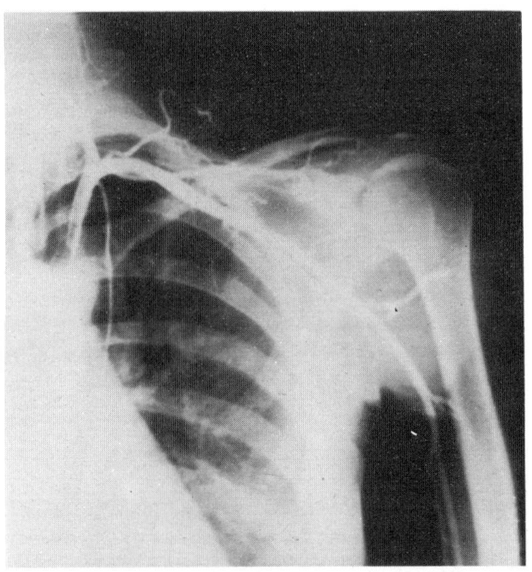

Fig. 1. Venogram of the left brachial, subclavian and external jugular veins, illustrating the tributaries entering at an acute angle and pointing always in the direction of blood flow. (Reproduced by kind permission of Mr S. Mottershead, MD, FRCS, Middlesbrough, and the Editor of the *British Medical Journal*.)

in the right atrium and pulmonary artery. They performed studies in heart failure, valvular heart disease and shock, and stimulated many other workers in this field around the world. For those who may be particularly interested, a definitive account of this period has been provided by Cournand (24).

The introduction of flexible polyethylene cannulas for intravenous feeding in children was introduced by Meyers (25) and Zimmerman (26) in 1945, and this innovation from the plastics industry heralded the beginning of an era in intravenous therapy and diagnostic intervention. Surgeons adapted the tubing with ingenuity; for example, the palliative treatment of obstructive hydrocephalus became a reality in May 1949, when Nulsen and Spitz established a valved shunt between the right lateral ventricle and the right internal jugular vein (27). They recognized the failure of the intravascular prosthesis caused by thrombosis inside the shunt and the jugular vein. The techniques derived from this procedure are now applicable for the direct cannulation of the internal jugular vein in the most difficult cases requiring parenteral nutrition.

The historical background to the individual techniques is provided in the relevant chapters which follow. The mass production of cannulas and central catheters consisting of polyvinyl chloride was inevitably followed by numerous clinical case reports and series describing local and systemic complications (28–32). Indar pointed out the problem of thrombosis which occurred when polyethylene catheters were used in the deep veins (33). Industry thus continued to research for improved inert materials for use as intravascular prostheses. Tetrafluoroethylene (FTE) and fluoroethylenepolypropylene (FEP) have been used and the incidence of thrombosis reduced as a result.

In 1960 Scribner, Dillard and Quinton jointly developed a Teflon and subsequently a Silastic arteriovenous shunt for use in haemodialysis (34). This advance has proved to be of tremendous significance in the achievement of safe chronic venous access. A Silastic intravenous catheter was introduced by Stewart and Sanislow in 1961 at Ann Arbor Hospital, Michigan (35). The tubing they used was extruded and cured at 480 °F for 16 hours, the cannula being connected to the intravenous administration set

by a 20 S.G. needle after the point had been removed by grinding. Herein lies a problem of the intertness of silicone, namely it is extremely difficult to bond the catheter to the hub securely. Mechanical catheter-related problems have now assumed importance in the care of patients receiving prolonged intravenous therapy (36). Design improvements are still needed in order to make further improvements in this aspect of patient care.

THE DEVELOPMENT OF PARENTERAL NUTRITION

During the past decade there has been a substantial increase in the number of patients who have received parenteral nutritional support in hospital. The terminology emerging from the scientific literature includes such new abbreviations as IVH (intravenous hyperalimentation), TPN (total parenteral nutrition) and, following the refinement of long-life silicone tunnelled catheters introduced by Scribner (37) and Broviac (38), HPN (home parenteral nutrition) has emerged as a reality for a few carefully selected patients. The infusion of energy substrates and nitrogen has been established as an integral feature of the supportive medical care of patients during severe medical or surgical illness.

The progress from the experiments by Sir Christopher Wren in 1656, when he infused wine, ale and opium into dogs, follows a fascinating path. John Hunter made some poignant observations throughout his surgical career; in his 'Treatise on the Blood, Inflammation and Gun-Shot Wounds' published in 1794 he discussed the aspect of wound healing which he termed 'Union by the First Intention'. The words he used then, and which have often been quoted since, are

> It will be proper to observe here that there is a circumstance attending accidental injury which does not belong to the disease, viz. that the injury done, has in all cases a tendency to produce both the disposition and means of cure (39).

Central venous catheters have played a vital role in current medical and surgical practice enabling clinicians to monitor, augment and support the efforts of the body to stabilize the circulation during (or following) major surgery and provide nutritional supplements in order to fire the 'disposition and means of cure'.

Following its isolation and purification, glucose was used intravenously in animals by Claude Bernard during 1843 (40). Thomas Latta of Edinburgh administered an infusion of water and saline to an elderly victim of cholera (41). Six pints were given intravenously in 6 minutes and the first complication of intravenous therapy recorded—circulatory overload! The populations of Asia, Europe and North America were intermittently attacked by epidemics of cholera and typhoid throughout the eighteenth century and some of the earliest crude attempts at providing fluids and nutrition were made on the unfortunate victims of this disease.

In 1859 Edward Hodder of Toronto suggested to his friend, James Bovell, that it would be 'proper and a probable success' to transfuse blood into cholera victims (42). Bovell pointed out that the supply would quickly run out in an epidemic as few people would be willing to part with their blood, and they could not be sure the blood itself would not be diseased. This is the first record of infusion contamination being contemplated as a hazard. Hodder felt that the nearest available analogue of blood in abundant supply was milk and he knew that it had been given intravenously to animals by Donné without a fatal result. Hodder and Bovell bided their time, and in 1873, the City Fathers of Toronto were just as unprepared for cholera as in 1859. An old shed in the hospital grounds was made ready and the first cholera victim brought in a state of circulatory collapse. Four other medical officers were consulted and agreed about the diagnosis and hopeless prognosis. On announcing his planned experiment, Hodder was told he would kill the patient. All but one of the medical officers refused to stay and observe the proceedings. A cow was brought to the shed, milked into a bowl, the milk was filtered through a gauze and 14 ounces injected through a tube inserted in a cut-down venesection from a warmed syringe. The effect was 'magical' and the patient recovered his pulse and survived. Two other patients had this form of treatment, rallied and died during Hodder's absence from the shed. Hodder and Bovell were the first to realize that the cost of the nutritional fluids and apparatus could be a limiting factor in the provision of

their treatment. They applied to the Corporation for a cow and a few items 'indispensably necessary for the comfort and well being of patients'; these were refused, and they thereupon sent in their resignation!

J. D. Malcolm, in 1893, published a classic description of 'The Physiology of Death from Traumatic Fever' and noted that shock was simply one of the phenomena caused by injury, whether surgical or otherwise, rather than a complication (43). His work stimulated the study of metabolic processes in shock. The value of glucose infusions for patients was not accepted immediately. The work of Pasteur in 1877 (44) had provided the impetus to produce sterile solutions for animal and clinical use. Sugar was first infused in man by Biedl and Kraus in 1896 (45) and Kausch first infused glucose for postoperative nutritional purposes in 1911 (46).

The concept of providing intravenous nutrition was furthered when, in 1913, Henriques and Andersen injected protein hydrolysate, glucose and salt solution into goats for 16 days (47). Murlin and Riche infused fat experimentally for the first time in 1916. (48). Four years later, Yamakawa was the first to use an intravenous infusion of fat in man (49). The significance of this early work was overlooked until 1937 when Elman and his colleagues performed their experiments. Several basic questions concerning the metabolic response to injury were being investigated by Sir David Cuthbertson during the 1930s. He made a teleological proposition that an injured animal in response to injury is faced with a diminished food supply, and he suggested that the rapid early catabolism of tissues could be associated with the first signs of regeneration of the injured part (50). He went on to perform outstanding investigations into many aspects of the catabolic response to injury (51, 52). He pointed out that a high protein and high calorie diet after fractures of the long bones was beneficial in attenuating the marked loss of body proteins (53). Cuthbertson introduced the terms 'ebb phase' and 'flow phase' for the initial depressed period of metabolism and the later period of increased metabolic rate after trauma (54).

In 1937, Elman demonstrated the effectiveness of a 5 per cent amino acid mixture derived from a sulphuric acid hydrolysate of casein to which tryptophan and cystine were added (55). In dogs depleted of their blood by acute haemorrhage, regeneration of the plasma proteins was evident after 6 hours in the group fed with 5 per cent amino acid and 5 per cent glucose; whilst the controls who were given 10 per cent glucose showed no evidence of plasma protein repletion after 6 hours and very little after 24 hours. In 1939, Elman and Weiner reported the first use of protein hydrolysate in man (56). Positive nitrogen balance was maintained in postoperative patients and in patients with inoperable carcinoma by providing 20 g of casein hydrolysate, tryptophan supplement, glucose and saline. The first artificial amino acid mixture used intravenously in man was described by Shol and Blackfan in 1940 (57).

During World War II the importance of this work was becoming apparent. It was recognized that intravenous therapy with protein hydrolysates and 5 per cent or 10 per cent glucose given through peripheral veins failed to provide sufficient non-protein calories to ensure that administered amino acids would be used for tissue protein synthesis and regeneration rather than for immediate energy purposes. The alternatives were to give large volumes of fluid or very concentrated solutions. Fat emulsions were a promising alternative source of energy. The observation that the body could tolerate the intravenous fat emulsion issuing from the thoracic duct provided the proof which stimulated Wretlind to search for a suitable alternative emulsion that could be manufactured. In the United States an emulsion derived from cotton seed oil (Lipomul) was associated with toxic reactions and all fat emulsions were removed from the market. Wretlind and his co-workers in Sweden embarked upon a long series of experiments using an animal test system to find a suitable emulsion. They finally developed a soybean oil and egg yolk phospholipid emulsion free of toxic reactions and the experimental dogs survived the 28-days test period (58). Patients were found to tolerate this compound (Intralipid), and in 1965 an adult patient with Crohn's disease was kept in a good nutritional state for 5 months, fed intravenously with amino acids, glucose, fat, electrolytes and vitamins (59). In the United Kingdom, Rickham and his colleagues started to use intravenous fat emulsions together with amino acids and sugar solutions in

paediatric surgical practice during the period 1962–67 for children who had required extensive intestinal resection (60). In 1966 Hadfield administered high calorie intravenous feeding in surgical patients whilst he was at the Radcliffe Infirmary, Oxford. He used Intralipid in combination with casein hydrolysates and noted reductions in the postoperative weight loss of patients undergoing partial gastrectomy and also improvements in the serum protein levels of patients with ulcerative colitis and severe intestinal malabsorption (61).

At the same time as these advances were being made in Stockholm and the United Kingdom, the use of concentrated glucose as an alternative energy source was being investigated in the USA. Following careful fundamental research into the metabolic care of surgical patients, Francis Moore in Boston described the use of the superior vena cava for the infusion of concentrated glucose (62). He also stated that 'patients on prolonged intravenous feeding rarely gain weight by tissue synthesis, yet it is conceivable that this might some day occur as intravenous hyperalimentation is perfected and concentrated'. In 1966 Dudrick et al. (63) reported that they could successfully perform total parenteral nutrition on Beagles and match orally fed controls in weight gain, development and growth. They went on to report similar results in man (64–66). They were able to achieve their remarkable results in free moving Beagle puppies by using fine catheters, which after insertion into the central veins were tunnelled subcutaneously for a distance to the back of the animal's neck. Such catheters were kept in place for periods of 72–256 days of intravenous hyperalimentation. The American investigators used concentrated glucose solutions in order to provide an adequate calorific intake, and for this to be accomplished without a high incidence of thrombosis or phlebitis, a central venous infusion system was developed.

The need to provide an adequate supply of protein, calories, vitamins and trace elements to patients undergoing major surgery, following severe trauma or recuperating from intercurrent disease is well recognized. In 1968 Peaston summarized the situation succinctly by stating:

> In recent years, materials have become available whereby intravenous nutrition can be adequately maintained. The therapeutic decision not to use them

is a positive action to starve the patient, and must in itself be justified unless the complications from their use outweigh the advantages conferred (67).

When nutritional support has to be provided by the intravenous route, as much as 1600 calories may be provided per day in an adult by peripheral venous infusion (68). This should be the route of choice in patients requiring short-term nutritional support. However, where prolonged therapy is required, the incidence of painful thrombophlebitis becomes unacceptable for most patients and central catheterization must be employed. The biochemistry and methodology of providing supplementary or total parenteral nutrition has steadily progressed and several comprehensive reviews have been produced.

During the past decade there has been an increasing awareness of the need to make an accurate assessment of the nutritional status of patients and the competence of their humoral and cellular immunological defence systems (69). Several groups of workers have been investigating a variety of parameters and developing the concepts of 'nutritional profiles' 'anergic metabolic profiles' and a 'prognostic nutritional index' in order to diagnose the type and degree of malnutrition (70–72).

These studies have shown definite correlations between a variety of parameters and operative morbidity and mortality in surgical patients. A considerable effort is now needed to elucidate the complex and interrelated metabolic events which take place in patients in whom severe sepsis, renal and hepatic impairment are established, so that the most beneficial and cost-effective combination of nutrients may be safely infused.

References

1. Franklin K. J.: *William Harvey, Englishman*. London: MacGibbon & Kee, 1961.
2. Wren C.: Cited by Dudrick S. J. and Rhoads J. E.: New horizons for intravenous feeding. *JAMA* 1971; **215**: 939–49.
3. Lower R., King E.: An account of the experiment of transfusion. *Phil. Trans.* 1662; **2**: 557–64.
4. Lower R.: Tractatus de Corde, 1669. In: K. J. Franklin (trans.): *Early Science in Oxford*, vol. IX. London: Oxford Press, 1932.
5. Major J. D.: *Chirurgia Infusorii*. Kilonia: Reumannus 1667.
6. Wheatley H. B.: *The Diary of Samuel Pepys*, vol. II. New York: Random House, 1966.
7. Birch T. (ed.): *The Works of the Honourable Robert Boyle in Five Volumes*. London: Millar, 1744.
8. Denys J. B.: *Lettres Touchant Deux Experiences de la Transfusions Fites sur des Hommes*. Paris: Cusson, 1667: 12–13.
9. Blundell J.: *Medico-Chirur. Trans.* 1818; **9**: 56–92.
10. Hales S.: Experiment 3. Statical Essays: Containing Haemastaticks. Quoted by White P. D.: *Heart Disease*, 3rd ed. New York: Macmillan, 1974: 92.
11. Hoff H. E., Guillemin R., Sakiz E.: Claude Bernard on animal heat. An unpublished manuscript and some original notes. *Perspect. Biol. Med.* 1965; **7**: 347–68.
12. Magnus G.: Über die im Blute enthaltenen Gase. Sauerstoffe, Stickstoff und Kohlensäure. *Ann. Phys. Chem.* 1837; **12**: 583.
13. Bernard C.: *Leçons sur la Chaleur Animale*. Paris: Librairie J.-B. Baillière et Fils, 1876: 42–81.
14. Chauveau A., Marey E, J.: Appareils et Expériences Cardiographiques Demonstration Nouvelle du Mécanisme des Mouvements du Coeur par l'emploi des Instruments Enregistreurs à Indications Continués. *Mem. Acad. Médé.* 1863; **26**: 268.
15. Rolleston H. D.: Observations on the endocardial pressure curve. *J. Physiol.* 1887; **8**: 235.
16. Porter W. T.: Researches in the filling of the heart. *J. Physiol.* 1892; **13**: 513.
17. Franck O.: Kritik der Elastischen Manometer. *Z. Biol.* 1903; **44**: 445.
18. Franck O.: Die Puls in den Arterien. *Z. Biol.* 1905; **45**: 441.
19. Cournand A., Ranges H. A.: Catheterisation of the right auricle in man. *Proc. Soc. Exp. Biol. Med.* 1941; **46**: 462.
20. Forssmann W.: Die Sondierung des Rechten Herzens. *Klin. Wochenschr.* 1929; **8**: 2085.
21. Bleichroeder F. *Berl. Klin. Wochenschr.* 1912; **49**: 1503.
22. Bleichroeder F. *Virch. Arch. Pathol.* 1904; **177**: 435.
23. Forssmann W.: Über Kontrastderstellung der Hohlen des Pebenden rechten Herzens und der lungenschlagadr. *Munch. Med. Wochenschr.* 1931; **78**: 489–92.
24. Cournand. A.: Cardiac catheterisation. Development of the technique, its contributions to experimental medicine, and its initital application in man. *Acta Med. Scand.* 1975; *Suppl.:* 7–32.
25. Meyers L. Intravenous catheterisation. *Am. J. Nurs.* 1945; **45**: 930–1.
26. Zimmerman B.: Intravenous tubing for parenteral therapy. *Science* 1945; **101**: 566–8.
27. Nulsen F., Spitz E. B.: Treatment of hydrocephalus by direct shunt from ventricle to jugular vein. In: Proceedings of 37th Clinical Congress of the American College of Surgeons, San Francisco, California. *Surg. Forum* 1952: 399–403.
28. Morris J.: Thrombophlebitis following intravenous infusions. *Lancet* 1955; **1**; 154.
29. Moncrief J. A.: Femoral catheters. *Ann. Surg.* 1958; **147**: 166–72.
30. Crane C.: Venous interruption for septic thrombophlebitis. *N. Engl. J. Med.* 1960; **262**: 947–51.
31. Doering R. B., Stemmer E. A., Connelly J. E.: Complications of indwelling venous catheters. *Am. J. Surg.* 1967; **114**: 259–66.

32. Neuhof H., Seley G. P.: Acute suppurative phlebitis complicated by septicaemia. *Surgery* 1974; **21**: 831–42.
33. Indar R.: The dangers of indwelling polyethylene catheters in deep veins. *Lancet* 1959; **1**: 284–6.
34. Quinton W. E., Dillard D. H., Scribner B. H.: Cannulation of blood vessels for prolonged haemodialysis. *Trans. Am. Soc. Artif. Int. Organs* 1960; **6**: 104, 1962; **8**: 236.
35. Stewart R. D., Sanislow C. A.: Silastic intravenous catheter. *N. Engl. J. Med.* 1961; **265**: 1283–5.
36. Fleming C. R., Witzke D. J., Beart R. W.: Catheter-related complications in patients receiving home parenteral nutrition. *Ann. Surg.* 1980; **192**: 593–9.
37. Scribner B. H., Cole J. J., Christopher G.: Long term total parenteral nutrition: the concept of an artificial gut. *JAMA* 1970; **212**: 457–63.
38. Broviac J. W., Cole J. J., Scribner B. H.: A silicone rubber atrial catheter for prolonged parenteral alimentation. *Surg. Gynecol. Obstet.* 1973; **136**: 602–6.
39. Hunter J.: *A Treatise on Blood, Information and Gunshot Wounds*. London: Nicol, 1794.
40. Bernard C.: Cited by Dudrick S. J. and Rhoads J. E.: New horizons for intravenous feeding. *JAMA* 1971; **215**: 939–49.
41. Latta T.: Injections of saline solution in extraordinary quantities into the veins of cases of malignant cholera (Letter). *Lancet* 1831–32; **2**: 243.
42. Hodder E. M.: Transfusion of milk in cholera. *Practitioner* 1873; **10**: 14–16.
43. Malcolm J. D.: *The Physiology of Death from Traumatic Fever*. London: Churchill, 1893.
44. Pasteur L., Joubert J. F.: Charbon and septicémie. *Compt. R. Hebd. Séanc. Acad. Sci. Paris* 1877; **85**: 101–15.
45. Biedl A., Kraus R.: Cited by Dudrick S. J. and Rhoads J. E.: New horizons for intravenous feeding. *JAMA* 1971; **215**: 939–49.
46. Kausch W.: Über intravenose and subcutane Ernahrung mit Traubenzucker. *Deutsch. Med. Wochenschr.* 1911; **37**: 8–9.
47. Henriques V., Andersen A. C.: Cited by Greenstein J. P., Winitz M.: *Chemistry of Amino Acids*, Vol. I., New York: Wiley, 1961: 332.
48. Murlin J. R., Riche J. A.: The fat of the blood in relation to heat production, narcosis and muscular work. *Am. J. Physiol.* 1916; **40**: 146.
49. Yamakawa S.: Parenteral nutrition. *Nippon Naika Gakkai Zasshi* 1920; **17**: 122.
50. Cuthbertson D. P.: The influence of prolonged muscular rest on metabolism. *Biochem. J.* 1929; **23**: 1328–45.
51. Cuthbertson D. P.: The disturbance of metabolism produced by bony and non-bony injury, with notes on certain abnormal conditions of bone. *Biochem. J.* 1930; **24**: 1244–63.
52. Cuthbertson D. P.: The distribution of nitrogen and sulphur in the urine during conditions of increased catabolism. *Biochem. J.* 1931; **25**: 236–44.
53. Cuthbertson D. P.: Further observations on the disturbance of metabolism caused by injury with particular reference to the dietary requirements of fracture cases. *Br. J. Surg.* 1936; **23**: 505–20.
54. Cuthbertson D. P.: Post-shock metabolic response. *Lancet* 1942; **1**: 433–7.
55. Elman R.: Intravenous injection of amino acids in regeneration of serum protein following severe experimental haemorrhage. *Proc. Soc. Exp. Biol. Med.* 1937; **36**: 867–70.
56. Elman R., Weiner D. O.: Intravenous alimentation with special reference to protein (amino acid) metabolism. *JAMA* 1939; **112**: 796–802.
57. Shol A. T., Blackfan K. D.: The intravenous administration of crystalline amino acids to infants. *J. Nutr.* 1940; **20**: 305–16.
58. Hakasson I.: Experiences in long-term studies on nine fat emulsions in dogs. *Nutritio et Dieta* 1968; **10**: 54–76.
59. Hallberg D., Schuberth O., Wretlind A.: Experimental and clinical studies with fat emulsion for intravenous nutrition. *Nutritio et Dieta* 1966; **8**: 245–81.
60. Rickham P. P.: Massive small bowel resection in newborn infants. *Ann. R. Coll. Surg. Engl.* 1967; **41**: 480–92.
61. Hadfield J.: High caloric intravenous feeding in surgical patients. *Clin. Med.* 1966; **73**: 25–30.
62. Moore F. D.: *Metabolic Care of the Surgical Patient*. Philadelphia: Saunders, 1959: 25–48, 49–68.
63. Dudrick S. J., Vars H. M., Rhoads J. E.: Growth of puppies receiving all nutritional requirements by vein. *Fortsch. Parenteral Ernahrung.* 1966; **2**: 16–18.
64. Dudrick S. J., Wilmore D. W., Vars H. M.: Long-term total parenteral nutrition with growth in puppies and positive nitrogen balance in patients. *Surg. Forum* 1967; **18**: 356–7.
65. Dudrick S. J., Wilmore D. W., Vars H. M. et al.: Long-term parenteral nutrition with growth, development and positive nitrogen balance. *Surgery* 1968; **64**: 134–42.
66. Wilmore D. W., Dudrick S. J.: Growth and development of an infant receiving all nutrients exclusively by vein. *JAMA* 1968; **203**: 140–4.
67. Peaston M. J. T.: Parenteral nutrition in serious illness. *Br. J. Hosp. Med.* 1968: 708–11.
68. Johnston I. D. A.: Parenteral nutrition in the cancer patient. *J. Human Nutr.* 1979; **33**: 189–96.
69. Leading Article: Parenteral nutrition before surgery? *Br. Med. J.* 1979; **2**: 1529.
70. Blackburn G. L., Kaminski M. V.: Nutritional assessment and intravenous support. In: Karran S. J., Alberti G. (eds.): *Practical Nutritional Support*. London: Pitman Medical, 1978.
71. Daly J. M., Dudrick S. J., Copeland E. M.: Intravenous hyperalimentation effect on delayed cutaneous hypersensitivity in cancer patients. *Ann. Surg.* 1980; **192**: 587–92.
72. Mullen J. L., Buzby G. P., Matthews D. C. et al.: Reduction of operative morbidity and mortality by combined preoperative and postoperative nutritional support. *Ann. Surg.* 1980; **192**: 604–13.

Chapter 2

Applied Anatomy

J. Jessop and C. Fisher

A knowledge of the anatomy of the venous system is essential for successful venous catheterization. The accurate application of surface anatomy enables deep veins to be localized precisely, and an awareness of the related structures should result in a reduced incidence of iatrogenic trauma. In addition, the presence of valves and tributaries which may obstruct the smooth passage of a catheter needs to be appreciated. The superficial veins are prone to variations in their position, but the deep veins follow a more constant pattern. This chapter deals with the anatomy of the various sites commonly used for central catheter insertion in the adult and child (*Fig.* 2.1).

ACCESS POINTS FOR CENTRAL VENOUS CATHETERIZATION

1. Antecubital fossa
2. Deltopectoral groove
3. Subclavian vein
4. External jugular vein
5. Internal jugular vein
6. Long saphenous vein
7. Scalp
8. Umbilical vein

Antecubital Fossa

The cephalic vein originates from the venous network on the dorsum of the hand and winds around the radial border of the wrist to run up the lateral aspect of the forearm. It may be cannulated as it crosses the roof of the 'anatomical snuff box' at the wrist joint. Just below the anterior aspect of the elbow it gives off a

median cubital vein, which usually receives a deep communicating vein and crosses medially to join the basilic vein. The median cubital vein is usually the largest vein at this site and it lies in front of the brachial artery and median nerve. Separating the vein from these important structures is the bicipital aponeurosis, traditionally called the 'Grace à Dieu fascia'. However, it can easily be penetrated, particularly in obese subjects where the vein is difficult to find with resultant arterial or nerve trauma. There is also a superficial ulnar artery occurring in 3 per cent of the population which can be cannulated by

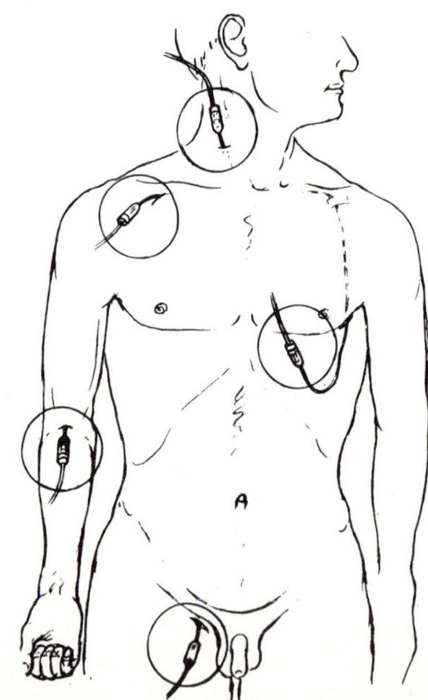

Fig. 2.1. Common approach routes for central venous catheter insertion.

the unwary novice. The vein is also related closely to the median cutaneous nerve of the forearm, injury to which has been implicated as a cause of troublesome neuralgia in blood donors (*Fig.* 2.2).

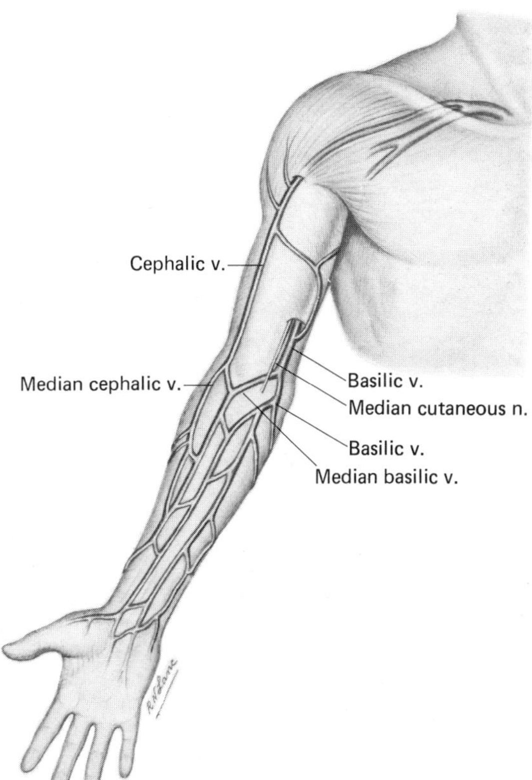

Fig. 2.2. Anatomy of the superficial veins of the arm and forearm (right).

The median vein of the forearm runs up the centre of the forearm and joins the median cubital or basilic vein. Sometimes it divides below the elbow into a medial and lateral branch which pass respectively to the basilic and cephalic veins (*Fig.* 2.2). There is often an accessory cephalic vein laterally, which joins the main vein at the elbow. The lateral cutaneous nerve of the forearm is an immediate deep relation of the cephalic vein.

Both the cephalic and basilic veins lie in the superficial fascia, forming the roof or the antecubital fossa. The basilic vein continues up the medial aspect of the arm and pierces the deep fascia medial to the biceps, midway between the

elbow and axilla. It is therefore the vein of choice for central catheter insertion. The cephalic vein, by contrast, continues superficially up the lateral aspect of the arm and pierces the clavipectoral fascia in the deltopectoral groove. Difficulty is often experienced manipulating long central venous catheters past this point. Abduction of the arm at the shoulder sometimes allows the catheter to pass.

Deltopectoral Groove

The cephalic vein runs up the arm lateral to the biceps to pass between pectoralis major and the deltoid. The vein then enters the infraclavicular fossa, passes behind the clavicular head of pectoralis major and pierces the clavipectoral fascia before joining the subclavian vein. Unfortunately, in some people, the cephalic vein above the elbow may be absent or small, particularly where the basilic vein is large (*Fig.* 2.3). The

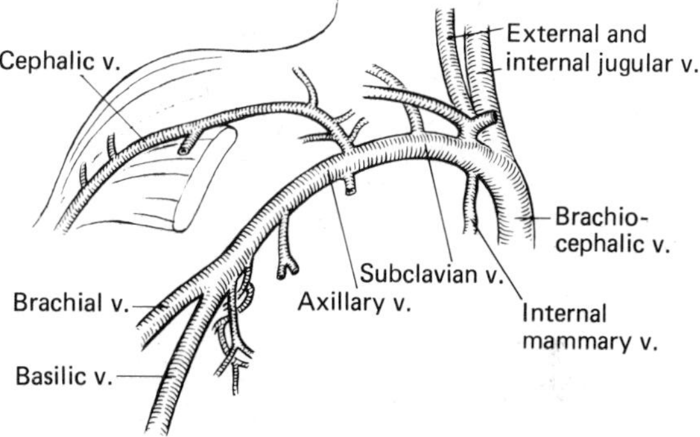

Fig. 2.3. Anatomy of the superficial veins of the shoulder and root of the neck (right).

acromiothoracic branch of the subclavian artery pierces the clavipectoral fascia above the pectoralis minor. A deltoid branch passes laterally and is related to the cephalic vein in the upper part of the groove. The cephalic vein receives acromial and pectoral tributaries which can complicate catheterization.

Subclavian Vein

The subclavian vein is the continuation of the axillary vein and starts, by definition, at the outer border of the first rib. It extends as far as the medial border of scalenus anterior, which is running obliquely upwards from the scalene tubercle on the medial border of the first rib to the anterior tubercles on the third to sixth cervical vertebrae (*Fig.* 2.4). The vein lies im-

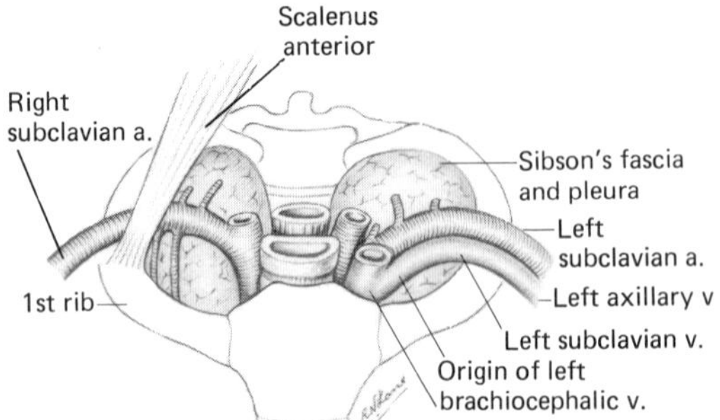

Fig. 2.4. Relationship of the subclavian vein, artery and pleura.

mediately behind the middle third of the clavicle, running upwards and slightly backwards and it unites with the internal jugular vein behind the sternoclavicular joint to form the brachiocephalic vein. Percutaneous catheterization can thus be achieved by infraclavicular or supraclavicular approaches and it is important to know the adjacent structures.

Above, the clavicle is covered by skin and the lowest fibres of platysma. The skin of this area is innervated by the supraclavicular branches of the third and fourth cervical nerves, and they traverse the posterior triangle (*Fig.* 2.5). Attached to the medial end of the clavicle is the clavicular head of sternomastoid. The clavicular head of trapezius is attached to the lateral end. Between them, and enclosing each muscle, is the deep investing fascia of the neck.

Below, the clavicle has the clavicular head of pectoralis major attached to its medial third. Immediately inferior to the clavicle is the subclavius muscle, enclosed in clavipectoral fascia. Behind, the subclavian vein lies in front of scalenus anterior with the phrenic nerve lying on the surface of the muscle. Talbot (1), in an elegant post-mortem anatomical study, found accessory phrenic nerves passing in front of the subclavian vein in 45 per cent of cadavers dissected at Charing Cross Hospital Medical School (*Fig.* 2.6). In rare instances, the phrenic nerve passed through the subclavian vein. Such abnormalities naturally predispose to nerve injury during catheterization procedures with

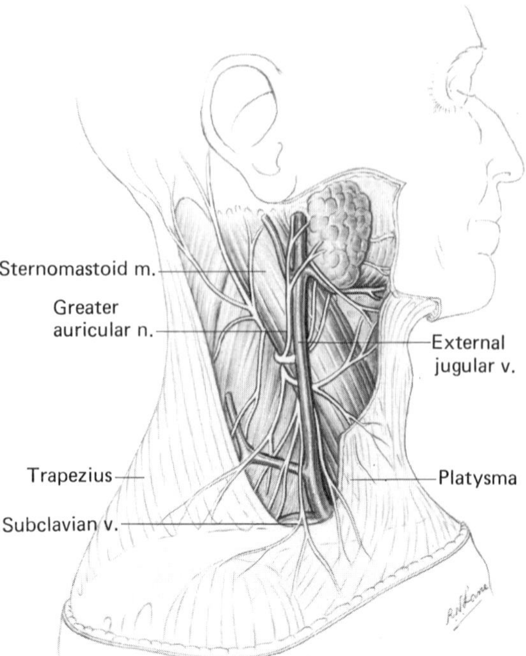

Fig. 2.5. Relationship of the external jugular and subclavian vein in the posterior triangle of the neck to platysma and cervical nerves.

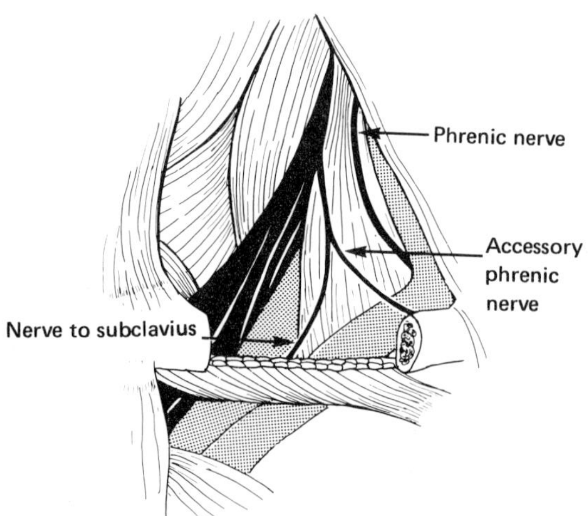

Fig. 2.6. The right subclavian vein and its relationship to the course of the phrenic nerve, accessory phrenic nerve and the nerve to the subclavius muscle. (Reproduced with the kind permission of Mr R. Talbot, FRCS and the Editor of the *Annals of The Royal College of Surgeons of England.*)

resultant diaphragmatic paralysis. The subclavian artery and its branches run behind and slightly above the vein, owing to the obliquity of the first rib. Behind the first part of the vein (medial to scalenus anterior) lies the lowest root of the brachial plexus, and more laterally, the trunks (*Fig.* 2.7). The vein rests on a groove in

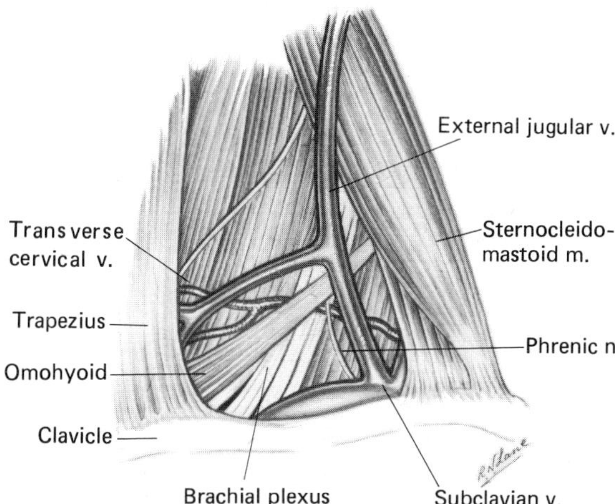

Fig. 2.7. The anatomy of the veins, brachial plexus and muscles in the inferior aspect of the posterior triangle of the neck (right).

the first rib and medially on the suprapleural membrane (Sibson's fascia), a dense layer passing from the medial border of the first rib to the transverse process of the seventh cervical vertebra. The cervical dome of pleura is attached to the underside of this membrane. Since the first rib slopes downwards, the cupola of the lung lies immediately below and behind the medial part of the subclavian vein, separated only by Sibson's fascia. This provides scant protection for the pleura from the sharp point of an errant catheter introducer (*see Fig.* 2.4).

Just lateral to scalenus anterior, the external jugular vein enters. At this point, on the left, the subclavian vein is also joined by the thoracic duct, and on the right by the right lymphatic duct. There is sometimes a pair of valves situated in the subclavian vein anterior to the scalenus muscle which may impede a central catheter.

External Jugular Vein

The external jugular vein is formed by the union of the posterior division of the retromandibular vein and the posterior auricular vein. It starts at the level of the angle of the mandible in or just below the parotid gland, and runs down the neck towards the middle of the clavicle. In doing so, it crosses sternomastoid obliquely and pierces the deep investing fascia 2·5 cm above the clavicle, before joining the subclavian vein in front of, or just lateral to scalenus anterior (*see Fig.* 2.5). Superficially, it is covered by skin and platysma, and is readily visible when filled with blood. It has two pairs of valves, one where it enters the subclavian vein and another 4 cm above the clavicle. Three small tributaries join the vein deep to the investing fascia and may obstruct the forward advancement of a catheter.

Internal Jugular Vein

The internal jugular vein is the continuation of the sigmoid sinus. It emerges from the jugular foramen and descends under the cover of the sternomastoid to join the subclavian vein behind the sternoclavicular joint. It runs in the carotid sheath accompanied medially by the internal carotid artery and then, below the upper border of the thyroid cartilage, by the common carotid artery, lying alongside the vein. In the root of the neck, the vein passes anterior to the artery. Between the two vessels, and somewhat posterior, is the vagus nerve. Posteriorly, the carotid sheath lies on the prevertebral fascia, covering the prevertebral muscles. The sympathetic chain runs down as a posterior relation of the sheath. The vein is surrounded by deep cervical lymph nodes. (*Fig.* 2.8).

It has a dilatation at each end—the superior and inferior bulb. The inferior bulb lies behind the depression which divides the sternal and clavicular heads of the sternocleidomastoid. There is often a valve just above this point.

The surface marking of the internal jugular vein is a straight line drawn from the lobule of the ear to the sternoclavicular joint. It is divided into three parts by the crossing of the posterior belly of the digastric muscle and superior belly of the omohyoid. The posterior belly of the digastric runs from the mastoid process to a fibrous sheath on the greater horn of the hyoid bone. Both bony points are palpable and the line taken can therefore be visualized. The omohyoid crosses the vein just below the level of the cricoid cartilage (which is also palpable).

Between the digastric and the omohyoid, the cervical plexus, consisting of the anterior primary rami of the upper four cervical nerves, emerges behind the vein. In front lies the ansa

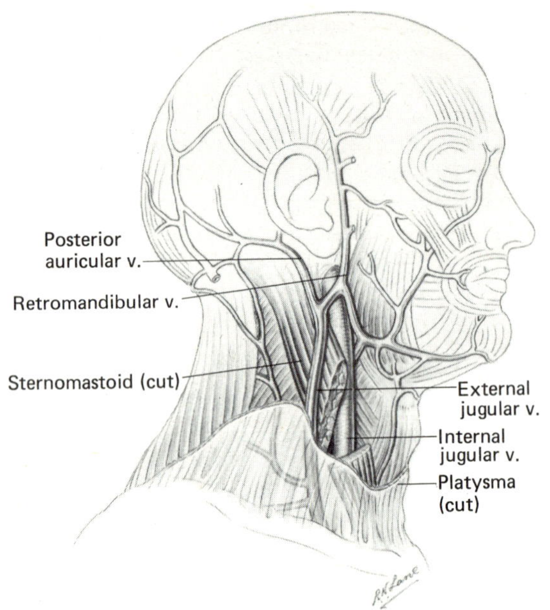

Fig. 2.8. Anatomical relationships of the internal and external jugular veins in the neck.

hypoglossi supplying the infrahyoid muscles. Below the omohyoid, the vein lies first on scalenus anterior and the phrenic nerve. Further down, it crosses the thyrocervical trunk (a branch of the subclavian artery), the vertebral vein and, finally, the first part of the subclavian artery before joining the subclavian vein. Superficially, it is crossed by the infrahyoid muscles, sternomastoid and the anterior jugular vein. Medially, it is related to the lateral lobe of the thyroid gland and the trachea. Running up alongside the trachea is the recurrent laryngeal nerve, which can be injured if the vein is transfixed during the insertion procedure.

Long Saphenous Vein

This large superficial vein originates from the medial marginal vein of the foot. It ascends 2·5 cm anterior to the medial malleolus of the tibia and passes up to the knee, running posteromedially to the medial condyles of the femur and tibia. The vein next runs along the medial aspect of the thigh into the femoral triangle. The vessel passes through the cribriform fascia to enter the common femoral vein at a variable angle. Just before the long saphenous vein meets the femoral vein, it receives a variable number of

tributaries. Commonly, there are five, namely the superficial epigastric vein, the superficial circumflex iliac vein, the superficial and deep pudendal veins and a vein draining the lateral aspect of the thigh (*Fig.* 2.9). The femoral vein and inferior vena cava can be cannulated

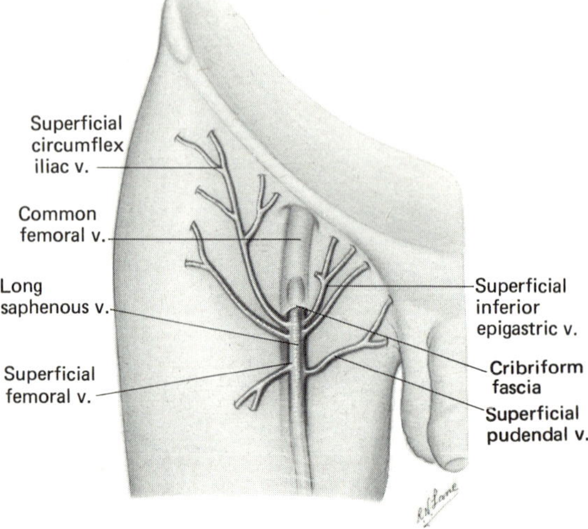

Fig. 2.9. Superficial and deep veins of the femoral triangle (right).

through one of these tributaries following exposure using a cut-down technique, percutaneously or using a modified Seldinger technique. This route is not recommended except as a last resort in view of the high rate of deep venous thrombosis encountered in the past. In rare instances, where the veins of the upper extremity or neck cannot be used because of burns, cellulitis or infection, fine silicone catheters may be inserted using this route. Preferably, these should be tunnelled subcutaneously to the anterior abdominal wall.

THE NEONATE

All the sites described for the adult may be used for the introduction of a central venous catheter in a neonate. Most clinicians do not attempt subclavian catheterization (except as a last resort). The advent of fine-bore silicone catheters has enabled central catheterization to be accomplished via the peripheral veins already mentioned. Two sites require special consideration—scalp veins and the umbilical vein.

Scalp

Small scalp veins can frequently be entered with specially designed 'scalp vein needles'. Their anatomy is shown in *Fig.* 2.8. In practice, the superficial temporal vein is most commonly used. The right side is preferable to the left. These veins may be distended by a temporary 'tourniquet' of rubber tubing fixed around the occipito-frontal plane of the head.

Umbilical Vein

Umbilical vein catheterization can be used for exchange transfusions, central venous pressure measurement, fluid infusions and for obtaining blood samples.

The umbilical vein passes in a cranial direction from the umbilicus lying for a short distance in the subcutaneous tissue. Then it turns back to run in the inferior (free) border of the falciform ligament, to reach the under surface of the liver. The vein ends by joining the left branch of the portal vein, after first giving off some small branches to the left lobe of the liver and the quadrate lobe.

The ductus venosus begins at the cranial aspect of the left branch of the portal vein, usually directly opposite the umbilical vein. It then passes cranially and dorsally to join the left hepatic vein just before it enters the inferior vena cava. Normally, the ductus venosus remains patent for 15–20 days after birth. The origin of the ductus venosus may be narrow or be situated to the right of the umbilical vein outlet. Catheters blindly introduced at this site are very likely to be incorrectly positioned; such catheters have found their way into the right or left branches of the portal vein. Catheters may bend backwards and pass along the right hepatic portal vein, portal vein and superior mesenteric vein. The catheter can be inadvertently advanced through a patent foramen ovale into the left atrium. Complications of such misplacement and infusion of fluid can include portal vein thrombosis leading to subsequent portal hypertension. Catheter misplacement and related sepsis has also been implicated in necrotizing enterocolitis in the neonate. It is essential that anteroposterior and lateral X-ray views of the abdomen and chest be obtained following catheterization. When the umbilical vein catheter is correctly placed, it takes a slight curve to the right of the mid-sagittal line at T12 before entering the ductus venosus. In the lateral view, the catheter takes a characteristic S-shaped line, the change in direction signifying the origin of the ductus venosus.

MEDIASTINAL VEINS AND PULMONARY ARTERY

The brachiocephalic veins are formed behind the sternoclavicular joints by the union of the internal jugular and subclavian veins. The right brachiocephalic vein is about 3 cm long, and descends behind the body of the manubrium, anterolateral to the brachiocephalic artery (*Fig.* 2.10). Running laterally between it and the

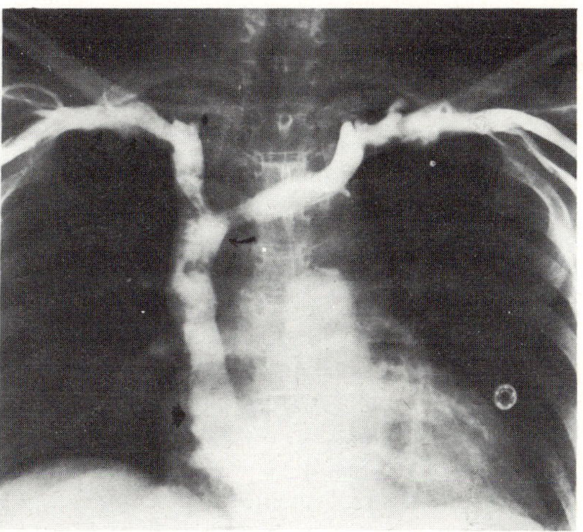

Fig. 2.10. Contrast venogram of the subclavian veins, brachiocephalic (innominate) veins, origins of the internal jugular veins and the superior vena cava, illustrating their relationships to the clavicle and first rib. (Reproduced by kind permission of Dr S. E. Mitchell and the Editor of the *American Journal of Roentgenology*.)

pleura is the right phrenic nerve. The left brachiocephalic vein is 6 cm long. It crosses obliquely behind the body of the manubrium and in front of the trachea and three large branches of the aortic arch. The brachiocephalic veins unite at the centre of the right border of the manubrium to form the superior vena cava, which descends vertically into the right atrium. In its lower half the superior vena cava is enclosed by the fibrous and serous pericardium (*Fig.* 2.11). Perforation by catheters below the pericardial reflection will lead to tamponade,

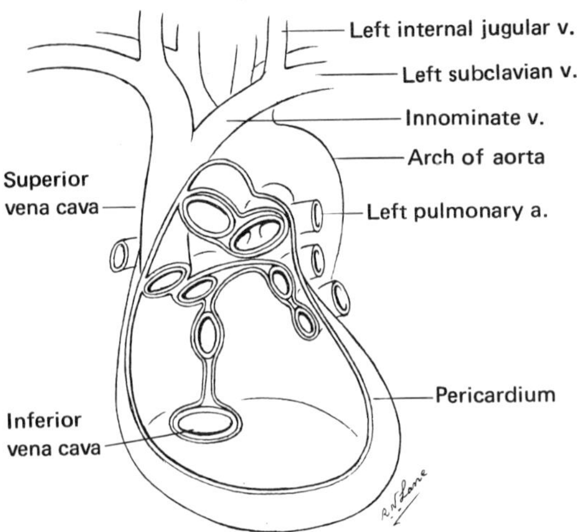

Fig. 2.11. Diagrammatic relationship of the pericardium and great vessels in the mediastinum.

Laterally lies the phrenic nerve, pleura and right lung; medially, the ascending aorta and brachiocephalic trunk. Behind is the hilum of the lung; in front, the lung, pleura and manubrium. Several anomalies of the brachiocephalic and superior vena cava occur, in such cases the post-insertion X-ray may show the central catheter travelling down the left lateral border of the manubrium on its way to the right atrium. If any doubt exists as to the correct intravenous placement of such a catheter, then its position should be checked by using contrast medium and fluoroscopic control whenever possible.

The right atrium is a thin-walled chamber forming the right border of the heart. Normally, a catheter passes, with the flow of blood, through the tricuspid valve into the right ventricle. But it may stray into one of three other potential openings—the inferior vena cava, entering the atrium from below; the coronary sinus; a patent foramen ovale.

From the right ventricle, the pulmonary trunk, about 5 cm long, ascends to the left of the ascending aorta, with which it shares a pericardial cuff. It then bifurcates into left and right pulmonary arteries in the concavity of the arch of the aorta. They lie along the upper borders of the atrium in front of the bronchi and inferior tracheobronchial lymph nodes which separate these vessels from the oesophagus. The lobar divisions of the pulmonary arteries pass into the

fissures between each lobe for a variable distance before being finally surrounded by the lung parenchyma. This point has an important bearing on the possibility of arterial rupture during Swan–Ganz catheterization. Whilst a small intrapulmonary haematoma may not be of consequence, a split in the artery outside of the lung tissue can cause a rapidly fatal haemothorax.

Congenital anomalies of the superior vena cava exist in approximately 0·3 per cent of the normal population and in 4·3 per cent of children born with congenital heart disease. This usually results from a failure of the left common cardinal vein to become obliterated, and may occur unilaterally or in conjunction with a normal right superior vena cava. If this failure occurs and is bilateral, there may or may not be a connection between the two venae cavae. Usually, blood from the left superior vena cava returns to the right atrium by way of the coronary sinus as shown in *Fig.* 2.12; thus it is

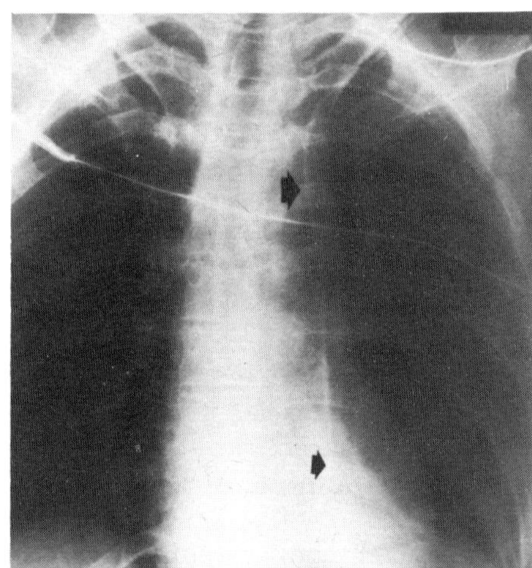

Fig. 2.12. Left superior vena cava. A left subclavian catheter has been inserted and is seen to course along the left paramediastinum (upper arrow) and left heart, then turn medially (lower arrow) into the coronary sinus. (Reproduced by kind permission of Dr S. E. Mitchell and the Editor of the *American Journal of Roentgenology.*)

important to be aware of this possibility when inserting a catheter via veins in the left upper limb or left side of the neck.

References

1. Talbot R. W.: Anatomical pitfalls of subclavian venepuncture. *Ann. R. Coll. Surg. Engl.* 1978; **60**: 317–19.

Chapter 3

Indications

J. L. Peters

Central venous catheterization must always be considered to be an invasive procedure, and strict criteria should be applied with each patient to decide whether its use is indicated. The function of the catheter and the predicted duration of use must be considered so that the most suitable device can be selected. There is no doubt that those hands experienced in the art can accommodate wide variations in the design of the needle, catheter and the anatomy of each individual; however, the house surgeon or physician with little experience can easily make an inadvertent error which will have disastrous consequences for the patient. Inexperience is a principal cause of morbidity associated with the procedure. Prior to embarking upon the operations, the following points must be considered:

Define the indication.
Decide upon the route of insertion.
Determine the choice of catheter.

There has been a steady growth in the applications for central venous catheters during the past decade. These may be conveniently listed and described alphabetically and historically as follows:

L   Long term infusions of inotropic drugs, hypertonic fluids, cytotoxic and antibiotic therapy
Liver biopsy by the transvenous route
M   Manometry and Monitoring
N   Nutrition (*see* Chapters 17–20)
O   Oximetry and cardiac output (*see* Chapter 10)
P   Plasmapheresis
Peritoneovenous shunts
Prevention of pulmonary embolism

LONG TERM INFUSIONS

As mentioned in Chapter 1, Werner Forssmann envisaged central catheters being used for the direct infusion of concentrated drugs into the heart. It is now well known that a wide variety of hypertonic fluids and vasoactive (e.g. 8·4 per cent sodium bicarbonate, adrenaline and noradrenaline) will cause tissue necrosis if subcutaneous infusion occurs from peripheral venepuncture sites (*Fig.* 3.1). Many parenteral nutrition fluids, especially amino acid solutions, although they may not give such a florid reaction, do cause a superficial thrombophlebitis, which is extremely painful. Where such infusions are planned, it is best to provide a means of central venous access. The massive skin loss depicted in *Fig.* 3.1 can only be replaced by grafting, and many patients who have suffered such mishap have taken recourse to litigation, even though their lives may have been saved by surgery or intensive care measures.

Many patients with acute leukaemia are now subjected to intensive regimens of chemotherapy, total body irradiation and, occasionally, bone-marrow transplantation from HLA-matched siblings. Invariably, they also require large doses of intravenous antibiotics during their illness in the attempt to obtain remission and cure. Furthermore, after the commencement of this treatment, diarrhoea, vomiting and anorexia often ensue, requiring large volumes of intravenous fluids and electrolytes. These patients also incur a profound catabolic state and their survival has been enhanced by the use of total parenteral nutrition, introduced early into their regimen of therapy. Such patients require

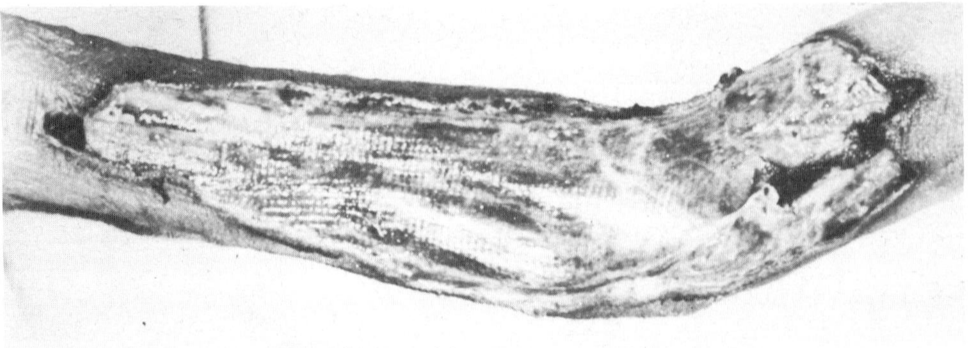

Fig. 3.1. Extensive skin necrosis following subcutaneous extravasation of hypertonic intravenous fluids into the ante cubital fossa. (Reproduced by kind permission of Mr N. R. Gaze, FRCS and the Editor of *The Lancet.*)

safe and efficient venous access for the administration of their drugs and subsequent whole blood, granulocyte, platelet and plasma protein fraction transfusions. Hickman and co-workers, in Seattle, conducted a prospective and randomized trial and the incidence of septicaemia in their patients, using an indwelling right atrial catheter, was less than in those treated with conventional venepuncture and drip techniques (1). Catheters with an internal diameter of 1·6 mm were used for all aspects of care, i.e. blood sampling, blood product transfusion and antibiotic administration. The patients did not have to suffer multiple injections or needle punctures, which are not only painful, but cause haematomas which themselves act as sources of sepsis in immunosuppressed patients. The effectiveness of this technique, using a slightly different silicone catheter, has been confirmed by Jacobs and colleagues in South Africa (2). It is interesting to remember that this multiplicity of uses for central catheters (i.e. blood letting and direct provision of drugs into the central circulation) was first suggested by Forssmann in his original paper. Central catheters can only be used in this way by adhering to a rigid aseptic and antiseptic protocol for the maintenance and management of the line. Prolonged and intermittent chemotherapy for lymphoma has been successfully carried out over a period of 1 year using a central catheter (3). Patients with such diseases often quickly run short of viable peripheral veins for venepuncture and infusion; consequently, the ability to maintain chronic venous access is likely to become important in the future, when, one hopes more effective treatments evolve.

Well-maintained central venous catheters provide an invaluable route for injecting high doses of antibiotics in episodes of overwhelming septicaemia and bacterial endocarditis. The infraclavicular subclavian route is the approach of choice (4). Very rarely in severe streptococcal infections of the face, neck and other extremities a silicone rubber catheter has to be inserted via one of the tributaries of the femoral vein in the groin, and this should be tunnelled away to a distant point on the anterior abdominal wall.

LIVER BIOPSY BY THE TRANSVENOUS ROUTE

It is of interest that Bleichroeder, perhaps the earliest pioneer of catheterization of the inferior vena cava, was intrigued by the biochemistry and pathology of cirrhosis; he is reputed to have used catheters to sample blood from the hepatic veins. More than 50 years later, in 1967, Hanafee and Weiner developed a transjugular technique for performing cholangiography for patients with an increased bleeding tendency (5). They also introduced the technique of transvenous (jugular) biopsy of the liver in 1970 (6). Their work was confirmed by Rösch in 1973 (7). Because of the obvious advantage in avoiding a potentially serious intraperitoneal haemorrhage in such selected patients, Gilmore, Bradley and Thompson have constructed an improved design for the biopsy needle (8). A similar attempt at needle improvement has also been reported by Henriksen et al. from Denmark (9). The catheter has to be guided into a hepatic vein under fluoroscopic control. Wedge and hepatic vein pressures can also be measured at the same time, if indicated.

MANOMETRY

Following the pioneering work of Cournand, Ranges and Richards referred to in Chapter 1, the technique of central venous catheterization for pressure recording slowly gained acceptance. The central venous pressure (CVP) is representative of the state of distension of the venous collecting system and the effectiveness of the pumping action of the heart in emptying the system. Landis pointed out how the CVP gives an indication of the composite effects of a homeostatically controlled dynamic reservoir (10). Underfilling or overdistension are alterations in the system recognizable by CVP measurement before clinical indications have developed. Accordingly, CVP monitoring has been accepted as an important index to record for both diagnosis and assessing the therapeutic effect of volume replacement in critical circulatory problems (11–14). The importance of measuring the pulmonary artery and wedge pressures is further emphasized in Chapter 11.

Peripheral Venous Pressure

Moritz and Von Tabora described the direct measurement of the peripheral venous pressure in 1910 (15). Starling studied the relationship between venous pressure, cardiac output and the energy of myocardial contraction between 1912 and 1918 at University College London; and ultimately developed his 'Law of the Heart' (16, 17). In 1912 Meek and Eyster found a poor correlation between blood volume in haemorrhage and alterations in peripheral venous pressure (18). Shenkin found transient and insignificant changes in peripheral venous pressure when up to one litre of blood was removed from human volunteers (19). Just prior to this, in 1943, Starr et al. found a poor correlation between right heart failure and peripheral venous pressure (20). In the same year, Warren et al. observed only transient increases in peripheral venous pressure after giving dogs up to ten times their estimated blood volume in the form of normal saline (21).

Central Venous Pressure Manometry

In 1942 Cournand, Ranges and associates measured the pressure of blood in the right atrium of animals and man as a part of their comprehensive series of experimental investigations, after siting their catheters under fluoroscopic control. Their experiments were performed in both normal patients and those in right heart failure (22).

The advent of cardiac surgery and of improved and simplified methods of central venous catheterization caused a renewal of interest in venous pressure measurement. In 1956 Gauer and co-workers (23) demonstrated a linear relationship between central venous pressure and blood volume changes in man when 6–8 ml/kg were transfused or withdrawn. Removal of larger amounts (10–15 ml/kg) resulted in subjective and objective evidence of circulatory stress. These workers could only correlate central venous pressure with right median basilic vein pressure at the elbow if the patient stayed in the right lateral position with the arm dependent and abducted at 90° so that there was an uninterrupted column of blood from the atrium to the elbow (23).

The venous circulation has been extensively investigated, and Guyton (24) developed a concept of mean systemic pressure (MSP), which is that pressure to which the entire vascular system would equilibrate if the heart were to stop suddenly and the blood were pumped rapidly from the arterial to the venous system until their pressures were equal. This approximates to 7 mmHg. At rest, the MSP is determined by the ratio of the blood volume to the capacitance of the circulation. The rate of venous return is:

$$F_v = \frac{(MSP - RAP)}{R}$$

where RAP is right atrial pressure and R is resistance to flow in the vein. The CVP is directly proportional to the venous return and inversely proportional to the myocardial competence or contractility. The venous return is regulated by the blood volume and the capacitance of the venous system. In crude terms, the central venous pressure is a measure of the effective circulating blood volume relative to the ability of the heart to handle that volume (*Fig.* 3.2).

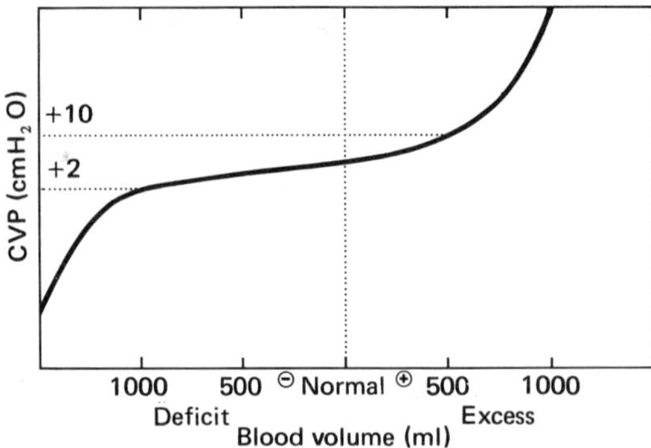

Fig. 3.2. Relationship of the central venous pressure (CVP in cmH$_2$O) to changes in the blood volume.

The CVP is not, however, a linear function of blood volume in clinical situations. Isolated CVP readings, unless high or low, are of little value. The continuous measurement of the CVP and correlation of changes with volume expansion or contraction are useful guides to intravenous fluid therapy. This measurement is merely an adjunct to other parameters and action should never be based upon a single facet of the patient's circulation. The correct interpretation of the measurement is particularly important when in the high range; the possibility of an acute obstruction affecting the right ventricular outflow tract by pulmonary emboli, or impairment of the heart's contraction by tamponade or pericardial constriction, must be considered in addition to myocardial failure and over-transfusion.

The technique, despite its physiological limitations, is invaluable for the monitoring and careful control of fluid replacement in conditions of (*a*) hypovolaemia; (*b*) myocardial failure; (*c*) acute renal failure; (*d*) septicaemia. In such circumstances, the careful and repeated measurement of right atrial, pulmonary artery and pulmonary capillary wedge pressures has been shown to be of great significance in the management of episodes of cardiopulmonary malfunction, especially in the elderly. In particular, the pressure of blood in the pulmonary capillaries is a basic factor in the shift of fluid into the interstitial tissues of the lung and the alveoli.

Starling first investigated the importance of the colloid or oncotic pressure of plasma in his efforts to find a suitable fluid for intravenous therapy during World War I. The normal plasma colloid osmotic pressure is 25–30 mmHg. Pulmonary oedema will occur if the pulmonary capillary pressure exceeds 30 mmHg. In many surgical patients the plasma colloid osmotic pressure may be diminished because of the dilutional effect of infused crystalloidal solutions. Hypoproteinaemia will also be associated with a more rapid development of pulmonary oedema, and this will occur at lower pressures in the pulmonary capillary bed. Recently, Weil has shown such a correlation between plasma oncotic pressure and the development of pulmonary oedema (25). The pulmonary capillary wedge pressure has proved to be a reliable indicator of left ventricular filling in patients without severe left ventricular failure and with normal mitral valve function. Starling's Law of the Heart applies to left ventricular function, and increases in stroke volume will occur with increasing left ventricular filling pressures measured at the end of diastole (*Fig.* 3.3).

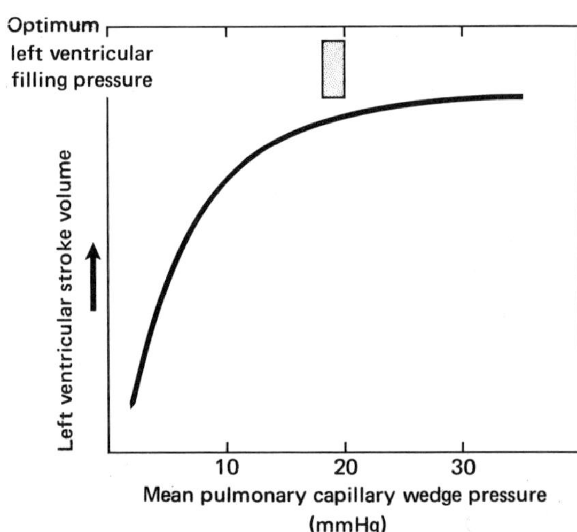

Fig. 3.3. The relationship between increasing left ventricular filling pressure and left ventricular stroke volume to illustrate Starling's Law of the Heart.

It can be seen from the graph that when the pulmonary capillary pressure exceeds 18 mmHg, further increases in this pressure by the infusion of excess fluid will have little effect on the stroke volume and pulmonary oedema will supervene.

Zero Reference Level

The need to establish a common reference level from which comparable values of the central venous system could be determined has long been recognized. It has been known that the pressure in the right atrium is virtually the same as that in the superior vena cava since the early work of Richards and his colleagues in the 1940s (22). Recent studies agree that the normal should range between 0 and 8 cmH$_2$O (12, 26). There is still a lack of uniformity concerning the choice of the extrathoracic reference point. The various methods used include:

1. A fixed distance from the anterior surface of the chest, e.g. suprasternal notch (27); costochondral junction of the fourth rib (15); angle of Louis.

2. A fixed distance from the posterior surface of the chest or operating table. Lyons selected a zero level 10 cm from the resting surface as a result of a fluoroscopic study of normal subjects (28).

3. A measure relative to the anteroposterior diameter of the chest. The 'phlebostatic axis' described by Winsor and Burch is the line of intersection between this plane (which has been shown on X-ray to be the point corresponding to the entrance of the caval veins into the right atrium) and a plane through the fourth intercostal space adjacent to the sternum (29).

An accurate and elegant study was performed by Pedersen and Husby in 1951 in order to find a plane that is easily determined using external landmarks and passes through the same level of the heart in all patients (30). They chose the middle of a line between the entrance of the superior vena cava and inferior vena cava into the right atrium. This was done with the patient lying horizontal during cardiac catheterization procedures under fluoroscopic control. The catheter was passed through the superior vena cava and right atrium and into the inferior vena cava. Lateral radiographs were taken and the levels were determined from the fourth intercostal space anteriorly. The anterior and posterior points through this plane were marked on the body surface with lead gum. A mean zero point was found of 0·43 times the depth of the chest below the anterior surface of the sternum on a level with the fourth intercostal space. The

mean deviation was only 3 per cent of the thoracic diameter (*Fig.* 3.4) (30).

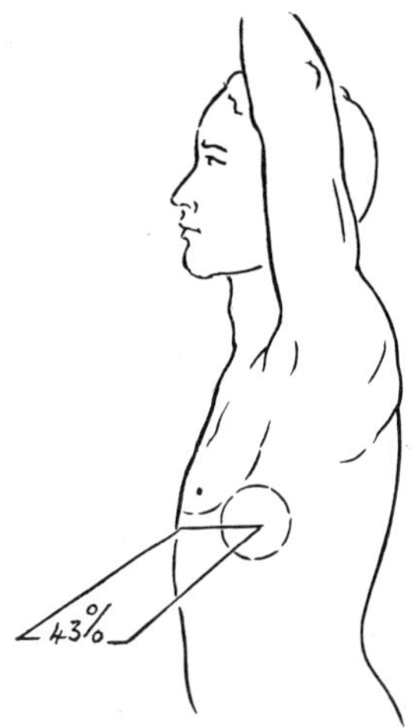

Fig. 3.4. Diagrammatic illustration to show the relationship between the zero reference point and the surface of the thoracic cavity.

Many clinicians now use a point on the mid-axillary line at the level of the fourth costal cartilage as a zero point. During surgery it is important to keep recalibrating readings on saline manometer sets with respect to this point before any therapeutic measures are instituted because the surgeon may have readjusted the height of the operating table.

Techniques for Calibrating Manometer Zero Reference Levels

The usual technique employed for measurement of central venous pressure is to connect the central catheter to a simple saline manometer linked to an administration set line via a three-way tap. The manometer tubing is usually fixed to a calibrated centimetre scale and some current sets are fitted with a telescopic arm fitted with a spirit level (*Fig.* 3.5). The level is extended and matched against the zero point selected on the patient's chest; this is either the intersection between the mid-axillary line and the anteroposterior plane from the fourth costochondral cartilage or the sternal angle itself. It is important to know which point individual members of the nursing staff may have used, because there is a difference of 6 cmH$_2$O between these points. Where no purpose-built level is available, a

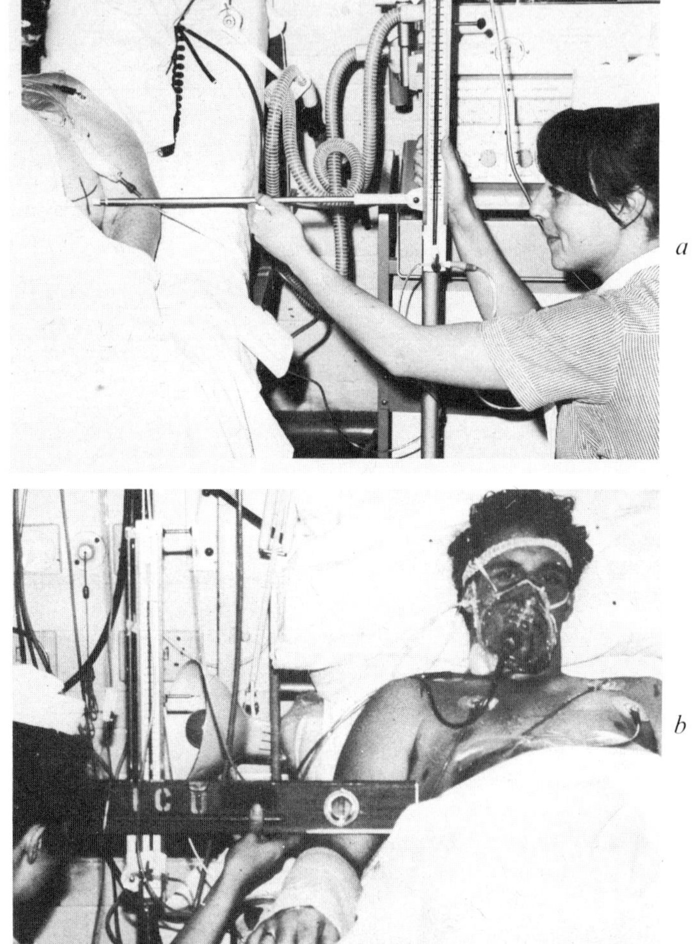

Fig. 3.5. Calibration of the central venous pressure manometer arm from the zero reference point on the chest wall using (*a*) an integral scale and spirit level and (*b*) a carpenter's spirit level.

carpenter's spirit level may be used. A further variation on this principle is shown in *Fig.* 3.6, in which an extending string or wire fitted with a small spirit level is used to determine the zero point. Notaras (31) introduced a simple technique for this purpose by utilizing a length of PVC tubing (e.g. from an intravenous administration set), filling it with coloured fluid or spirit and arranging it as a closed loop. This acts as an effective 'spirit level' and may be easily hung up on the drip stand between readings (*Fig.* 3.7).

Some intensive care units simply use a length of PVC intravenous tubing fixed to a wooden or plastic ruler which is inserted into the main line using the port of a three-way tap. The mano-meter line is primed by manipulating the tap and the zero point of the ruler is held directly against the reference level on the patient's chest wall. The three-way tap is then turned to close off the main intravenous line and the fluid in the mano-meter slowly falls, swinging with respiration and oscillating in synchrony with atrial activity until it equilibrates with the central nervous pressure.

Although these are the techniques most widely used, it should be apparent that mano-meter systems are open to the risks of air embolism and bacterial contamination of the infusion line or catheter should the nurse or clinician inadvertently leave the three-way stop-cock open. Conversely, in those manometer systems that are fitted with an air filter or small

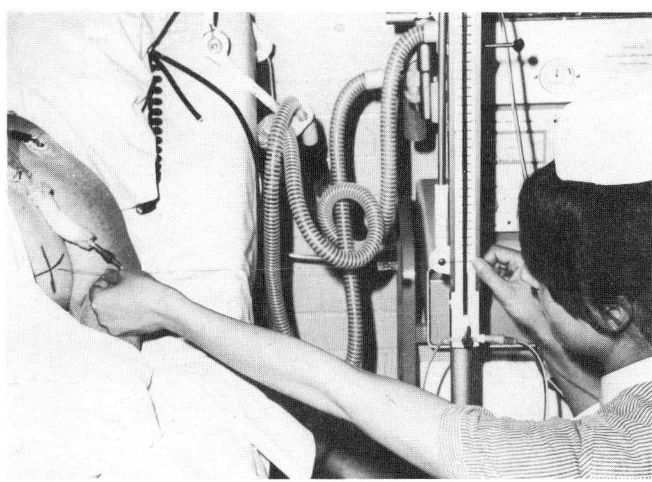

Fig. 3.6. Calibration of the central venous pressure manometer to the zero reference level using a home-made spirit level. The fluid capsule can be mounted on a piece of string, nylon or a Seldinger guide-wire.

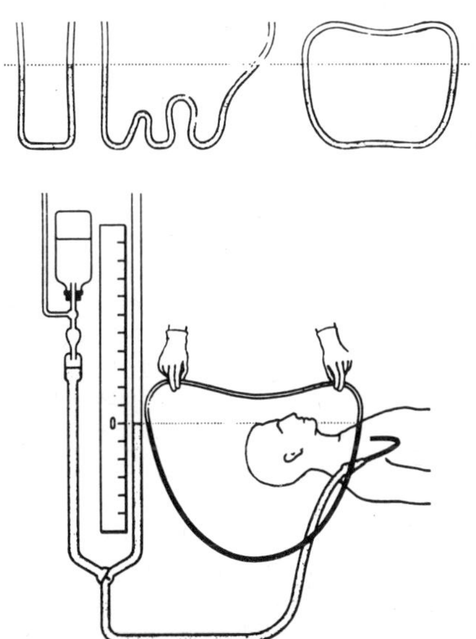

Fig. 3.7. Another useful variation of a 'spirit-level' which can be easily constructed in the ward situation. (Reproduced by kind permission of Mr M. J. Notaras, FRCS and the Editor of *The Lancet*.)

plug of sterile cotton-wool, if these become wet then the manometer will not work efficiently, and indeed falsely high readings of CVP may be obtained. Closed systems involving transducers and oscilloscopes are usually only employed in operating theatres and intensive care units at present. Perhaps in time a more sophisticated system will be developed for routine ward use.

Normal Levels

At birth the right atrial pressure is low ($0\,cmH_2O$). Occasionally, if there has been a large transplacental transfusion, it may reach $+5\,cmH_2O$, although this effect quickly subsides. In the newborn wide swings of between 5 and $12\,cmH_2O$ often occur, presumably as a result of the higher intrapleural negative pressure (32).

In adults at rest the normal right atrial pressure is approximately $7\cdot7\pm1\cdot5\,cmH_2O$ (mean $\pm$ s.d.), whilst the normal left atrial pressure is $5\cdot3\pm2\cdot7\,cmH_2O$ higher and is never lower than the pressure in the right atrium (33). Whenever measurements are made the zero reference point must be determined, since variations in the patient's position will obviously cause inaccuracy, especially if a sternal angle zero point is used. Falsely high readings of the central venous pressure will be obtained if the catheter is in the jugular vein, has looped or kinked or has advanced into the right ventricle, or if the lumen has become partially occluded by fibrin. There should be a free and easy fall of the saline manometer meniscus before any reliance can be placed on individual pressure readings.

Factors causing *elevation of CVP* include:
1. Intermittent positive pressure ventilation
2. Open chest—due to a loss of negative intrathoracic pressures

3. Myocardial failure
4. Cardiac tamponade
5. Constrictive pericarditis
6. Pulmonary embolism
7. Tension pneumothorax, hydromediastinum, hydrothorax
8. Overtransfusion and right ventricular failure
9. Chronic obstructive airways disease and cor pulmonale
10. Tricuspid incompetence

Factors causing *diminished CVP* include:
1. Hypovolaemia due to haemorrhage, plasma or extracellular fluid losses
2. Septic shock—with peripheral vasodilatation
3. Spinal anaesthesia

Thus, any developing abnormality in the central venous pressure should be rechecked and stimulate a further thorough appraisal of the cardiovascular and respiratory state of the patient. The exact reason for an elevated central right atrial pressure may be deduced from known preceeding events in an individual case, and from carefully examining the heart and peripheral circulation. When an elevated level is recorded, the reason should be diagnosed by arranging further appropriate investigations as necessary, e.g. an ECG, chest X-ray, echocardiogram and by reappraising the fluid infusion therapy. After cardiac surgery the onset of tamponade can be insidious and the central venous catheter itself should be considered as a cause of mediastinal superior vena cava or cardiac perforation. This can easily be ruled out by taking a chest X-ray after injecting a small volume of Conray 280 or Hexabrix (May & Baker Ltd) diluted with sterile saline through the catheter lumen.

In the presence of right ventricular failure, the cardiac output can be improved by an increase in right atrial pressure (RAP), an improvement of ventricular performance brought about by adjustment of autonomic nervous activity or the infusion of appropriate inotropic drugs. Thus, multiple levels of ventricular performance can be achieved, and this has become known as the Frank–Starling mechanism (*Fig*. 3.8) (34). It is possible by judiciously controlling the RAP or pre-load, the rate and force of myocardial con-

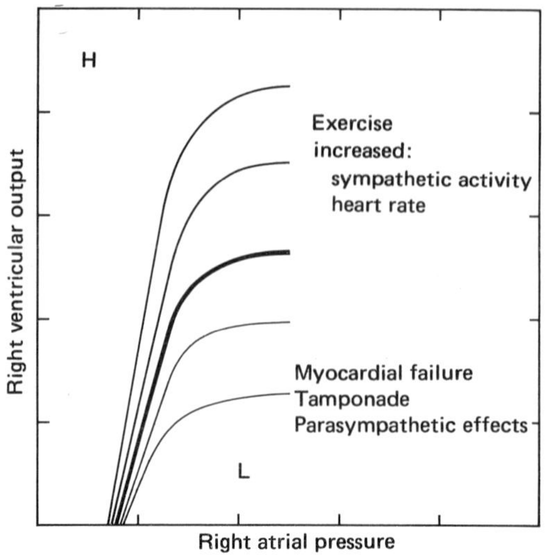

Fig. 3.8. The relationship of the right ventricular output and increasing right atrial pressure with varying levels of cardiac performance, e.g. Frank–Starling curves. Heart performance: H = high; L = low.

tractility and by reducing the after-load (i.e. the pulmonary or peripheral resistance) to achieve considerable therapeutic improvement.

A low CVP reading invariably means hypovolaemia due to haemorrhage, plasma or extracellular fluid losses. The action to be taken must of course depend upon the individual clinical situation. The central venous pressure is a good early indicator of acute upper gastrointestinal haemorrhage and may give prior warning of further haemorrhage by as much as 2 hours before the pulse or blood pressure changes. However, if the haemorrhage is severe the patient should undergo the appropriate emergency surgery rather than have a vain struggle instituted in order to restore the CVP to normal levels by blood transfusion. In these circumstances, resuscitation should proceed simultaneously with movement of the patient to theatre and induction of anaesthesia.

Central venous pressure estimations can be extremely helpful in the situation in which there is a low cardiac output state yet a CVP which lies within the normal range. There may be a relative hypovolaemia or primary myocardial failure and in such circumstances a fluid challenge can be used to assess cardiac performance (35, 36). In an adult 100–200 ml of fluid is infused at 25–50 ml/min. If a rise of more than

3 cmH$_2$O in the CVP persists, this indicates that the heart is unable to respond and the low output state is due to impaired myocardiac contractility. Experience has shown that CVP measurement is not a truly reliable guide in the prevention of overtransfusion and resultant pulmonary oedema. The value of measuring pulmonary capillary wedge pressure is further discussed in Chapter 11. For those wishing to read further into the subject, Russell has provided an excellent monograph and literature review (37).

MONITORING FOR AIR EMBOLISM DURING SURGERY

The problem of air entrainment into the venous system is not new or confined to neurosurgical procedures. Until 10 years ago, the single most sensitive diagnostic aid was the stethoscope (38). Prior to the introduction of Doppler ultrasound, air embolism was detected during neurosurgery in 5–14 per cent of patients (39, 40). With the advent of ultrasound, the incidence has increased to 33 per cent (41). Whether a central venous catheter can be used for the successful evacuation of air from the atrium is doubtful, but it is an essential instrument for calibrating the Doppler monitoring system. The intraoperative situation is depicted in *Fig.* 3.9.

The Doppler detects a 0·1 ml injection of carbon dioxide through the central catheter, and suitably insulated instruments are now available so that diathermy interference is eliminated. Maroon and Albin have been able to diagnose air embolism before pathophysiological changes in the heart rate, arterial or venous blood pressure, ECG or expired gases have occurred. The anaesthetist calibrates and correctly sites the Doppler probe over the praecordium using a minute injection of air or carbon dioxide. The classic echoes are heard through the ear-phones, and similar sounds are listened for during the surgery. The value of monitoring in this way for early detection of air embolism is illustrated in *Fig.* 3.10.

PLASMAPHERESIS

This term was first used by Abel, Rowntree and Turner of the Johns Hopkins University Pharmacology Department in 1914 (42) to describe 'the withdrawal of quantities of blood from an animal without apparent injury that exceeded several times the maximum quantity of blood that can be safely drawn by the usual method of venesection provided that the corpuscular elements of the blood suspended in Locke's solution (0·6 per cent NaCl) be returned to the vascular system after each bleeding'. They applied their technique to dogs who had undergone bilateral nephrectomy. They observed a marked improvement in their clinical condition and improved survival rates over control dogs.

The technique was used for the collection of plasma in 1944 (43) and first used in a blood bank in 1950 (44). The authors of the latter report also described the use of plasmapheresis in patients suffering from essential and renal hypertension. With the advent of more sophisticated plastic collection systems, Kliman and Schwab, in 1961, described a technique involving a collection system that included integrated and linked bags and tubes so that blood could be withdrawn, centrifuged and the plasma transferred to the infusion container without disconnecting the system (45). Today continuous

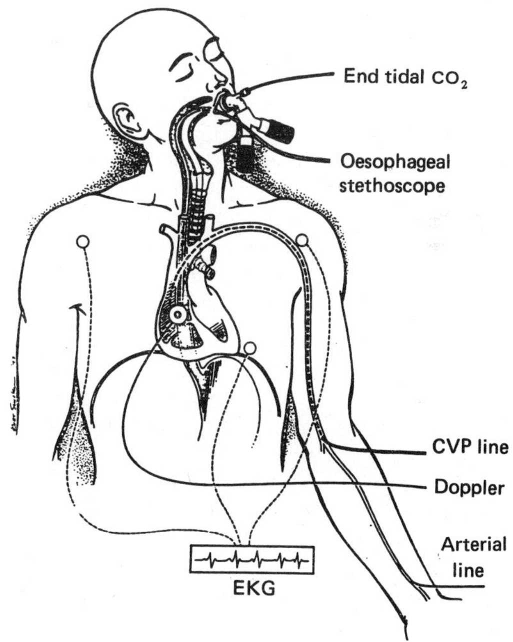

Fig. 3.9. An illustration of the intraoperative monitoring situation used during neurosurgery to detect air emboli using Doppler ultrasound. (Reproduced by kind permission of Dr H. M. Shapiro, MD and Dr L. Marsh, MD, San Diego, California, USA, from their monograph *Bubble, Bubble, Toil and Trouble.*)

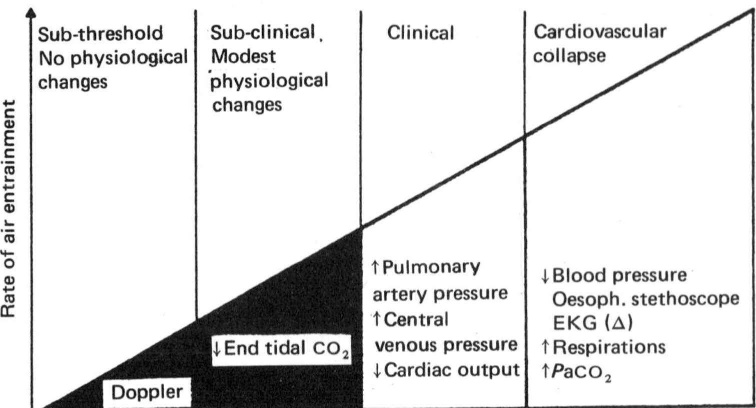

Fig. 3.10. The clinical spectrum of events associated with an increasing rate of air entrainment and the effective role of Doppler ultrasound and other monitoring procedures. (Reproduced by kind permission of Dr H. M. Shapiro, MD and Dr L. Marsh MD, San Diego, California, USA, from their monograph *Bubble, Bubble, Toil and Trouble.*)

flow cell separators are able to remove and process blood at 50 ml/min and can totally exchange 5000 ml of a patient's plasma for fresh frozen plasma or plasma substitute in 3 hours.

Although the process can be performed using peripheral veins, if repeated procedures are envisaged satisfactory long term venous access must be provided. This may be either an external arteriovenous (Scribner) shunt or an internal arteriovenous fistula or, alternatively, blood may be collected from a large calibre Hickman central venous line. Each of these techniques has a place in management of individual patients. In certain immune complex diseases, peripheral vascular disease may co-exist and rule out the shunt procedures because of the risk of digital gangrene. Also, episodes of hypotension may cause shunts to thrombose, hence the need for central venous access techniques.

During the past 5 years plasmapheresis has been used increasingly by physicians in the management of autoimmune disease. Experimental evidence suggests that immune complexes or specific autoantibodies are the principal initiators of glomerular injury. However, the damage to the basement membrane in nephritis is mediated by many humoral and cellular factors involved in the inflammatory response. Pinching (46) maintains that plasma exchange provides 'the opportunity for control of a hostile internal macromolecular environment, either by the selective depletion of abnormal substances and excessive levels of normal plasma factors (by exchange with fresh frozen plasma) or by the depletion of all plasma proteins except albumin (by exchanging for plasma protein fraction)'.

The removal of complement factors and kinins probably also has an immediate anti-inflammatory action. In this field of immune complex disease plasmapheresis is used in combination with immunosuppressive agents and corticosteroids. The technique is used in the management of the hepatic coma found in Reyes' syndrome, hepatitis and biliary cirrhosis (47); in the management of Goodpasture's syndrome and autoimmune disease in which antibodies develop against glomerular and pulmonary basement membranes (48) and in hyperviscosity states and malignant paraproteinaemias (49). The technique is also used to obtain plasma from normal donors. The limiting factor is the donor's ability to restore plasma proteins. Normally, about 10 g of plasma albumin and 2 g of plasma gamma-globulin are replaced each day (50). During intensive plasmapheresis Kliman found that up to 49 g of protein were replaced daily, suggesting that the liver was capable of a fivefold increase in the rate of synthesis of serum proteins (51). Cohen and Oberman reported no abnormality in donors who had given a plasma equivalent of up to 4 units of blood each week (52). Williams has succinctly stated, in an excellent review of the technical considerations (53), that this procedure represents a modern-day reincarnation of blood letting, practised from pre-Hippocratic times to the middle of the nineteenth century, when it fell out of favour due to the ill-effects of anaemia caused by its excessive use.

PERITONEOVENOUS SHUNT PROCEDURES

The principle of diverting body fluid directly into the venous system was established by Nulsen and Spitz (54) for the treatment of obstructive hydrocephalus when they published their work in 1952. In 1974, LeVeen et al. introduced a similar technique for the management of intractable ascites (55). As in the treatment of hydrocephalus, a one-way valve had to be developed so that a uni-directional flow of peritoneal fluid could be achieved from the abdominal cavity into a central vein. The intra-thoracic pressure falls with the descent of the diaphragm and the intra-abdominal pressure rises, so that a differential pressure provides the force required to propel ascitic fluid into the superior vena cava. LeVeen devised a valve that opens at a pressure of $3\,cmH_2O$. The peritoneum is drained through the valve and the fluid passes upward via a silicone tube to the superior vena cava. The valve is situated deep to the oblique muscles of the abdominal wall and superficial to the peritoneum at a site just below the liver's edge. The silicone peritoneal catheter is inserted into the peritoneal cavity, whilst the tube for insertion into the internal jugular vein is tunnelled subcutaneously using long alligator biopsy forceps. A venotomy is made into the internal (or external) jugular vein and this vessel is tied off distally and proximally around the catheter. The initial experience with this form of treatment in selected patients has been encouraging and satisfactory palliation has been achieved (56). Careful electrolyte control has to be maintained, and in some patients sudden return of fluid to the circulation has precipitated heart failure requiring diuretic therapy. In some case reports dramatic improvements have resulted; when the procedure has been performed for ascites in association with malignant disease, dissemination of the tumour has been reported. LeVeen points out that a technical failure of the device is indicated by the absence of haemodilution and diuresis in the early period after insertion. Late blockage is associated with a recurrence of the patient's ascites. This invariably responds to replacement of the valve and the peritoneal tube alone. Other reported complications have been sepsis and disseminated intravascular coagulation (57). An unusual complication of air embolism occurring via a LeVeen shunt has also been reported. This event occurred following perforation of the caecum after colonoscopy with polypectomy and cautery of a bleeding ascending colon lesion. Despite resuscitation, the patient died and was found to have suffered an air embolism which had entered the circulation via the LeVeen shunt (58).

PREVENTION OF PULMONARY EMBOLISM—CAVAL FILTERS

Central venous and, more recently, balloon flotation catheters have been used for many years to cannulate the pulmonary artery and perform angiography. If a major pulmonary embolism is diagnosed the catheter can be left in place and used to infuse heparin, streptokinase or urokinase as indicated by the clinical situation. During the past decade devices have been developed in the United States of America for insertion using a transvenous approach, via either the internal jugular or femoral vein, which interrupt the passage of thrombi from the iliac and femoral veins to the heart. Naturally, these are only used in patients at risk from recurrent pulmonary embolism where the presence of a major life-threatening iliofemoral deep venous thrombosis has been established, and moreover where the introduction of effective anticoagulation therapy would be contraindicated. In 1968, Eichelter and Schenk proposed the transvenous approach for partial occlusion of the inferior vena cava using local anaesthesia (59). The intraluminal devices which evolved were initially pioneered by Mobin-Uddin at the University of Miami Hospitals in 1968, and these techniques can be accomplished under local anaesthesia using fluoroscopic control (60). Several serious complications have been subsequently reported, including improper insertion into the common iliac and renal veins, migration and embolization of the 'umbrella' to the right atrium, ventricle or pulmonary artery. These complications have persisted despite increasing the diameter of the devices. In addition, complications have arisen from retroperitoneal haemorrhage, perforation of the duodenum and ureter and the formation of thrombus on the device itself proximal to the filters. The Mobin-Uddin umbrella has also been associated with thrombotic occlusion of the inferior vena cava below the device in 60 per cent of patients, and this naturally is associated with limb oedema.

Subsequently, Greenfield and his colleagues developed a stainless steel conical device with small hooks for fixation in the caval wall and designed for introduction through either the femoral or the jugular vein (61). In a small series these workers subsequently reported a 92 per cent patency rate at up to 3 years for the inferior vena cava and filter, and a 2·7 per cent incidence of recurrent embolization was noted. This group have also reported a technique of extracting emboli from the pulmonary artery using a specially designed large catheter introduced via the femoral vein, which is guided into the pulmonary artery. A balloon is then inflated close to the tip of the catheter, which has the shape of a suction cup, and with the pulmonary artery temporarily occluded, contrast medium can be injected down the main lumen of the catheter in order to outline the thrombus. The thrombus itself is then aspirated on to the suction cup and after deflation of the balloon, the catheter and embolus are then withdrawn simultaneously (62). The place of this procedure in the management of major pulmonary embolism has yet to be established. Indeed, at the present time, transvenous insertion techniques of umbrellas and filters are restricted to a very few select patients since the majority of patients are still managed with conventional anticoagulant therapy.

CHOICE OF CATHETER

There are many varieties of catheter now available from the medical plastics industry. None of these devices is suitable for all the previously mentioned clinical applications and it is important that the same care should be given by the clinician to the creation of the infusion system as is accorded to the selection of the fluids and the drugs administered through the lumen of the extra-corporeal auxiliary plastic appendage which he has linked to the patient's circulation.

Individual clinicians develop preferences based on the shape of the tip, the stiffness of the shaft, the chemistry of the material, the configuration of the hub and the method of introduction provided by the manufacturer. It is important that the catheter selected should suit the route of insertion and due regard should be given to the length of time for which the device is likely to be in position. The choice of a device should also take into account the known complications that have been documented.

Accordingly, it is the author's opinion that central venous catheters introduced using a through-needle technique are obsolete and should not be used, regardless of whether the needle has a splitting configuration or not. The risk of catheter embolization is not one that should be accepted by the clinician on behalf of the patient. The safest techniques involve either a through-cannula introducing cannula, in which there is always only a plastic-to-plastic juxtaposition and hence the definitive central line cannot be sheared, or a Seldinger wire technique. Similarly, home-made catheters which have 'disconnecting hubs' are likely to be a source of hazard for patients. The union between catheter and shaft is a potential source of bacterial contamination from the body surface and can now be eliminated by suitable chemical and mechanical bonding processes. Furthermore, the fixed hub provides extra security against the catheter inadvertently snaking into the circulation. Such reservations are based upon reported cases in the world literature.

The advent of silicone rubber has made long term venous cannulation a reality, and either this material or a variant of Teflon should be used when it is intended to leave the catheter in place for more than a few days. Experience has shown that PVC is unsuitable for long term cannulation in man.

In adults, for the approaches using the arm, a 60–70 cm catheter is necessary, for the subclavian route, 30–35 cm and for the internal jugular route, 12–15 cm. The correct choice of length is sometimes important and *Fig.* 3.11 illustrates the problem of malposition which may occur when a subclavian catheter is inserted via the internal jugular vein. Conversely, the majority of the short Teflon over-needle jugular catheters are inappropriately 'stiff' when introduced via the subclavian route. The risk of

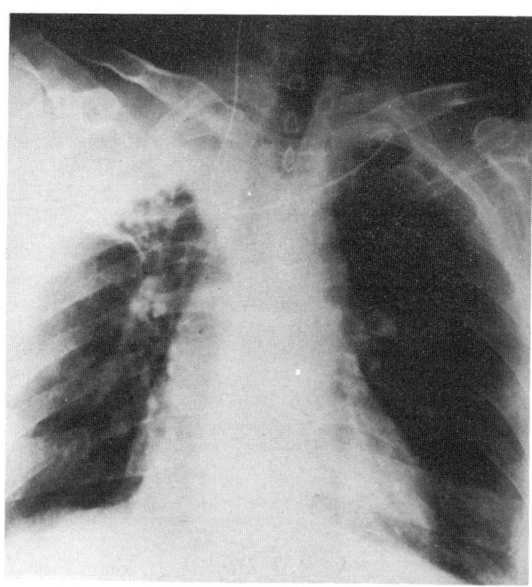

Fig. 3.11. Catheters which are too long and flexible may be inappropriate for the jugular route and are easily misplaced.

perforation of the superior vena cava or innominate vein is thus increased because the catheter has to assume the curves of the great veins in the superior mediastinum. Movement of the patient's shoulder or infusion line will cause a to-and-fro movement of the relatively rigid catheter tip against the endothelium of the vein.

The various tunnelling techniques naturally require catheters with different specifications and at the present time these are usually 90–110 cm in length. The hubs of these devices are also more resilient for their intended long term placement. The advent of these catheters is a welcome sign that the companies involved in this area of supportive patient care are willing to design more appropriate devices for use in the central venous circulation. There are subtle but important differences in the physiology of the central veins as compared with their peripheral tributaries. The great veins are subjected to an intermittent negative intrathoracic pressure which is exacerbated during episodes of hypovolaemia, tachypnoea, shock or periods of mechanical ventilation. There is an obvious need to change the characteristics of the hub in order to assist the nursing profession and patients during the changing of the administration set when the risks of bacterial contamination and air entrainment are ever present.

References

1. Hickman R. O., Buckner C. D., Clift R. A.: A modified right atrial catheter for access to the venous system in marrow transplant recipients. *Surg. Gynecol. Obstet.* 1979; **148**: 871–5.
2. Jacobs P., Jacobson J.: A practical method for ensuring long-term venous access. *J. R. Soc. Med.* 1979; **72**: 263–5.
3. Riella M. C., Pasquini R.: Atrial catheter for prolonged chemotherapy. *Lancet* 1977; **1**: 658.
4. Oakley C. M.: Infective endocarditis. *Br. J. Hosp. Med.* 1980: 232–43.
5. Hanafee W., Weiner M.: Transjugular percutaneous cholangiography. *Radiology* 1967; **88**: 35–9.
6. Weiner M., Hanafee W. M.: A review of transjugular cholangiography. *Radiol. Clin. North Am.* 1970; **8**: 53–68.
7. Rosch J., Lakin P. C., Astanovic R. et al.: Transjugular approach to liver biopsy and transhepatic cholangiography *N. Engl. J. Med.* 1973; **289**: 227–32.
8. Gilmore I. T., Bradley R. D., Thompson R. P. H.: Improved method of transvenous liver biopsy. *Br. Med. J.* 1978; **2**: 249.
9. Henriksen J. H., Matsen P., Christoffersen P. et al.: Improved transvenous liver biopsy needle. *Scand. J. Gastroenterol.* 1979; **14**: 593–8.
10. Landis E. M., Hortenstine J. C.: Functional significance of venous blood pressure. *Physiol. Rev.* 1950; **50**: 1.
11. Wilson J. N., Grow J. B., Demomg C. V. et al.: Central venous pressure in optimal blood volume maintenance. *Arch. Surg.* 1962; **85**: 563–70.
12. Weil M. H., Shubin H., Rosoff L.: Fluid repletion in circulatory shock. *JAMA* 1965; **192**: 668.
13. Longerbean J. K., Vannix R., Wagner W. et al.: Central venous pressure monitoring. *Am. J. Surg.* 1965; **110**: 220.
14. Brisman R., Parks L., Benson D. W.: Pitfalls in the clinical use of central venous pressure. *Arch. Surg.* 1967; **95**: 902.
15. Moritz F., Von Tabora D.: Ueber einer methode beim Menschen der druck in oberflachlichen venen exakt zu bestimmen. *Deutsch. Arch. Klin. Med.* 1910; **98**: 475.
16. Patterson S. W., Starling E. H.: The mechanical factors which determine the output of the ventricles. *J. Physiol.* 1914; **48**: 358.
17. Starling E. H. *The Linacre Lecture on the Law of the Heart.* London: Longmans, 1918.
18. Meek W. J., Eyster J. A. E.: Reactions of haemorrhage. *Am. J. Physiol.* 1921; **56**: 1.
19. Shenkin H. A., Cheney R. H., Govans S. R. et al.: The diagnosis of haemorrhage in man. *Am. J. Med. Sci.* 1944; **208**: 421.
20. Starr I., Jeffers W. A., Mead R. H.: The absence of conspicuous increments of venous pressure after severe damage to the right ventricle of a dog, with a discussion of the relation between clinical congestive cardiac failure and heart disease. *Am. Heart J.* 1943; **26**: 291.
21. Warren J. V., Merrill A. J., Stead E. A.: The role of the extravascular fluid in the maintenance of normal plasma volume. *J. Clin. Invest.* 1943; **22**: 635.
22. Richards D. W., Cournand A., Darling R. C. et al.: Pressure of blood in the right auricle in animals and

man: under normal conditions and right heart failure. *Am. J. Physiol.* 1942; **136**: 115.

23. Gauer O. H., Sieker H. O.: The continuous recording of central venous pressure from an arm vein. *Circn. Res.* 1956; **4**: 74.

24. Guyton A. C.: Cardiac output and its regulation. In: *Circulatory Physiology*. Philadelphia: Saunders, 1963.

25. Puri V. K., Weil M. H., Micheals S. et al.: Pulmonary oedema associated with reduction in plasma oncotic pressure. *Surg. Gynecol. Obstet.* 1980; **151**: 344–8.

26. Hardaway R. M.: *Clinical Management of Shock.* Springfield, Ill.: Thomas, 1968: 163.

27. Lewis T.: Remarks on early signs of cardiac failure of the congestive type. *Br. Med. J.* 1930; **1**: 849–52.

28. Lyons R. H., Kennedy J. A., Burwell C. S.: The measurement of venous pressure by the direct method. *Am. Heart J.* 1938; **16**: 675.

29. Winsor T., Burch G. E.: Phlebostatic access and phlebostatic level; reference levels for venous pressure measurements in man. *Proc. Soc. Exp. Biol. Med.* 1945; **58**: 165.

30. Pedersen A., Husby R.: Venous pressure measurement: (i) choice of zero level. *Acta Med. Scand.* 1951; **141**: 317–30.

31. Notaras M. J. Aid to central venous pressure measurement. *Lancet* 1971; **1**: 214.

32. Cottom D., Young M.: Venous pressure in exchange transfusion. *Arch. Dis. Childh.* 1965; **40**: 323.

33. Braunwald E., Brockenbrough E. C., Frahm C. J. et al.: Left atrial and left ventricular pressure in subjects without cardiovascular disease. Observations in eighteen patients studied by transeptal left heart catheterisation. *Circulation* 1961; **24**: 267–9.

34. Sarnoff S. J.: Myocardial contractility as described by ventricular function curves: observations on Starling's Law of the Heart. *Physiol. Rev.* 1955; **7**: 102–22.

35. Sykes M. K.: Venous pressure as a clinical indication of the adequacy of transfusion. *Ann. R. Coll. Surg. Engl.* 1963; **33**: 185–97.

36. Weil M. H.: Progress in the bedside management of shock. *J Trauma* 1969; **9**: 154–6.

37. Russell W. J.: *Central Venous Pressure: Its Clinical Use and Role in Cardiovascular Dynamics.* London: Butterworths, 1974; 1–75.

38. Michenfelder J. D., Terry H. R., Daw D. F. et al.: Air embolism during neurosurgery, a new method of treatment. *Anaesth. Analges.* 1966; **45**: 390–4.

39. Marshall B. M.: Air embolism in neurosurgical anaesthesia, its diagnosis and treatment. *Can. Anaesth. Soc. J.* 1965; **12**: 255–61.

40. Michenfelder J. D., Martin T. J., Altenburg B. M. et al.: Air embolism during neurosurgery. An evaluation of right atrial catheters for diagnosis and treatment. *JAMA* 1969; **208**: 1353–8.

41. Maroon J. C., Albin M. S.: Air embolism diagnosed by Doppler ultrasound. *Anaesth. Analges.* 1974; **53**: 399–402.

42. Abel J., Rowntree L. G., Turner B. B.: Plasma removal with return of corpuscles (plasmapheresis). *J. Pharmacol. Exp. Ther.* 1914; **5**: 625.

43. Cotui F. C., Bartter F. C., Wright A. M. et al.: Red cell reinfusion and the frequency of plasma donations. *JAMA* 1944; **124**: 331.

44. Grifols-Lucas J. A.: Use of plasmapheresis in blood donors. *Proc. Soc. Exp. Biol. Med.* 1952; **80**: 377.

45. Kilman A., Schwab P. J.: Plasmapheresis with simple equipment. *Am. J. Clin. Pathol.* 1961; **36**: 379.

46. Pinching A. J.: Plasma exchange. *Br. J. Hosp. Med.* 1978; **20**: 552.

47. Strauss R. A., Kling T. F., Livinsohn M. W. et al.: Facilitation of exchange transfusion with Scribner shunts in Reyes' syndrome. *Am. J. Surg.* 1976; **131**: 772.

48. Lockwood C. M., Pearson T. A., Rees A. J. et al.: Immunosuppression and plasma exchange in the treatment of Goodpasture's syndrome. *Lancet* 1976; **1**: 711.

49. Pineda A. A., Brzica S. M., Taswell H. F.: Continuous and semicontinuous flow blood centrifugation systems. *Transfusion* 1977; **17**: 407.

50. Peters T.: The biosynthesis of serum proteins. In: Sunderman F. W. and Sunderman F. W. jun. (ed.): *Serum Proteins and Dysproteinaemias*. Philadelphia: Lippincott, 1964: 9.

51. Kliman A., Carbone P. P., Gaydos L. A. et al.: Effects of intensive plasmapheresis on normal blood donors. *Blood* 1964; **23**: 647.

52. Cohen M. A., Oberman H. A.: Safety and long term effects of plasmapheresis. *Transfusion* 1970; **10**: 58.

53. Williams R. A.: Vascular access for cancer chemotherapy, chronic intravenous medication and plasmapheresis. In: Wilson S. E. and Owen M. L. (ed.): *Vascular Access Surgery*. Chicago: Year Book, 1980: 53–65.

54. Nulsen F., Spitz E. B.: Treatment of hydrocephalus by direct shunt from ventricle to jugular vein. *Surg. Forum* 1952; 399–403.

55. LeVeen H. H., Christoudias G., Ip M. et al.: Peritoneovenous shunting for ascites. *Ann. Surg.* 1974; **180**: 580–91.

56. Wapnick S., Grosberg S., Kinney M.: LeVeen continuous peritoneo-jugular shunt. *JAMA* 1977; **237**: 131–5.

57. Matsesche J. W., Beart R. W., Bartholomew L. G. et al.: Fatal disseminated intravascular coagulation after peritoneo-venous shunt for intractable ascites. *Mayo Clin. Proc.* 1978; **53**: 526–8.

58. Jacobsen W. K., Briggs B. A., Thorpe R. et al.: Air embolism in association with LeVeen shunt. *Crit. Care Med.* 1980; **8**: 659–60.

59. Eichelter P., Schenk W. G.: Prophylaxis of pulmonary embolism. A new experimental approach with initial results. *Arch. Surg.* 1968; **97**: 348.

60. Mobin-Uddin K., McClean R., Bolooki H. et al.: Caval interruption for prevention of pulmonary embolism. *Arch. Surg.* 1969; **99**: 711.

61. Greenfield L. J., McCurdy J. R., Brown P. P. et al.: A new intracaval filter permitting continued flow and resolution of emboli. *Surgery* 1973; **73**: 599.

62. Greenfield L. J., Reif M. E., Guenter C. E.: Haemodynamic response to transvenous pulmonary embolectomy. *J. Thorac. Cardiovasc. Surg.* 1971; **62**: 890.

Chapter 4

Equipment

J. V. Farman

The equipment needed for central venous catheterization consists of the catheter and its introducer, a sterile tray or set for the insertion procedure and a suture set; dressings and a CVP manometer or administration set; the appropriate extensions, manifolds and infusion apparatus. A constant evolution of design is taking place in this field of intravenous technology.

CATHETERS AND INTRODUCERS

The design of an individual catheter will depend on the way in which it is intended to be introduced. To attempt to introduce a catheter except in the way intended may prove difficult or even dangerous. Some types of catheter are more suited to one route of introduction than to another. The subject will be discussed from the clinician's standpoint, bearing in mind these considerations.

Methods of Introduction

Through a Cannula

An ordinary type of cannula is introduced into the vein, the needle is withdrawn and the catheter is passed in its place and advanced up the vein. The greatest advantage of this technique is that the needle never comes into contact with the catheter so there is no risk of damage or shearing (1). It is possible to employ a safe flexible catheter with either a well-smoothed end or a blind tip and side holes (2). This is the least complicated method of introduction and is strongly recommended for general purposes.

Catheters are usually packed in sterile sets with introducers but some are available alone.

The latter may be introduced via a cannula of another make, although care must be taken to ensure that the catheter will pass through before putting the cannula into the vein.

Special purpose catheters such as the Swan–Ganz may require special introducers. One such is the Desilet venous dilator (*Fig.* 4.1) which employs a Seldinger technique to insert a large cannula through which the catheter may be introduced. The Intralet is a similar double cannula, introduced over a needle (*Fig.* 4.2). An alternative method for inserting special catheters such as the Swan–Ganz employs a 12 G Medicut polyproplyene cannula and a disposable stitch cutter (3). The cannula is removed from its introducer needle, split longitudinally (*Fig.* 4.3) and then replaced on the needle and pushed into the vein, the material being sufficiently stiff to retain its shape. While spillage of blood is prevented by pressure over the tip of the cannula, the needle is removed. The catheter may be lubricated with sterile glycerine or silicone oil. It can then be passed in the usual way although it may stretch the cannula in the process. Once the catheter is in place, the cannula can be withdrawn, split apart and removed (*Fig.* 4.4). The ability to remove the introducing cannula would be a desirable improvement in future central venous catheter systems. At the present time, when the definitive central line hub is locked on to or fitted in the introducing cannula, a small but significant film of blood often remains which can act as a nidus for bacterial contamination.

The current available sterile through-cannula catheters together with their materials and dimensions are listed in Table 4.1.

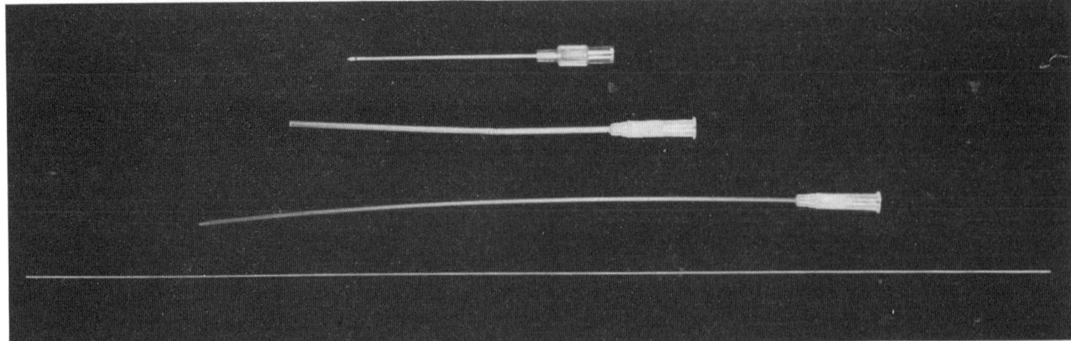

Fig. 4.1. The Desilet venous dilator and central catheter introducer kit. *From above:* the introducer, outer cannula, inner cannula (vein dilator) and guide wire.

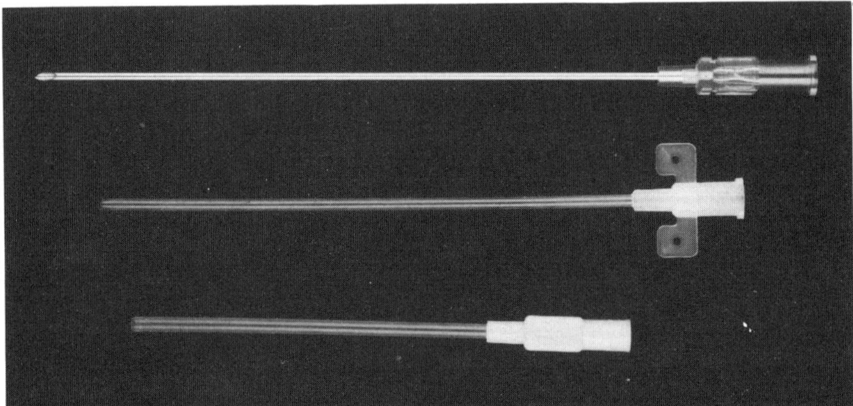

Fig. 4.2. The Intralet catheter introducer: *from above,* the introducer needle, inner cannula and outer cannula.

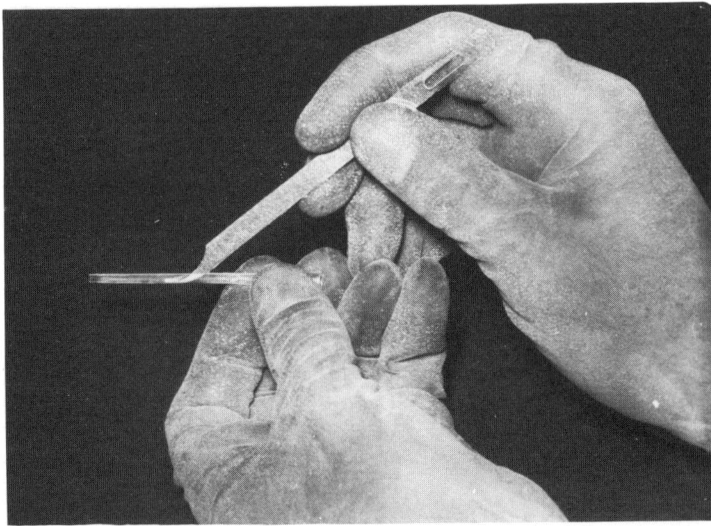

Fig. 4.3. Splitting a large Medicut cannula (Sherwood–Argyle) with a sterile stitch-cutting scalpel blade to create an alternative catheter introducer.

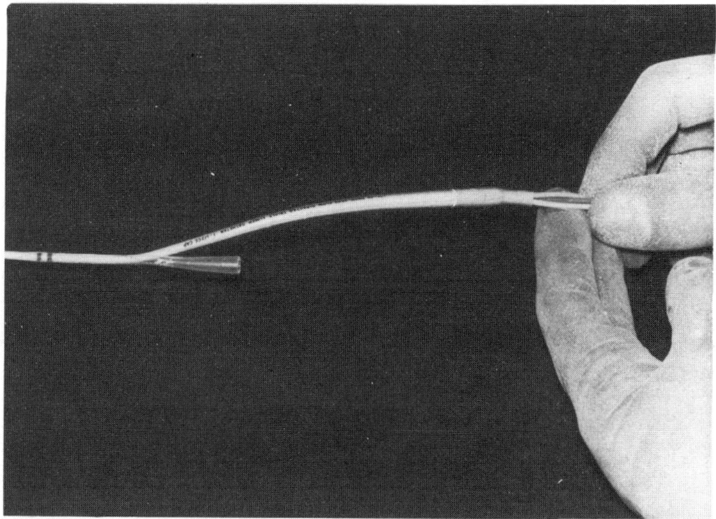

Fig. 4.4. Removing a split Medicut cannula from a Swan–Ganz catheter after insertion. The Medicut is then discarded.

Table 4.1. **Through-cannula catheters**

Type	Maker	Material	Lengths (mm)	Bores (mm)
Advanset	Bard	FEP Teflon	230, 300, 600	0·3, 0·8, 1·1
Cardioflex	Vygon	Polyethylene	1250	0·6, 1, 1·5
Centrasil	Travenol	Silicone	216	1·1
Intramedicut	Sherwood	Polyethylene	200, 300, 700, 1050	0·9, 1·1, 1·5, 1·9
I. V. Cannula*	Portex	Nylon	300, 600, 760	0·4–1·8 (7 sizes)
Piggy-Back PBP	Wallace	Polyester based polymer	200, 660	1·1
Piggy-Back S	Wallace	Silicone	200	0·8
Piggy-Back FEP†	Wallace	FEP Teflon	330, 660	0·84
Pulmoball*	Vygon	PVC	1250	1·7, 2·3 o.d.
Surcath	Vygon	Polyethylene	300, 500, 750	0·5, 1·2
Steriflex*	Vygon	Polyethylene	300–1500	0·3–3·0
Swan–Ganz*	Edwards	Polyethylene	1100	1·7, 2·0, 2·3 o.d.
XRO Silicone	Vygon	Silicone	350, 600	1·0, 1·2, 1·5, 2·0

o.d., outside diameter.
* Supplied without introducer.
† No longer available.

Over a Needle

This technique is essentially the same as that used for the ordinary short cannula. The needle sticks out of the end of the catheter which is tapered to fit closely to it. One advantage is that the smallest possible hole is made in the venous wall. The whole unit is passed into the vein, the needle withdrawn and the catheter is advanced. Some versions are in effect extra-long cannulas and these short central catheters are widely used for cannulation of the internal jugular vein using a percutaneous technique (Chapter 6). Others, such as the E–Z Cath (originally invented by Dr J. S. M. Zorab of Bristol) and the Trocaflex, have a wire to pull out the needle (*Fig.* 4.5).

The long type is best suited to the median cubital route because it may be difficult to tell when the needle has entered the vein, although in 1972, Savege described a modification to improve the flashback of blood (4). Another disadvantage is that these catheters are made of

Table 4.2. **Over-needle catheters**

Type	Maker	Material	Lengths (mm)	Bores (mm)
Abbocath T.	Abbott	FEP Teflon	140	1·1, 1·5
A-Cath	Bard	TFE Teflon	150	1·0, 1·4
Angiocath	Deseret	TFE Teflon	135	1·1, 1·5
E–Z Cath*	Deseret	TFE Teflon or PVC	215, 300, 600	0·8, 1·1, 1·5
Intranula	Vygon	Polypropylene	120	0·7, 1·1, 1·4, 1·0
Intralet	Vygon	Polypropylene	75	1·7, 2·0
I. V. Cannula	Wallace	FEP Teflon	137	1·0, 1·5
Longdwel	Becton, Dickinson	FEP Teflon	100, 150, 200	0·8, 1·1, 1·5
Medicut	Sherwood	Polypropylene	170	1·8
Steritex	Molnlycke	Teflon	50, 150	1·1, 1·4, 1·7, 2·2
Trocaflex*	Vygon	PVC	300	1·2, 1·45
Vena Subclavia Cannula	Stille	TFE Teflon	165	1·45, 1·75, 2·2

* Wire-located needle.

a fairly stiff material that can stand being pushed through the skin, and the resulting hard sharp end may damage the vein (*see below*).

The commonly available sets of over-needle catheters together with their materials and dimensions are shown in Table 4.2.

Over a Guide

By this method, first described by Seldinger in 1953 for arterial cannulation (5), a guide (usually wire) is inserted into the vein through a needle which is then withdrawn. The catheter is then passed into the vein over the guide (this, of course, must be longer than the catheter to allow its removal) which in turn is withdrawn. The benefits are that the catheter never comes in contact with the needle and only a small hole is made in the vein. The drawbacks are that the guides (if made of spiral wire) are expensive and that the catheter tip must be stiff and tapered to follow the guide through the skin and the venous wall and so has a rather sharp end (*Fig. 4.6*).

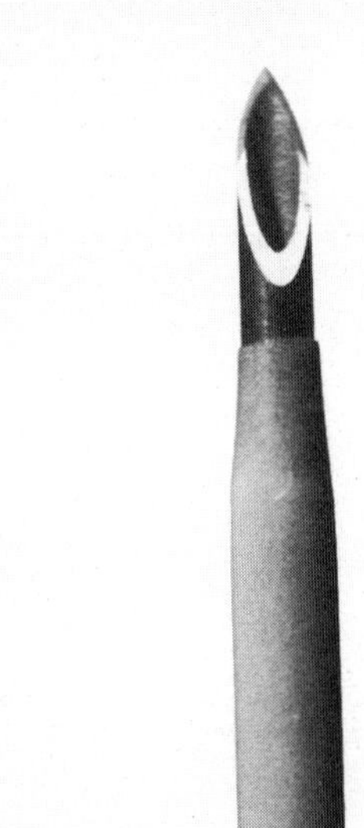

Fig. 4.5. The tip of the E–Z catheter in position on its introducer needle. The tapered tip fits closely to the needle and assists skin penetration.

Table 4.3 gives the currently available sets of sterile over-guide catheters with their materials and dimensions.

Table 4.3. **Seldinger catheters**

Type	Maker	Material	Lengths (mm)	Bores (mm)
Arrow	Arrow	Polyurethane	127, 152, 300, 450	1·0, 1·4
Atrial suction catheter	Cambridge	PVC	800	0·8
Desilet	Vygon	Polypropylene	—	1·2–3·0
Haemaquet	USCI	Teflon	90	1·6, 2·0, 2·3, 2·6
Leadercath	Vygon	Polyethylene	80, 180, 250, 300	0·8, 1·0, 1·2, 1·45

The Cut-down Technique

This safe technique is indicated when a patient's veins are too empty for percutaneous catheterization. The catheters used are essentially the through-cannula type.

Through a Needle

The first venous catheters to become widely available were introduced through needles that were merely withdrawn to lie outside on the skin. Special plastic protective devices (purses) were provided in an attempt to prevent the sharp edges of the needles cutting the catheters. At one time accidents due to shearing of through-needle catheters were so common that the Department of Health and Social Security issued a warning against their use (6). The British Standard excludes such catheters on the grounds of safety. Now that more satisfactory and safer alternatives are available *there is no justification for the use of through-needle catheters.*

Sterility

Although at one time it was common practice to buy non-sterile catheters and to 'sterilize' them before use, nowadays single-use, pre-sterilized catheters and equipment are almost universally used. However, there are still exceptions in the case of expensive or special-purpose devices such as thermistor catheters and transducers and their taps for pressure recording. Physical cleaning of many devices is often difficult or impossible. The amount of re-sterilizable equipment should always be minimized. Materials vary in their tolerance of sterilization, and may deteriorate if an unsuitable method is employed. The common methods are autoclaving, dry-heat sterilization, or use of ethylene oxide, ionizing radiation or other chemical methods.

The British Standard for Intravascular Catheters

The British Standards Institution has been preparing a specification for intravascular catheters to be published shortly. It covers catheters and introducer devices (needles, cannulas and guides). There are, or will be, separate standards for cannulas (short catheters, BS 4843: 1972), radiodiagnostic catheters (BS 5322: 1976) and cardiac catheters. Size designation, materials, finish, sterility, packaging and labelling are included. More importantly, BS 5616: 1981 details the preferred shapes of catheter tips, size of side holes and shape of introducer needles, cannulas and guides.

The standard includes a test which requires that flow should not be unduly restricted (by more than 40 per cent) when the catheter is bent through 90° around a 12 mm diameter bar. The hub security test demands that the catheter should not immediately become detached when a 2·5 kg weight is applied. The catheter has to be cured for 2 hours beforehand in a water bath at 37 °C and may be supported by a mandril. The first leakage test requires the catheter and hub to withstand a pressure of 300 kPa for 30 s. The second leakage test detects entry of air on aspiration. Radio-opacity is verified by placing the catheter beneath an aluminium step wedge. After exposure to X-rays at 70 kV with a focal distance of 1 m the thickness of aluminium through which the catheter is distinguished gives an indication of its radio-opacity.

The eventual aim is for all catheters to conform to the British Standard, so giving the user the assurance of certain qualities. Several catheters at present on the market would not meet these requirements (*see below*).

Materials

Venous catheters are made from flexible polymers. Early examples were usually manufactured from polyethylene, PVC or nylon (polyamide). These materials have proved to be either thrombogenic (7, 8) or rather stiff. Polypropylene appears to be both stiff and thrombogenic (9, 10). Fluorocarbons were introduced in a search for less thrombogenic polymers. Tetrafluorethylene (Teflon TFE) seems to be some improvement on the earlier materials and Teflon FEP, a co-polymer of hexfluoropropylene and tetrafluorethylene, is much better and is now widely used for cannulas (11), although it is really too stiff and liable to kink for catheters. (Note that both these materials are called by the trade name Teflon, a cause of considerable confusion.) One maker uses a polyester-based polymer which combines flexibility with satisfactory implant characteristics. Silicone elastomer has long been recognized as non-thrombogenic (12), but is so pliable as to be difficult to insert, although use of a suitable stylet overcomes this problem.

Apart from their chemical properties, stiff catheters tend to generate thrombus by pressure on the venous walls (7). Because flexible catheters float in the bloodstream and are unlikely to lie against vessel walls, they cause less damage (8).

The British Standard requires simply that 'neither the catheter nor any part of the set that may come into contact with the body fluids and tissues shall yield particles of materials or toxic substances'. Most plastics contain additives which may leach out once they are within the body. As much as half the material may consist of plasticizers, stabilizing agents, anti-oxidants and colouring (13). In addition, materials for venous catheters include an X-ray contrast medium which is usually a barium or tungsten salt. The only way to test for toxicity is by implant testing. With this technique, Lawrence et al. in 1969 found that about one-third of their examples of plastic tubing gave toxic responses due to the leaching out of constituents (14). A British Standard on biological implants is in preparation. Most British and American manufacturers now employ tested materials, but

Table 4.4. **Performance of through-cannula catheters**

Type	% flow, bent	Aspiration test	300 kPA leak test	2·5 kg pull test	X-ray opacity
Advanset	100	+	+	+S	+
Centrasil	100	+	+	+S	+
Intramedicut	96	+	+	+S	+
I.V. Cannula (Portex)	89	+	+	−	−
Piggy-Back PBP	93	+	+	+S	+
Piggy-Back S	98	+	+	+S	+
Piggy-Back FEP	100	+	+	+S	+
Surcath	93	+	+	−S	+
XRO Silicone	94	+	−	−S	+

+, Passed; −, failed; S, stretched.

Table 4.5. **Performance of over-needle catheters**

Type	% flow, bent	Aspiration test	300 kPA leak test	2·5 kg pull test	X-ray opacity
Abbocath T	94	−	+	+S	+
A-Cath	96	+	+	+	+
Angiocath	96	+	+	+	+
E–Z Cath	93	+	+	+S	+
Intranula	97	+	+	+	+
I.V. Cannula (Wallace)	98	+	+	+S	+
Medicut	22	+	+	+	−
Longdwel	98	+	+	−	+
Trocaflex	93	+	+	+	−
Vena Subclavia	99	+	+	+	+

* Wire-located needles; both needles withstood 2·5 kg.
+, Passed; −, failed; S, stretched.

Table 4.6. **Performance of Seldinger catheters**

Type	% flow, bent	Aspiration test	300 kPA leak test	2·5 kg pull test	X-ray opacity
Atrial suction catheter	94	+	+	+S	−
Leadercath	97	+	+	+S	+

+, Passed; −, failed; S, stretched.

many unsuitable substances remain in use, particularly in catheters of foreign origin.

An example of each catheter available in the United Kingdom at the time of writing was tested. The results are given in Tables 4.4, 4.5 and 4.6. The majority showed little or no reduction in flow when bent round a 12 mm rod. Teflon, nylon and polypropylene catheters had to be moulded by hand (which is impossible after insertion) otherwise they kinked. The polyethylene catheter was notably softer at 37 °C, the only one to behave in this way, and bent easily. The silicone catheters were very flexible. The 2·5 kg pull test was difficult to apply with some materials. Polypropylene and nylon catheters hardly stretched at all; Teflon, polyester-based polymer, PVC and polyethylene catheters all stretched indefinitely, and silicone catheters sprang back when the weight was removed. Further details of these tests are given under appropriate headings.

Complications Associated with Catheter Design

There have been a horrifying number of complications reported in the literature, with many cases ending fatally. In spite of the flood of reports in the past 15 years, representing only a small proportion of the actual numbers involved, deaths due to catheterization are still occurring (15). It cannot be too strongly emphasized that every possible safety precaution must be taken. The subject is fully discussed in Chapters 12, 13 and 14.

Damage during Introduction

Stiff catheters may fail to follow the course of a vein and if force is applied during introduction

the venous wall can easily be pierced or the endothelium stripped.

Late Trauma

Over-needle catheters have tips especially tapered to fit tightly around their introducer needles. When the needle is withdrawn a sharp edge is revealed which is capable of eroding the wall of a vein and even penetrating the myocardium. The tip of an over-needle catheter is shown in *Fig.* 4.5. Catheters designed to be introduced over guides by the Seldinger technique also have quite sharp ends (*Fig.* 4.6). Any catheter made of stiff material is capable of eroding vessels or the heart, even if the tip is rounded or square-cut, and bevelling the end increases this risk (16).

There are innumerable reports of penetration of the heart and great vessels by indwelling catheters, often with fatal results. Perforation is often delayed for 24–48 hours after insertion, suggesting that rhythmical movement of the catheter tip with the respiratory and cardiac cycles eventually erodes the vessel wall. When the tip lies in a subclavian or innominate vein or in the superior vena cava, erosion of the vein leads to hydromediastinum or, quite commonly, hydrothorax (17, 18). If the tip is allowed to remain within the right atrium or ventricle, erosion produces a pericardial effusion and tamponade, which is frequently fatal (15). This complication can be prevented by correct location and by use of a soft catheter.

Kinking

Catheters of stiff material or with thin walls kink easily; if the material is very flexible, they may also become compressed. Catheter design involves a compromise between a number of desirable properties and in general PVC, poly-

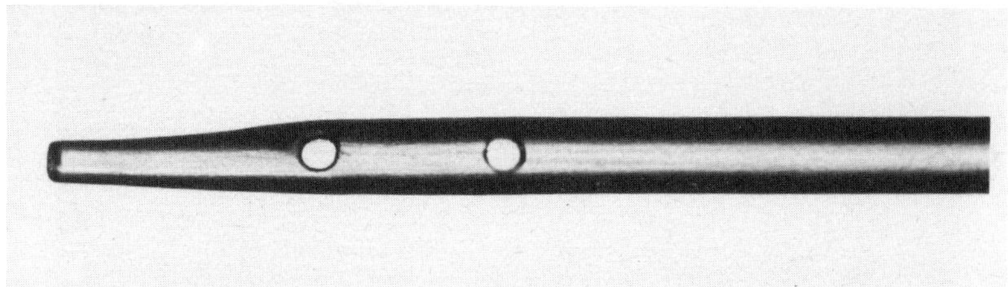

Fig. 4.6. Tip of the Cambridge atrial suction catheter. This is tapered to fit a wire introducer guide and so assists skin penetration.

ethylene and polyester catheters are fairly flexible; Teflon, nylon and polypropylene are rather stiff and so may kink, while silicone is very pliable indeed and can be compressed. Naturally, when kinks are not attended to, the flow of infused fluids will be impaired, central venous pressure measurement inaccurate and the catheter may subsequently split with resultant intraluminal bacterial contamination or even catheter embolism.

Shearing

This complication occurs typically with through-needle catheters and many such events have been reported in the literature. In 1963 Taylor and Rutherford (19) had 5 deaths out of 11 cases, while in a review of the literature Bennett found 5 deaths in 8 cases (20). The causes were either failure of the plastic sheaths to protect the catheters or attempts by users to pull the catheters back through the needle. Catheters with faults may break spontaneously (21); the author has seen two silicone catheters break under minimal stress, fortunately without harm to either patient.

Another common site of breakage is immediately next to the hub, which is fortunately nearly always exterior to the patient. No make of catheter is immune. This complication can only be prevented by meticulous care in securing the catheter hub. If the insertion site cannot be changed and is otherwise intact, a temporary repair can be effected by inserting a venous cannula into the open end (the tapered polypropylene Medicut is most suitable for this purpose). An alternative is to remove the catheter and replace it with a new one, either through the introducer cannula or over a guide.

Fibrin Formation

It is now recognized that as long as a catheter lies within a vein, a sheath of fibrin forms on the device (7, 8). Fibrin deposition usually begins at the point of entry or of intimal damage from the catheter tip and spreads along the vein. The amount of thrombus deposited increases with time. The materials used for catheters differ in their thrombogenicity as a result of variations in surface smoothness. Hecker has demonstrated this relationship particularly in radio-opaque catheters in which crystals of contrast medium obtrude from the surface (22).

Thrombophlebitis

This appears to result from a combination of fibrin thrombus with chemical and physical irritation from the presence of the catheter. The former is due to leaching of chemical substances or to irritating infusion fluids and is in any case more common with stiff catheters (*see above*). Thrombophlebitis does not necessarily imply the presence of infection. Welch et al. (23) observed organizing thrombus in the jugular veins of dogs with implanted polyethylene catheters but not in those with silicone elastomer ones. This was attributed in part to the stiffness of the material, and so may equally apply to the Teflon and nylon catheters.

Individual Catheters

Through-cannula Catheters

These have become the most popular type because of their safety and ease of insertion. They are also suitable for the cutdown technique

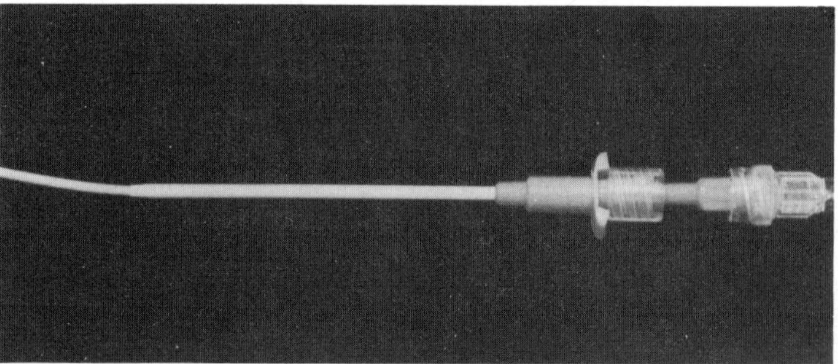

Fig. 4.7. New through-cannula catheter with a locking ring to prevent separation from the introducer and provide extra strength and stability of a hub–shaft junction. (Reproduced by courtesy of H. G. Wallace.)

and the Portex and the Vygon-Steriflex models are designed specially for this purpose. For inserting pulmonary artery catheters, a split Medicut cannula as described above or an Intralet or Desilet (*see above*) can be used. Note that for subclavian cannulation an introducer measuring 60–70 mm is needed, so that makers offer more than one introducer size. For general purposes, catheters of polyethylene, polyester-based polymer or silicone are preferred because of their flexibility; the latter material is the least toxic but the most expensive. The two Teflon FEP catheters (Advanset and Piggy-Back FEP), with their square-cut ends and stiff material, were occasionally difficult to advance. The new Wallace 66 mm FEP through-cannula device has a smoother tip to facilitate atraumatic intravenous advancement. Furthermore, the central venous catheter hub has been fitted with a locking ring which engages the introducing catheter and provides increased strength and stability of this junction whilst preventing inadvertent separation of the components (*Fig.* 4.7). The tips of several types of through-cannula central catheters are shown in *Fig.* 4.8.

Details of the through-cannula catheters are provided in Table 4.4. All passed the aspiration test and none leaked at the hub connection. However, one example of the Vygon silicone catheter leaked from a hole half-way along and broke at this point during the pull test. These catheters had a detachable hub secured by a plastic purse, and the joint is secure as long as this is in place. The hub has now been re-designed with a cone and screw lock which appears to be very effective, but this version was not available for test at the time of writing. One example of the Portex IV cannula had its hub detached by the 2·5 kg weight. The Surcath stretched and then broke at the hub during the pull test. No example of Cardioflex or Steriflex was available for testing. The balloon catheters (Swan–Ganz and Pulmoball) were not tested because of their multi-lumen construction.

Over-needle Catheters

The longer E–Z Cath and Trocaflex have sterile sheaths which permit their insertion by a no-touch technique and which are removed afterwards. No means of adjusting the length within the patient is needed because the catheter is

simply withdrawn until the correct amount is inside. They have wire-located introducer needles. The attachment of the needle was tested in each case and withstood a 2·5 kg pull.

The other catheters were in effect longer versions of the ordinary short cannula. They are suitable for internal jugular catheterization, although because of their stiff materials and sharp ends, they should not be left in place for long periods. The Abbocath T permitted a stream of air to pass between the catheter and the hub during the aspiration test and it was

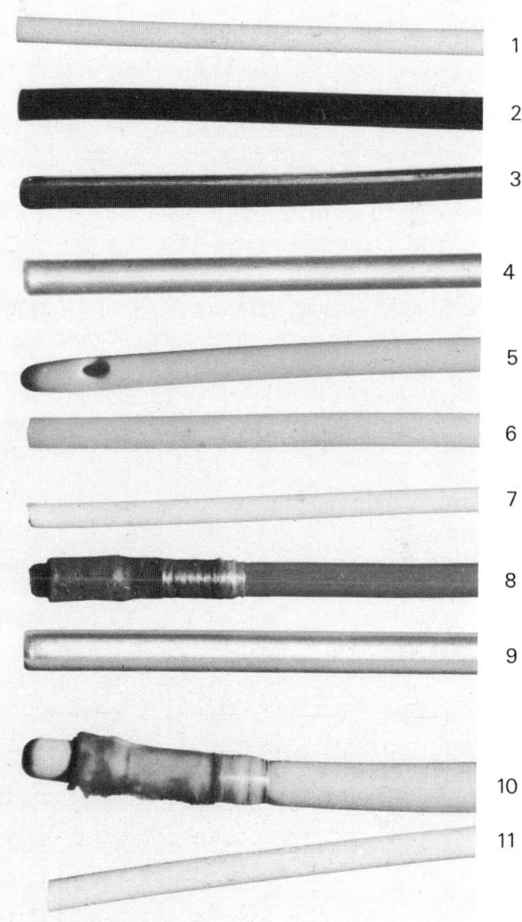

Fig. 4.8. Tips of some common catheters. **1.** Advanset (Bard). **2,** Centrasil (Travenol). **3.** Intramedicut (Sherwood). **4,** Nylon I. V. (Portex). **5,** Piggy-Back (Wallace). **6.** Silicone Piggy-Back (Wallace). **7,** FEP Teflon (Wallace, now withdrawn). **8,** Pulmoball (Vygon). **9,** Surcath (Vygon). **10,** Swan–Ganz (Edwards, with balloon damaged by the author). **11,** Silicone (Vygon).

possible to move the catheter up and down in the hub. The hub of the Longdwel came off in the pull test. The Medicut kinked when an attempt was made to bend it round a 12 mm rod. These results are summarized in Table 4.5.

Seldinger Catheters

These are frequently used, and may be invaluable in special circumstances. Table 4.6 gives details of the types available. The Cambridge atrial suction catheter (*see Fig.* 4.6) is designed for the aspiration of air embolus during neurosurgical operations and is therefore only intended for short term use. It is not radio-opaque and must be located by the injection of contrast medium, or by use of an ultrasound technique. The Leadercath is radio-opaque and, although the hub stayed on during the pull test, the catheter itself stretched and broke. The Desilet and Haemaquet venous dilators and catheter introducer are inserted over guides and so are included here.

EQUIPMENT USED IN INSERTING THE CVP CATHETER

The insertion of a central venous catheter is a sterile procedure. The risks of introducing infection are considerable (*see* Chapter 13) in the type of patient usually encountered. A strict aseptic technique should be used on all occasions.

Most hospitals prepare suitable sterile packs in the central sterile supply department. Towels are needed to shield non-sterile areas, swabs and forceps for skin cleaning, and a container is required for the skin preparation solution. Sterile gloves are worn. Local anaesthesia requires needles and syringes. The catheter will need to be stitched in place. Silk is preferred, being more 'grippy' than nylon. The inexpert surgeon will find that size 0 (3·5 mm) is strongest and easiest to handle, in combination with an atraumatic cutting needle. A list is given in Table 4.7. For cutting-down, a knife with a No. 15 blade, toothed tissue forceps and small retractors will be needed. An ampoule of physiological saline is used for filling the catheter before insertion in certain circumstances. Lastly, a sterile dressing is required, either a transparent sheet—Op-Site (Smith & Nephew) or similar—

Table 4.7. **Equipment needed for central venous catheterization**

Iodine aerosol or tincture of iodine
Gloves
Glove towel
Sterile central venous catheterization set
    Catheter
    Introducer needle and cannula
    Guide wire (if required)
3 towels or drapes
Swabs
Forceps
2 × 10 ml syringes
Orange (25 G); green (21 G) or cream (19 G) hypodermic needles
1% w/v lignocaine
10 ml Hepsal, 10 i.u./ml (Weddell Pharmaceuticals) or 10 ml 0·9% saline
3/0 or 0 silk suture with straight or curved atraumatic cutting needle
Op-Site I.V. dressing (6 cm × 8·5 cm); or wound (10 × 14 cm) or medium (28 × 30 cm); or large (28 × 45 cm) (Smith & Nephew)
Flushing device
Extension or manifold
CVP manometer (if required)
Solution infusion set
Filter (if required), e.g. Pall Ultipore

to cover the whole insertion site or a small dressing for the skin puncture.

ASSOCIATED EQUIPMENT

Infusion Sets

A basic requirement will be an infusion set. Unless blood products are to be given, a solution giving set with 3 mm tubing (to BS 2463) will be sufficient. For blood and blood products, a filter or filter set is required to remove clots and microaggregates. The ordinary blood giving set has a filter of 170–200 µm mesh and so does not trap microaggregates. There are a number of suitable microaggregate filters on the market (24). A microaggregate filter is recommended when fresh blood is not used. The bore size of the tubing is actually immaterial in this context as the flow rate will be limited by the narrow catheter. Note that some infusion pumps require special giving sets.

In view of the danger of air embolism occurring via catheters in the central veins, drip-sets with locking Luer connectors should be used. Unfortunately, this is not always possible at the present time because many of the manufacturers do not provide this safeguard on their manometer sets.

Central Venous Pressure Manometers

The common type of manometer consists of a column calibrated directly in centimetres, as shown in *Fig.* 4.9. It is controlled by a three-way

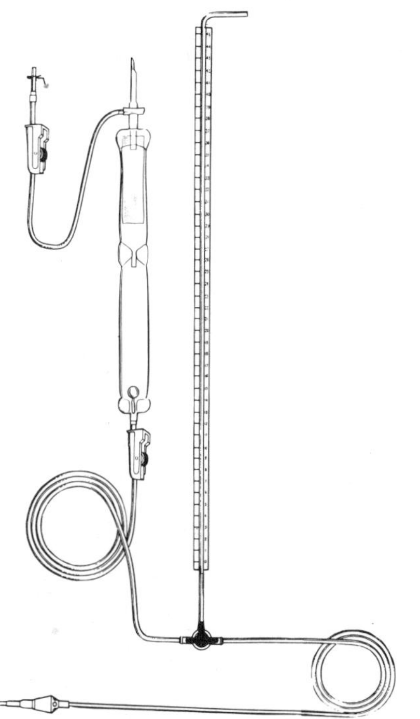

Fig. 4.9. Basic central venous pressure manometer, with administration dripset, three-way stopcock, manometer side arm and centimetre scale.

tap which is used to fill the column and then to connect it to the venous catheter. A spirit level is used to ensure that the column zero is at the correct level with reference to the patient. The level of fluid (usually 0·9 per cent saline or dextrose/saline) falls until the height of the fluid in the column is equal to the pressure in the vein. There are a number of variations on this basic theme.

Extensions and Manifolds

There are two great advantages in using some sort of extension or manifold. First, it is possible to include the catheter hub within the sterile dressing, so that changes of infusion set can be made without disturbing the catheter, its suture or the skin puncture site. This will reduce the chance of these becoming infected. Secondly, the flexible extension is able to move with the minimum disturbance of the catheter. The ordinary giving set is heavy enough to pull the catheter out of position, hurting the patient and disturbing the dressings.

There are a number of extensions available, such as the Abbott anaesthesia extension set, the Abbott T-connector (which incorporates an injection site) and devices from Viggo and Stille-Werner which have the additional safety advantage of locking Luer hubs. Manometer lines with Luer hubs (Portex and Vygon) make excellent extensions where low flows are acceptable and are available in various lengths.

A manifold allowing a number of connections is very useful in the intensive care unit where a number of different fluids may be infused simultaneously. Parts which are not in use are closed with sterile locking occluders. Examples of such devices are shown in *Fig.* 4.10. Vygon make two-way manifolds to which additional locking Y-connectors can be added; these are closed with lock-on occluders with rubber injection ports. Three-way taps may be used where a line must be turned off altogether, but should not be used as intermittent injection devices. Taps should be changed at regular intervals because of the high risk of bacterial contamination in the interstices of the mechanism.

Flushing Systems

To ensure that the venous catheter remains clear, it must be continuously flushed; 5 ml/h is generally sufficient. This can be achieved with a simple gravity system if the head of pressure is sufficiently high above the patient (over 1 m) and the flow rate is controlled carefully. It is difficult to measure such low flows with a standard giving set, but the majority of patients require larger intakes of fluid, and there is usually no problem keeping the catheter open. For minimal flows a high-resistance device which passes 3–5 ml/h (from Intraflo, Norton, AHS, Wallace) when the fluid-containing bag is compressed to 150–300 mmHg by a pressure infusion device, e.g. a Fenwall bag contained in a Norfolk

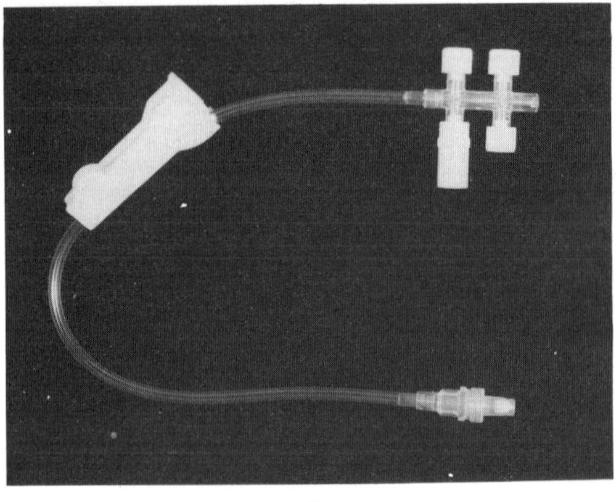

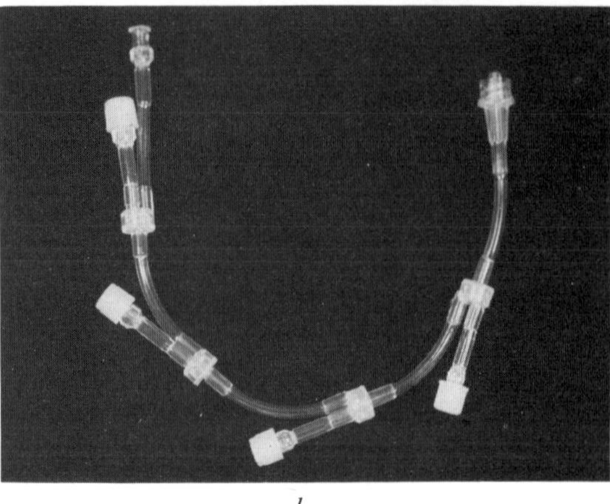

a   *b*

Fig. 4.10. *a,* Braun pre-sterilized four-branch manifold. *b,* Van Leer Medical manifold with integral non-return valves on each side arm.

and Norwich infusion box (*Fig.* 4.11) (25). Other auxiliary flow control devices are now available to protect the patient with gravity-fed infusion systems when large volumes or potent pharmacological agents are being used, e.g. the Dial-a-Flo device (*Fig.* 4.12, Abbott–Sorensen).

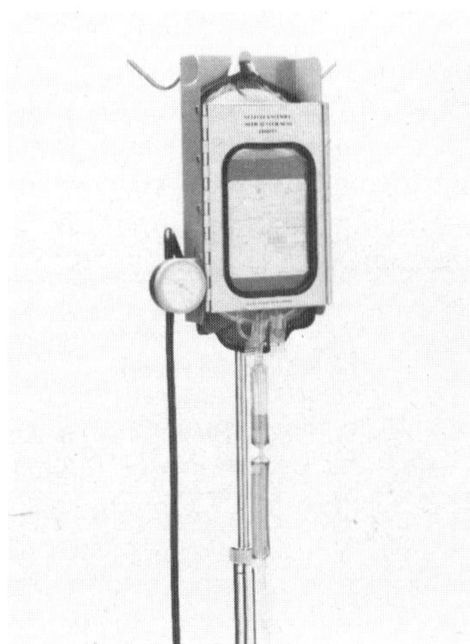

Fig. 4.11. The Norfolk and Norwich infusion box.

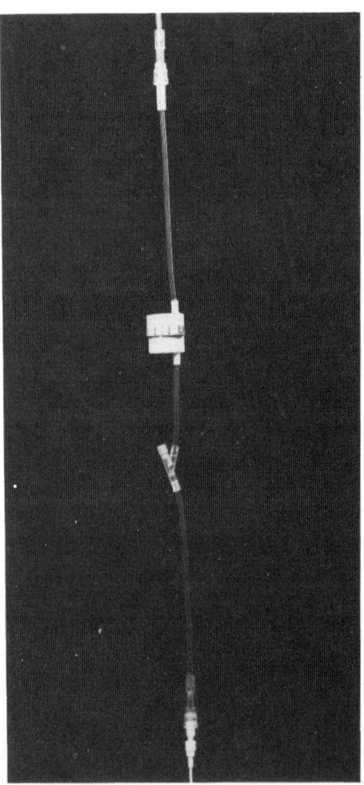

Fig. 4.12. The Abbott–Sorensen Dial-a-Flo device.

Syringe Pumps

By using a syringe pump to give a minimal flow the venous catheter can be kept clear of clot. It may not be justifiable to use a pump solely for this purpose, but if the need arises to give a drug by continuous infusion, this is the most convenient and economical way of doing so. A 50 or 60 ml syringe will accommodate 10–12 hours' dose which is injected in a volume of diluent at a rate of around 5 ml/h. This will be the method of choice for inotropes, heparin, insulin, potassium—indeed any potent agent. The greatest advantage is that a large volume infusion is not needed in order to achieve fine control of the dosage. There is a minimal risk of injecting air.

Most syringe pumps are electrically powered and must conform to current safety regulations (HTM8 or IEC standard). The best pumps can be controlled to 0·1 ml/h. The controls should have a positive action and be immune from inadvertent alteration. Clockwork pumps are portable and electrically safe, but only generate very low flows. High pressures can be generated by these pumps, but most modern designs give warning and cut-out automatically when this happens. Examples are the Sage, the Harvard and the Meltec; the author's unit uses Vickers Treonic IP3 pumps, which have proved highly satisfactory. A battery pump is made by Graseby Dynamics.

Composite Pumps

These pumps employ special syringes or cassettes which refill automatically from an ordinary infusion container. They combine the accuracy of the syringe pump with the large capacity of the conventional infusion pump. Examples are made by Imed, Ivac, Kontron and Valleylab.

Infusion Pumps

This type of pump may be used in conjunction with a central venous catheter. It works with infusion sets and bottles or packs, the pump acting on the drip tubing, using either the roller, sigamotor or delta principles. The roller pump has three rollers which compress the drip tubing against a circular track. An example is the Watson–Marlow pump. Sigamotor or peristaltic pumps have a series of fingers which bear on the tubing in turn, 'milking' the liquid contents along; examples are made by Graseby Dynamics, Braun, Ivac, Imed and Medishield. The delta pump uses three bars on a wheel, over which the drip tubing is stretched; as the wheel rotates the liquid is milked along the tubing by the moving bars. An example is the Vickers Treonic DC2 pump. This type cannot generate dangerously high pressures.

Very high pressures can be generated by some of these pumps, capable of disrupting ordinary Luer connectors, or even of ballooning and bursting a kinked catheter. A danger also exists with an open system, with an air inlet into a rigid container, that air may be pumped into the patient. All new models of infusion pumps are designed to stop pumping automatically in these events. Economy of drugs can be achieved by using a small-volume pack (e.g the Viaflex, 100 ml size).

References

1. Farman J. V., Powell D.: The performance of disposable intravenous catheters, needles and cannulae. *Br. J. Hosp. Med. (Equip. Suppl.)* 1968–69; **1–2**: 37–45.
2. Farman J. V.: A new central venous catheter. *Lancet* 1976; **1**: 780.
3. Farman J. V.: Which central venous catheter? *Br. J. Clin. Equip.* 1978; **3**: 210–14.
4. Savege T. M.: Cannulation of the internal jugular vein. *Lancet* 1972; **2**: 602.
5. Seldinger S. I.: Catheter placement of the needle in percutaneous arteriography. *Acta Radiol.* 1953; **39**: 368–76.
6. John G. E.: D.S. (Supply). Hazard Notice (HN 6). London: DHSS, 1972.
7. Indar R.: The dangers of indwelling polyethylene cannulae in deep veins. *Lancet* 1959; **1**: 284–5.
8. Hoshal V. L., Anuse R. G., Hoskin P. A.: Fibrin sleeve formation in indwelling subclavian central venous catheters. *Arch. Surg.* 1971; **102**: 353–5.
9. Wyatt R., Gloves I., Cooper D. J.: Cannulation of the radial artery. *Lancet* 1974; **2**: 156.
10. Fraser I. M., Eke N., Laing M. S.: Is infusion phlebitis preventable? *Br. Med. J.* 1977; **2**: 232.
11. Thomas E. T., Evers W., Raez G. B.: Post-infusion phlebitis. *Anaesth. Analges.* 1970; **49**: 150.
12. Fletcher R. F.: Silicone-rubber tubing for transfusion. *Lancet* 1956; **1**: 509–10.
13. Mitchell D. C. *Info 75* (Abbott Laboratories Ltd). 1975: no. 12.
14. Laurence W. H., Turner J. E., Autian J.: Re-evaluation of plastic tubings currently used in medical and paramedical applications. *J. Biomed. Mat. Res.* 1969; **3**: 291–303.
15. Czanky-Treels J. C.: Hazards of central venous pressure monitoring. *Anaesthesia* 1978; **43**: 172.
16. Galbert M. W., Kay J. E.: Perforation of the right innominate vein by central venous polyethylene catheter. *Br. J. Anaesth.* 1971; **43**: 713.
17. Adar R., Mozes M.: Fatal complication of central venous catheters. *Br. Med. J.* 1971; **3**: 746–7.
18. Rudge C. J., Bewick M., McColl I.: Hydrothorax after central venous catheterisation. *Br. Med. J.* 1973; **3**: 23–5.
19. Taylor F. W., Rutherford C. E.: Accidental loss of plastic tube into venous system. *Arch. Surg.* 1963; **86**: 177.
20. Bennett P. J.: Use of intravenous plastic catheters. *Br. Med. J.* 1963; **2**: 1252.

21. Parulkar D. S., Grundy E. M., Bennett E. J.: Fracture of a float catheter: a case report. *Br. J. Anaesth.* 1979; **50**: 201.
22. Spanos H. G., Hecker J. F.: Thrombus formation on indwelling venous cannulae. *Anaesth. Intensive Care* 1976; **4**: 217–24.
23. Welch G. W., McKeel D. W., Silverstein P. et al.: The role of catheter composition in the development of thrombophlebitis. *Surg. Gynecol. Obstet.* 1974; **138**: 421–5.
24. Walker A. K. Y.: Blood microfiltration: a review. *Anaesthesia* 1978; **33**; 35–8.
25. Chapman R. B., Keep P.: The Norfolk and Norwich infusion box. *Anaesthesia* 1980; **35**: 1211–14.
26. Ross S. M., Freedman P. S., Farman J. V.: Air embolism after accidental removal of intravascular catheter. *Br. Med. J.* 1979; **1**: 987.

Chapter 5

Insertion Routes: Peripheral Placement Techniques

J. L. Peters

There are many satisfactory approaches for gaining access to the central veins with a catheter. Whilst, theoretically, all venous tributaries link eventually with the great intrathoracic veins, it is only practical to use a few selected routes. The vagaries of anatomy prevent the smooth and safe advancement of catheters from many peripheral veins. Prior to attempting central venous catheterization, the clinician should consider which is the safest procedure for the patient and for how long the device will be required.

The possible alternatives in an individual patient may have been limited by previous peripheral cannulas causing thrombophlebitis. The routes of insertion that are usually considered are discussed in this and subsequent chapters under the two broad categories of insertion—by percutaneous and by surgical exposure or cut-down techniques.

1. Percutaneous technique
Scalp vein
Internal jugular vein
External jugular vein
Subclavian vein
Cubital fossa veins
Femoral veins

2. Surgical exposure techniques
Anterior facial vein
External jugular vein
Internal jugular vein
Cephalic vein
Cubital fossa veins
Umbilical veins
Long saphenous veins

Some of these routes are obviously primarily of value in the neonate and infant (umbilical, scalp, anterior facial and long saphenous veins). Conversely, the risk of pneumothorax from attempting to puncture the subclavian vein should rule this out as a route of choice in children unless other approaches have been eliminated because of burns or cutaneous infection. The internal jugular is a satisfactory vein to cannulate for short periods of manometry or therapeutic infusions, and the percutaneous techniques are described by Dr English in Chapter 6. The external jugular vein may be safely cannulated using a cut-down technique in children, and undoubtedly the safest techniques in this age group for the inexperienced practitioner are those peripheral techniques described in Chapters 17 and 18.

PERCUTANEOUS TECHNIQUES

In the adult the choice for the tyro faced with the need to assess the central venous pressure should be a left antecubital fossa approach to the median basilic vein either by a percutaneous or by a direct exposure technique. Similarly, the external jugular vein should be considered by junior house officers; with the patient in a 20° head-down Trendelenburg tilt this vein becomes engorged and is easily cannulated (*Fig. 5.1*). Some commercial kits are now supplied with a short J-wire which enables a Seldinger technique to be used on the external jugular vein in order that the catheter can be manipulated into the subclavian vein and superior vena cava. The main disadvantage of this route is the occasional difficulty in negotiating the catheter through the

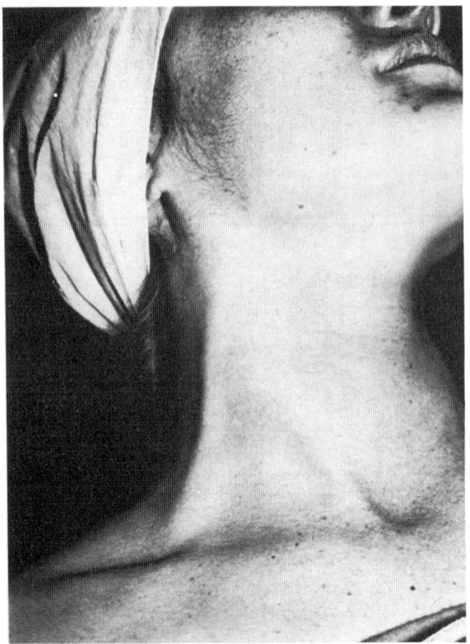

Fig. 5.1. The external jugular vein distended by placing the patient in a 20° head-down Trendelenburg tilt.

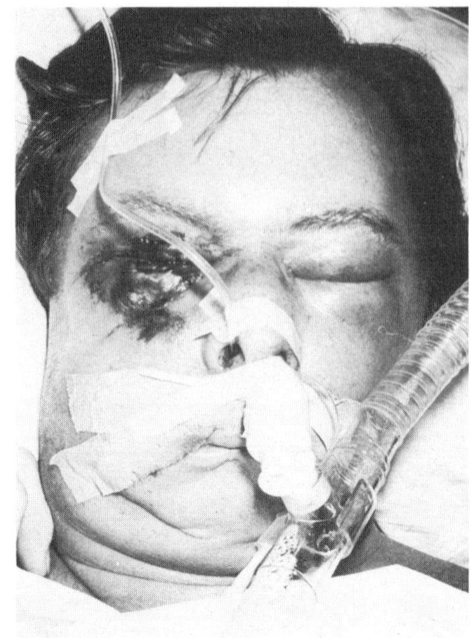

Fig. 5.2. This man, who was receiving a low dose of corticosteroids, developed a fulminating streptococcal cellulitis of the face following a minor abrasion; this spread rapidly to the neck and upper thoracic tissues. A silicone Broviac catheter was tunnelled down from his anterior abdominal wall and inserted via a tributary of his left long saphenous vein in order to provide venous access for his antibiotic therapy.

valves and past tributaries near the confluence with the subclavian vein.

With increasing experience, the next safest route of insertion is the right internal jugular vein, and percutaneous subclavian catheterization should only be attempted after instruction and under supervision. When prolonged catheterization of the central venous system is contemplated, consideration should be given to direct surgical exposure of the cephalic or external jugular veins, with the creation of the subcutaneous tunnel to a distant site. Very rarely, the subclavian or internal jugular vein, rather than their more convenient tributaries, many require direct exposure and catheterization. The need for such procedures usually only arises after numerous periods of prolonged cytotoxic treatment and chemotherapy via Hickman catheters in patients with leukaemia who have had several phases of remission induced.

Although the femoral vein is not usually cannulated because of the increased risk of iliofemoral deep venous thrombosis and infection, the approach may have to be used when the upper extremity veins have thrombosed,

been destroyed by burns or involved in cellulitis (*Fig.* 5.2). The initial disappointing experience in the early 1960s involved PVC catheters, and the insertion site care was not so meticulous. Bozetti in Milan (1) has shown that the femoral vein can be a satisfactory route for the inexperienced, provided that scrupulous attention to aseptic technique and catheter care is maintained. Catheters can also be tunnelled away from the site of insertion to the anterior abdominal wall.

Common Sense v. Iatrogenic Misadventure

For the patient with established shock or a severe illness, there is no greater risk to his or her recovery than an inexperienced practitioner making repeated and inaccurate attempts to puncture veins in the root of the neck. Moreover, if the doctor's determination to succeed with the procedure overrides natural caution, then a tragic sequence of events will follow, of which the sequelae are documented in Chapter 12. The lethal combination of surgical arrogance and a relative ignorance of the anatomy or pathophysiology has been responsible for many distressing case reports from throughout the world in this field of supportive patient care.

Examples and anecdotes abound, e.g. a fatal attempt to perform a percutaneous subclavian puncture upon a patient who had already undergone a contralateral pneumonectomy, resulting in a fatal tension pneumothorax; patients have died from pneumothorax after attempts to puncture the subclavian vein have been made on the contralateral side to a traumatic haemopneumothorax. Bilateral pneumothorax has been induced because the doctor omits to exclude the possibility of a pneumothorax and changes sides for a further attempt. Not all patients who are hypovolaemic need to have a central venous catheter inserted immediately for the purpose of fluid replacement. One or more peripheral infusions can be established, resuscitation achieved and, if surgery is contemplated, the safest route should be chosen for the insertion of a manometer line. A cautious attitude on behalf of the clinician and the application of common sense in the selection of the most appropriate route of insertion will avert clinical tragedies.

The Peripheral Vein Approach via the Cubital Fossa

This route, first selected by Forssmann, is deservedly popular for short periods of catheterization. The relatively high incidence of local thrombophlebitis and axillary vein thrombosis is the principal limiting factor in the use of this approach. In normal circumstances, the axillary and subclavian vein are kept patent during abduction and other movements of the shoulder by a concomitant rotation of the clavicle (*Fig. 5.3*). One can also see in this illustration that simultaneous elbow flexion and shoulder abduction must cause any intravascular prosthesis to undergo considerable to-and-fro movement. The piston effect and the long length of catheter in contact with the arm vein no doubt initiate the thrombophlebitic process which invariably occurs within 10 days when Teflon or PVC

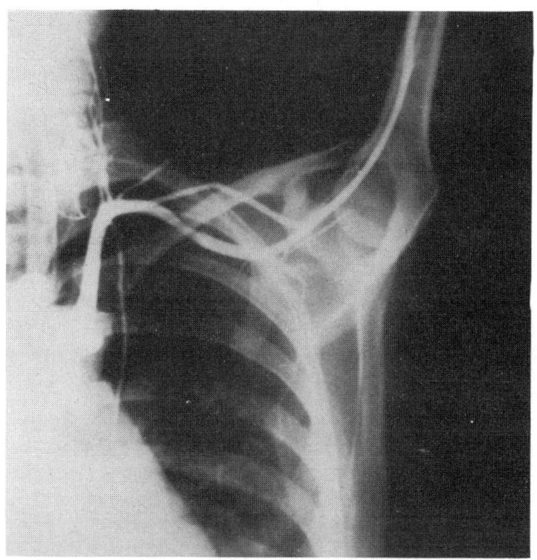

Fig. 5.3. A contrast venogram of the left cephalic, axillary and subclavian veins showing that the vessel remains patent during abduction and is not occluded by the clavicle or first rib. (Reproduced by kind permission of Mr S. Mottershead, FRCS, Middlesbrough, and the Editor of the *British Medical Journal*.)

catheters are used. This complication should not be dismissed lightly, because should suppurative bacterial thrombophlebitis become established in the axillary or subclavian vein, the prognosis is extremely poor and death from septicaemia can occur. Silicone catheters, although more difficult to insert, have been left *in situ* for slightly longer periods before they too cause thrombophlebitis. Another practical problem which arises with these long lines is that sometimes during the course of their clinical life the catheters gradually slide out of the arm. The consequence of this may be that hypertonic fluids are infused into the axillary vein and therefore cause a thrombosis to be propagated. Thus, catheters inserted via this route should preferably be removed after 7 days and care should be taken to ensure that the tip is sited in the central veins while hypertonic solutions are being administered. Despite these drawbacks, this route of insertion is safe, devoid of the risks of pneumothorax and injury to other important structures in the neck. It should be the route of choice for the inexperienced junior doctor, with patients who require short term central venous manometry. The freedom from the risk of pneumothorax also makes this approach of particular value in patients known to have impaired pulmonary function and for those about to undergo surgery with a period of intermittent positive pressure ventilation.

Preparation

The procedure is the least traumatic for the patient. A full and satisfactory explanation should be provided, except in emergency situations, and reassurance given to the patient in order to allay anxiety. The sight of 70 cm of plastic tubing gradually disappearing into their arm will cause concern to most people, and this aspect of the procedure should not be overlooked.

The patient should lie supine, with the selected arm positioned close to the appropriate edge of the bed, trolley or operating table. It is useful, but not essential, to have an arm-board available so that the shoulder is slightly abducted. Care should be taken in selecting the site for insertion because some of the veins in the antecubital fossa may have been obliterated by previous peripheral intravenous cannulations. The best tributary is the median basilic vein on the left, followed by the right median basilic, and finally the median cephalic, veins at the elbow. The passage of long central venous catheters through these tributaries leading into the cephalic vein is not generally preferred because of the difficulty in negotiating the segment of vein situated in the deltopectoral groove as it penetrates the layers of fascia before entering the subclavian vein. Successful placement is achieved most often by using the simpler and more direct median basilic route.

It is usually unnecessary to place the patient in a head-down Trendelenburg position; however, in severely shocked or tachypnoeic patients, once the tip of the catheter reaches the subclavian vein it is subjected to the negative intrathoracic pressure. Therefore, there should be no undue delay in connecting the catheter to the intravenous administration set and the catheter hub should not be left open to the atmosphere. If there is delay on the part of the nurse or assistant in assembling the infusion line or manometer, then a sterile syringe containing heparinized saline (e.g. Hepsal; Weddell Pharmaceuticals, 10 i.u./ml) should be placed into the hub in order to keep the lumen patent and eliminate the risk of air embolism.

Because of the serious sequelae which may arise if a septic thrombophlebitis becomes established, it is essential that a scrupulous aseptic and draping technique should be used in all cases except the most dire emergency. It is unsatisfactory simply to wipe the skin once or twice with a medicated spirit swab or sponge and then proceed. The operator, after completing a thorough handwashing procedure, should wear a gown and gloves; an assistant must be available to provide the necessary accessories. The important of this ritual in the prevention of catheter-related sepsis should not be underestimated. Howie and Cumming in 1962 (2) were able to reduce significantly their incidence of thrombophlebitis after cut-down venepuncture procedures by adopting a more disciplined approach to their aseptic and antiseptic procedures.

The patency of the median basilic vein at the elbow should be checked and the venous anatomy delineated by inflating a sphygmomanometer cuff around the arm to a pressure between diastolic and systolic. This should be placed high up the arm so that it does not encroach on to the draped area. Some may prefer to use an elastic tourniquet cuff which can be undone by operating the quick release mechanism through the drapes or towels. Occasionally it is necessary to pat the tissues gently with the flat of the hand and encourage the patient to flex the forearm muscles in order to fill the superficial veins. On rare occasions it is helpful to warm the limb in a water bath to achieve a satisfactory filling of the vessels. If the patient is shocked and the veins are collapsed, then a cut-down procedure should be considered first rather than destroy a valuable route of venous access by multiple unsuccessful percutaneous puncture attempts.

Requirements

Individual hospital practices vary a great deal. At the present time in the United Kingdom it is not uncommon for the house officer and nurse to be left to themselves to assemble the equipment. A great deal of time can be saved if this can all be collected before the procedure is embarked upon. The following list includes most items required:

Trolley and skin preparation solution

Dressing pack: sterile gauzes, sponges, cotton-wool and galley pots, sterile drapes/towels

Op-Site incise drape (28 × 15 cm, No. 4986, Smith & Nephew)

Disposable syringes: 5 ml and 10 ml

Hypodermic needles: 19 G, 21 G and 23 G

Lignocaine 1% w/v

Scalpel blade: No. 11

Central venous catheter (60–70 cm, 14 G or 16 G) and introducing cannula/syringe assembly

Heparinized saline 5 ml (e.g. Hepsal 10 i.u./ml, Weddell Pharmaceuticals)

Atraumatic silk suture: 3/0

Povidone-iodine spray (Disadine, Stuart Pharmaceuticals)

Op-Site I.V. Dressing (6·0 × 8·5 cm), Smith & Nephew)

Procedure

Before starting the procedure, the surgeon should ensure that the chosen intravenous administration set or manometer is primed with the selected solution and placed on a stand within easy reach of the assistant, and that the trolley is in a suitable position with all the equipment at hand. The antecubital fossa should be generously cleaned (and shaved when necessary) using povidone-iodine, iodine in 70 per cent spirit or a mixture of chlorhexidine in 70 per cent spirit for at least 3 minutes and allowed to dry or the excess cleaned from the skin using a sterile swab. If the procedure has to be performed in the patient's bed, it is useful to place a polythene-backed absorbent pad, e.g. Uri-Pad or incontinence pad, beneath the arm so that if spillage of blood should occur, the bed linen is not soiled and the work of the nursing staff is correspondingly reduced. The linen or paper drapes should then be arranged to leave the cubital fossa exposed and the elbow in a position of extension. The drapes always have a tendency to slip and it is wise to use an adhesive transparent polyurethane film incise drape (e.g. Op-Site) to keep the operative towels in order for the duration of the procedure. It is still worth while to take these precautions even though many of the current central catheters are dispensed from no-touch plastic sleeves.

The skin overlying the vein should be infiltrated with 0·5–2 ml of lignocaine 1 per cent w/v using a 25 SG needle; with experience this can be placed into the subcutaneous plane without raising a large weal which obscures the vein. Whilst the anaesthesia is taking effect, if the area of infiltration is gently compressed with a sterile swab this also disperses the fluid from around the vein. Once the technique has been mastered, and especially in patients with well-defined venous anatomy where there is little subcutaneous fat, a short subcutaneous tunnel can be created by infiltrating the local anaesthetic solution down a track away from the proposed site of venous entry to a more distal point on the forearm where skin puncture will occur (*Fig.* 5.4). The assistant should next inflate the

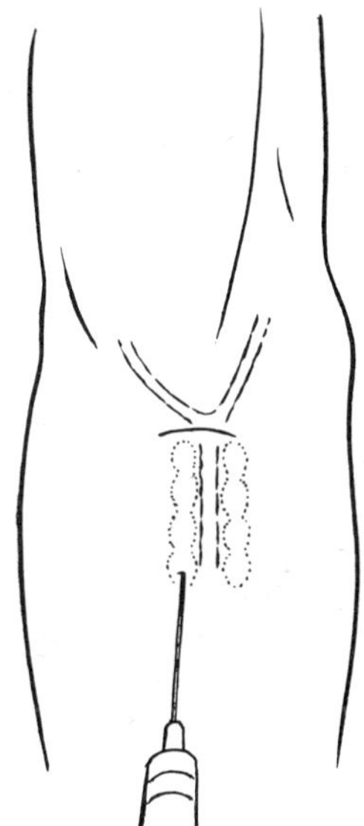

Fig. 5.4. The site immediately over the forearm vein has been infiltrated with local anaesthetic solution and, in addition, a short anaesthetized tunnel has been created prior to percutaneous puncture.

sphygmomanometer cuff or adjust the tourniquet and the patient should be encouraged to fill the superficial veins by intermittently making and releasing a fist. Following this, the introducing cannula and syringe assembly, together with the central catheter, should be dispensed from the manufacturer's sterile packet by the assistant on to the trolley; care should be taken at this point not to drop any of these components on to the floor.

A small nick may usefully be made in the skin with a No. 11 scalpel blade to facilitate the penetration of the introducing cannula and needle. A right-handed operator will find the left median basilic vein easiest to cannulate. The syringe should be completely emptied and the needle/cannula assembly advanced through the skin and moved initially parallel to the vein for approximately a centimetre before the vein is penetrated at an angle of 15–20°. The needle bevel should be facing upwards during this manoeuvre. When a short tunnel is to be created, the needle is advanced subcutaneously from a point 5–7 cm away from the vein and along the anaesthetized track until the vein is reached. After the needle has successfully entered the vein and a free reflux of blood into the syringe obtained, the assembly should be advanced a further half-centimetre into the lumen, the cannula rotated and the needle simultaneously withdrawn into the cannula lumen. When this has been achieved, the cannula may be then advanced up the vein without further trauma (*Fig.* 5.5).

The assistant should next release the sphygmomanometer cuff or tourniquet strap; at this time the operator can prevent undue spillage of blood by pressing lightly over the tip of the cannula with an index finger and placing a sterile gauze swab under the hub. Some may prefer to connect a 2 ml syringe loaded with heparinized saline to the cannula hub whilst the central catheter is prepared for insertion through the lumen. If one corner of the Op-Site sheet is turned back on itself when initially placed, this portion acts as a useful adhesive strip or 'third hand' to which a syringe can be temporarily fixed (*Fig.* 5.6). The central catheter should next be fed into the lumen of the introducing plastic cannula and, whenever possible, a no-touch technique should be used. This is not always possible if the cannula adheres to the PVC dispenser sheath. Most manufacturers now provide this sheath with a locking collet so that the introduction procedure can be theoretically accomplished without exposure of the central line. The definitive central catheter should be advanced along the vein, slowly and without force. If obstruction to the catheter's progress should be encountered, then it may be withdrawn a fraction and a further attempt made. Often, gentle rotation of the catheter around its long axis will help to negotiate a valve or tributary. It may occasionally be necessary to abduct the shoulder in order to negotiate the axillary vein; this is especially the case if the cephalic vein has been chosen. Once the desired length of catheter has been introduced, the plastic dispensing

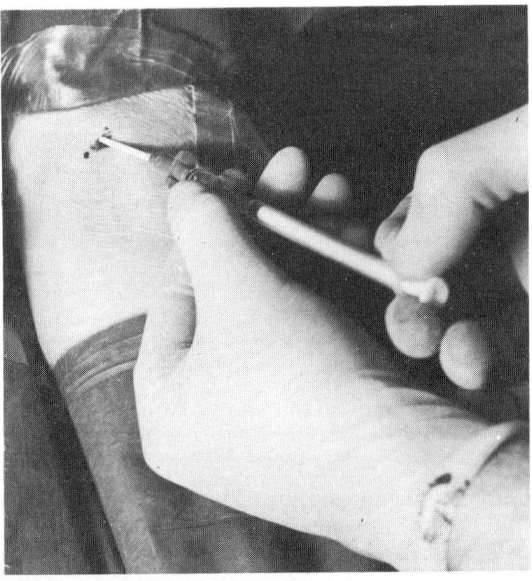
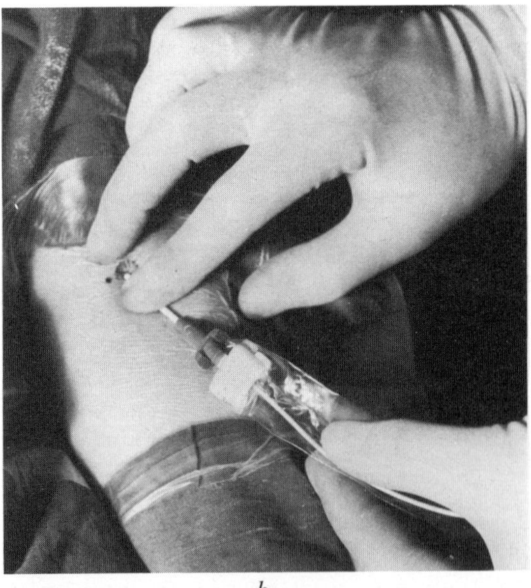

a   b

Fig. 5.5. Percutaneous cannulation of a left antecubital fossa vein (*a*), and subsequent no-touch introduction of a central venous catheter from its sterile sheath (*b*).

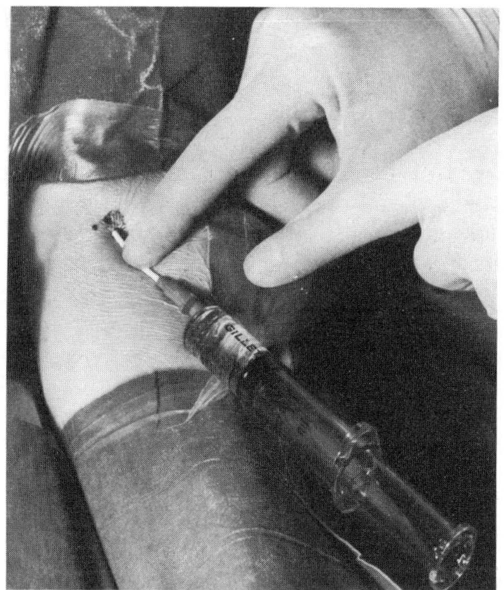

Fig. 5.6. The tourniquet cuff has been released and the introducing cannula hub protected by a syringe containing heparinized saline (Hepsal). Note the application of a folded corner of the Op-Site sheet as a 'third-hand'.

sheath can be removed, the introducing cannula withdrawn back over the central catheter shaft and approximated to the central venous catheter hub. Some catheters are fitted with a central plastic mandril which provides a degree of stiffness for the insertion procedure and also prevents the entry of air. This should be removed and the central catheter linked to the administration set by the assistant. Alternatively, whilst the dressing and suturing procedure is being performed, the catheter hub can be closed off by a syringe containing heparinized saline (e.g. Hepsal, 10 i.u./ml). This can be used intermittently to flush the lumen. During this time the mandril or plastic sheath may be used to assess roughly the suspected position of the catheter tip by using these components as a form of tape measure against the chest wall. A chest X-ray must still be performed to confirm the exact position of the catheter tip.

Fixation

Some may prefer to secure the catheter by inserting a 3/0 silk suture mounted on an atraumatic needle to the skin. This should be performed carefully lest the silk bites into the

catheter shaft material and initiates the development of a fracture. Because of this, many prefer to rely simply on the careful application of a dressing which also provides a degree of adhesive fixation to the skin. The checks that need to be performed in order to ensure the correct placement of the line in the central veins are described later in this chapter. The skin puncture site should be dressed, and the author finds the use of a dry povidone-iodine spray (Disadine) followed by the application of an Op-Site intravenous dressing to be satisfactory. The transparent dressing may be used either alone or in combination with a small, dry sterile gauze suitably cut to enclose the catheter shaft. Further Op-Site sheeting may be applied to the catheter shaft in order to provide further fixation to the skin surface and security against gradual dislodgement out of the vein. This auxiliary dressing should be separate from the skin puncture site dressing, so that this can be inspected and changed as described in Chapter 15. The introduction of this form of transparent polyurethane dressing allows inspection of the catheter entry site by the medical and nursing staff to be performed easily and without unduly disturbing the patient.

SURGICAL EXPOSURE OR CUT-DOWN TECHNIQUES

The ability to perform a cut-down at the wrist or ankle on to the cephalic or long saphenous vein should have been achieved by every newly qualified doctor. Similarly, the veins in the antecubital fossa can be expeditiously exposed and cannulated by a well-motivated clinician. The cut-down procedure has in the past been subject to criticism and associated with increased incidences of thrombophlebitis (3). Furthermore, the need for the procedure has naturally declined with the development of efficient cannula assemblies designed for the percutaneous introduction of intravenous devices. Because of these factors, many junior doctors are unwilling to consider performing this procedure. The operation still has an important place in the management of the obese patient in whom the veins may be obscured and difficult to cannulate, the patient in shock with no palpable peripheral veins at the elbow and the elderly patient possessing extremely fragile veins. It has been suggested that many of the poor results in the past have occurred because the house officer or resident has been attempting the procedure in the general ward without assistance, using inadequate aseptic techniques and poor lighting facilities (4). This report also showed that the employment of a meticulous technique, and the creation of a tunnel so that the cannula did not enter the vein directly through the skin incision, significantly reduced the occurrence of undesirable complications.

The same basic skin preparation and draping procedure should be followed as for the percutaneous technique, the only exception to this being that a greater area of the anterior aspect of the forearm should be shaved and left exposed so that a tunnel may be easily created. A sphygmomanometer cuff or tourniquet strap should be positioned around the upper part of the arm in readiness for application at the appropriate time in the operation.

Requirements

In addition to the items listed for percutaneous insertion, a small selection of instruments should be prepared. Most hospitals provide these in a separate intravenous cut-down tray from their CSSD, and this usually contains:

> Scalpel handle and No. 10 and 11 blades
> Gillies' fine-toothed forceps
> McIndoe's non-toothed forceps
> Fine scissors
> Mosquito artery forceps (4), curved and
>   straight
> Kelly's artery forceps (4), curved and straight
> Skin hooks
> Gauze swabs
> Chromic catgut or silk ligatures (3/0)
> Fine silk or nylon atraumatic skin suture (5/0
>   or 6/0)

Procedure

Under a good light, a diamond-shaped area of skin overlying the vein in the cubital fossa below the elbow should be anaesthetized by infiltration with 5 ml lignocaine 1 per cent w/v and an anaesthetized track made down the anterior aspect of the forearm as shown in *Fig.* 5.4. When this has become effective, the procedure may be

started. After instructing the assistant to inflate the sphygmomanometer cuff or apply the tourniquet strap, the vein will usually become palpable and this simplifies the dissection. A transverse 1·5–2·5 cm incision (according to the degree of obesity) should be made over the median basilic vein just distal to the flexural crease of the elbow joint. The vein may also be exposed above the elbow, where it is accompanied by the medial cutaneous nerve of the arm and forearm (*Fig.* 5.7). If this site is chosen, it is particularly important that the vein alone

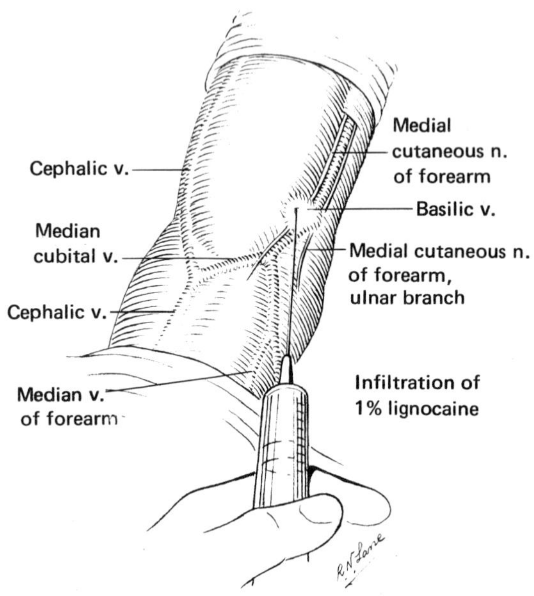

Fig. 5.7. Infiltration of local anaesthesia prior to cannulation of the basilic vein just above the elbow. Note the position of the medial cutaneous nerve of the forearm.

should be dissected out in case these nerves become included in a ligature. The incision should extend through the skin and just into the fat, which is oedematous with the anaesthetic solution. The next part of the dissection should be performed using the non-toothed forceps to hold the subcutaneous layer, whilst the fat is separated by using a pair of curved artery forceps; this is best performed by gently opening the forceps in the line of the vein (*Fig.* 5.8). When the vein is exposed, fine dissection scissors should be used to incise the peri-adventitial tissue plane around the vein. Once this layer has been defined, an artery forceps can be slipped

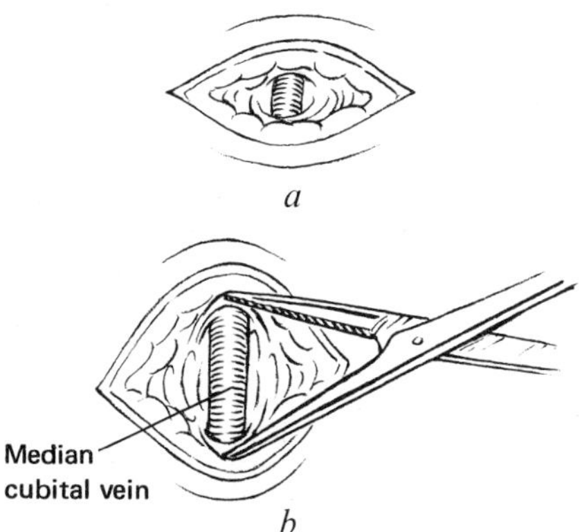

Fig. 5.8. Venous cut-down procedure at the elbow with incision of the skin and subcutaneous fat (*a*) and exposure of the vein by blunt dissection of the peri-adventitial venous tissue (*b*).

under the vein without difficulty and a catgut or fine silk ligature brought back under the vessel. This ligature can be brought through as a loop and divided at its mid-point, so that one-half may be moved proximal and the other distal in order to secure and control the vessel. The distal ligature should be tied and clipped with a forceps under slight traction to the drape or Op-Site. The proximal ligature should have a single throw made and run down to within a centimetre of the vein; this can also be clipped to the towels (*Fig.* 5.9).

Once the vein has been prepared, the assistant should release the tourniquet or sphygmomanometer cuff. Any haemorrhage from small vessels in the fat can be controlled by gentle pressure with gauze swabs during the procedure.

The 60–70 cm central catheter and introducing cannula/needle assembly should be gently delivered on to this sterile trolley by the assistant. It is always wise to create a tunnel down the forearm and this takes no extra time. A tunnel can be created by picking up the fat of the distal wound flap with fine-toothed forceps and sliding the introducing cannula and needle through the cut-down wound and under the skin for several centimetres along the anaesthetized track. After the needle is removed, the central catheter can be passed up the cannula lumen to the main wound. Only a short length of the central catheter should be passed out of its protective sheath at this time. The introducing cannula is then withdrawn from over the central catheter as shown in *Fig.* 5.10. The author has on occasions created a longer tunnel by using a fine hollow metal venotomy sucker passed in a similar retrograde fashion down the forearm and the central catheter is passed back through this device as shown in *Fig.* 5.11. Naturally, a longer zone of anaesthesia must be provided and a small cut should be made with a No. 11 blade so that the sucker can be slipped through the

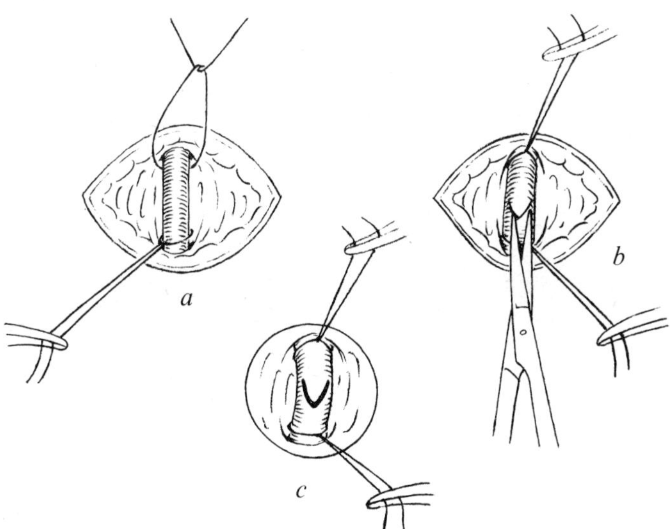

Fig. 5.9. Venous cut-down procedure showing (*a*) proximal and distal encircling Dexon or catgut ligatures carrying a single throw; (*b*, *c*) a venotomy being performed with scissors whilst the vessels are controlled and angulated by clipping the ligatures with forceps to the Op-Site drape.

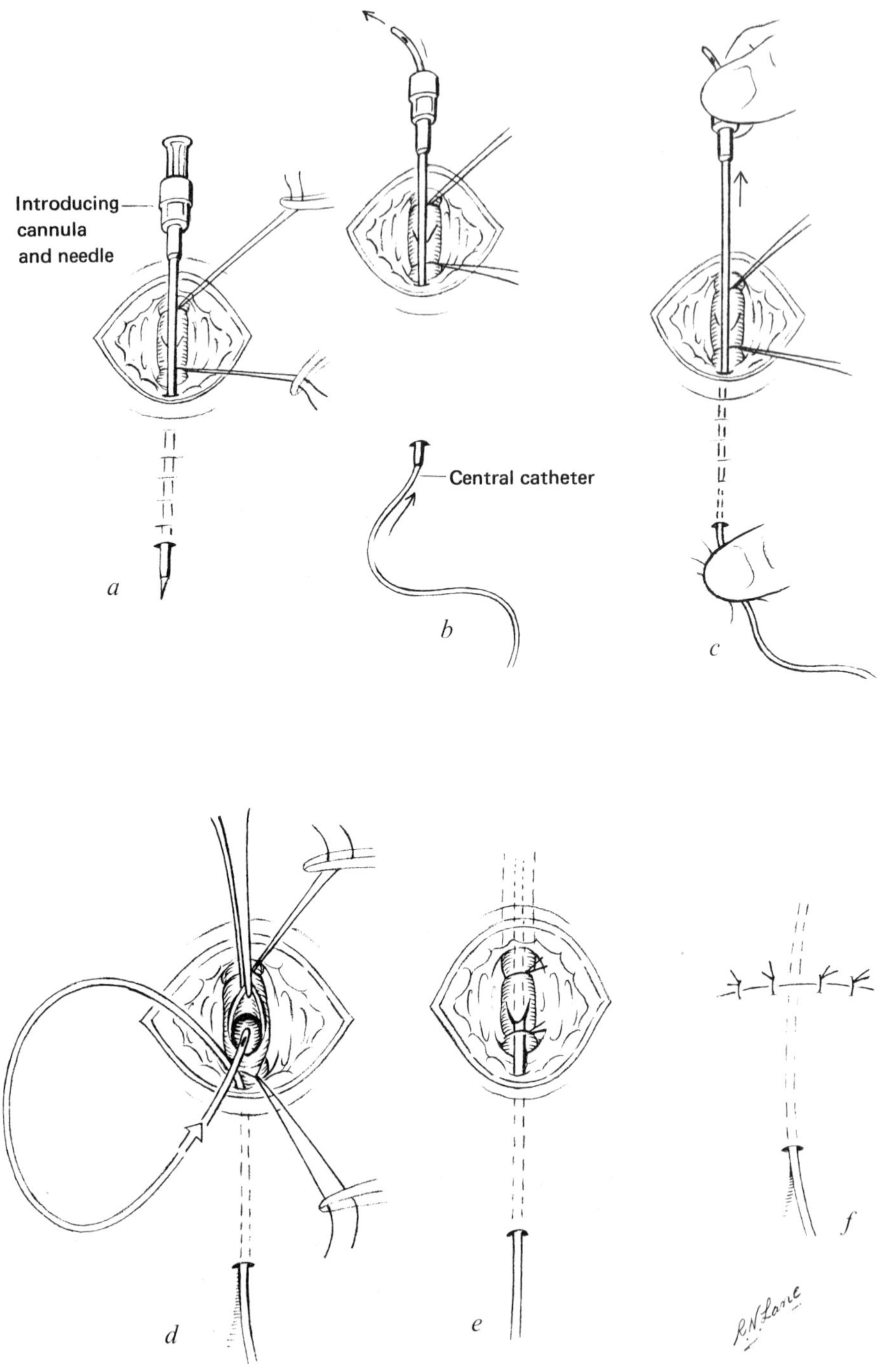

Fig. 5.10. Venous cut-down procedure showing the creation of a 6–7 cm tunnel using a Wallace 66 cm Piggy-Back smooth-tipped catheter. The introducing cannula and needle are passed in a retrograde fashion (*a*); the central catheter is passed through to the venotomy wound (*b*); the introducing cannula is then withdrawn (*c*); the catheter is then inserted through the venotomy into the vein and secured by the proximal and distal ligatures (*d, e, f*).

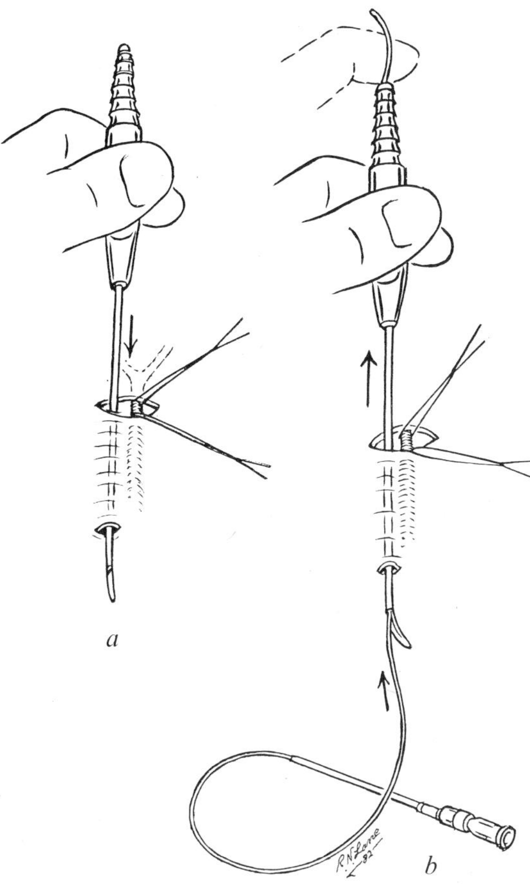

Fig. 5.11. A long forearm tunnel can be created using a venotomy sucker to introduce the central catheter.

skin as shown in *Fig.* 5.11. The tip of the central catheter should be sited in readiness for insertion into the vein. By applying gentle traction on the distal and proximal ligatures, the vein can be controlled whilst the anterior wall is grasped with fine non-toothed forceps and a neat V-shaped cut made with the scissors. Often the vessel may have constricted because of spasm and the lumen can be gently stretched by inserting a closed, curved artery forceps. Alternatively, the venotomy sucker can be slipped into the vein and this provides an archway through which the catheter may be introduced. The central catheter should then be guided up through the venotomy using forceps and past the proximal ligature which should be transiently released. The catheter should be gradually

delivered from its plastic sheath, through the tunnel and passed up the vein until the desired length has been inserted. Any central mandril in the lumen can be withdrawn and a 5 or 10 ml syringe containing heparinized saline (Hepsal, 10 i.u./ml) placed into the hub and used to flush the catheter intermittently whilst the wound is closed and dressed. The proximal ligature should then be tied around the catheter and the knot cut short. It is important that the vessel is not transfixed by a ligature as shown in *Fig.* 5.12 since this state of affairs could under rare circumstances lead to the entrainment of air into the circulation alongside the catheter (5).

Wound Closure and Dressing

The skin should be closed neatly using fine silk or nylon mattress sutures mounted on an atraumatic cutting needle, and if the patient is obese, a subcutaneous layer of fine interrupted 4/0 Dexon sutures (polyglycolic acid) should be used to obliterate unnecessary dead space. The skin sutures should be placed 0·5 cm apart and it is useful to align the wound correctly using skin hooks in order to obtain the best cosmetic result. The arm should be completely cleaned of any surface blood using hydrogen peroxide; the limb may then be dried and the wound sprayed with Op-Site or painted with mastic before applying a ribbon of gauze and an Op-Site dressing. It is useful to keep the cut-down wound and the catheter entry sites separate for future nurse dressing procedures. Many surgeons prefer to fix the central catheter at its entry site with a single suture, placed about a centimetre away from the actual wound and knotted carefully around the shaft. The entry site should then be treated with a dry povidone-iodine spray (Disadine) and an Op-Site intravenous dressing placed firmly over the junction between skin and catheter.

Finally, the catheter should be arranged on the forearm in a gentle curve and fixed with additional adhesive dressings. These precautions prevent kinking of the catheter during the period of infusion or manometry. A primed administration set fitted with a Luer-lock connector should then be inserted on to the hub and fixed in place. This junction should also be sprayed with Disadine and completely wrapped with a single sterile gauze swab and this should

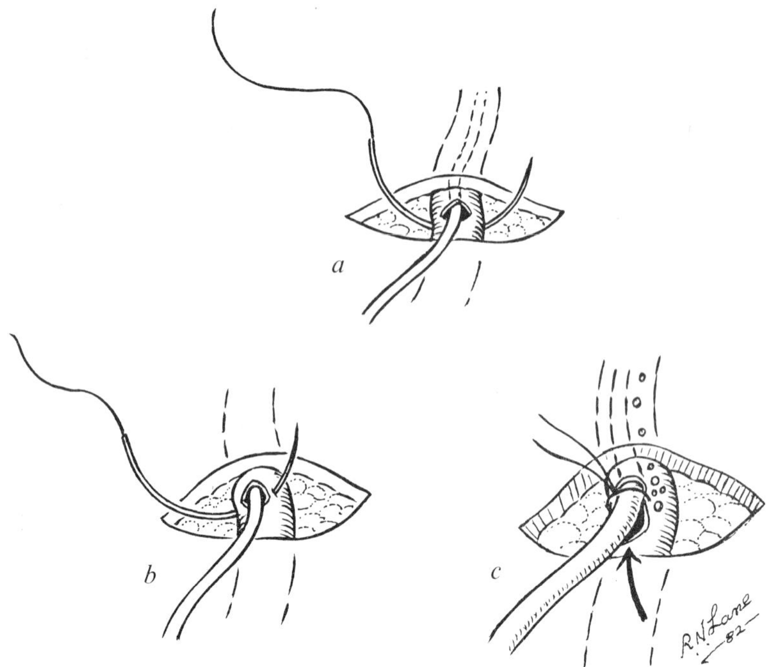

Fig. 5.12. Care must be taken when passing ligatures mounted on needles behind superficial veins so that the back wall is not transfixed. The correct procedure is shown in (*a*). If the needle is inadvertently passed through the vein (*b*) then air entrainment into the circulation could occur alongside the catheter (arrowed), as shown in (*c*).

be also strapped to the skin (*Fig.* 5.13). The time spent ensuring the integrity and patency of the line on the body surface is well spent and it is essential for the doctor to maintain a high standard in order to continually educate the changing nursing staff. When the technique used to insert a catheter is seen to be meticulous, the nursing staff respond by providing a corresponding degree of care in their daily management of the patient's infusion.

Placement Checks

After the insertion of a central venous catheter, it is vital to ensure that there has been correct intravenous placement. The tip should be in the appropriate position with regard to the function of the catheter and there should be no malposition, looping or knotting of the line.

Pitfalls

Although the catheter mandril or plastic dispensing sheath may be used as a rough guide as to how far the catheter has advanced, it does not accurately reflect the final position of the catheter tip; nor indeed will malposition, looping, knotting or translocation to the opposite innominate vein be identified. Similarly, the use of the catheter as an exploring electrode attached to an ECG recorder is not accurate enough when long term use of the device is contemplated. Attempts have been made to locate catheter tips by using Doppler ultrasound probes placed over the praecordium in order to detect the disturbance created by aliquots of sterile normal saline squirted through the catheter. This has not been found to be a reliable guide because detectable changes can be identified using the ultrasound probe when the catheter tip is as far as 30 cm from the right atrium (*Fig.* 5.14) (6). This technique deserves further evaluation with respect to placement which has been verified by chest X-ray.

It is not safe to rely upon the observation of fluctuations in the fluid pressure recorded by a manometer. Such pressure variations can be recorded from catheters which have their tips sited in the mediastinal tissues (7).

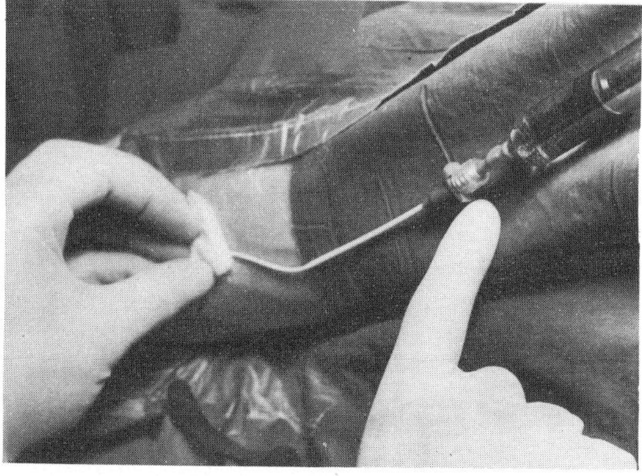

a

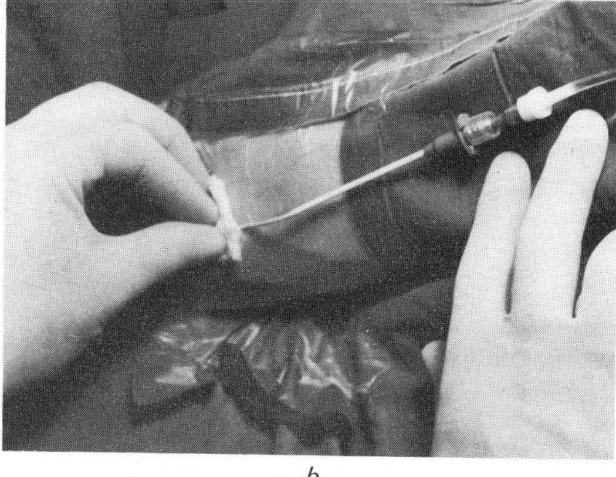

b

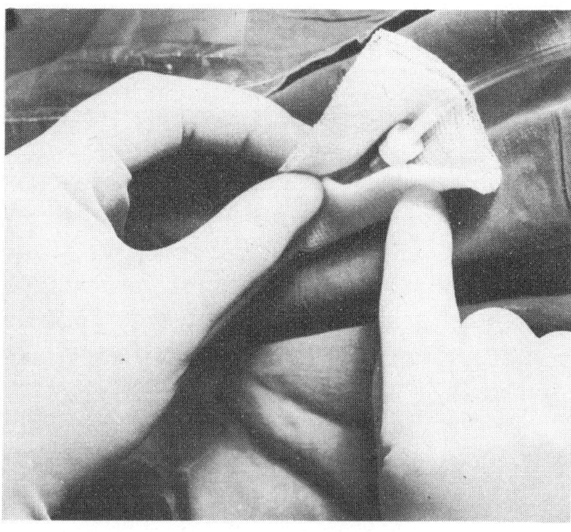

c

Fig. 5.13. The central catheter after insertion is locked to the introducing cannula (*a*); a Luer-lock administration set connection is attached (*b*) and this area sprayed with povidone-iodine and dressed (*c*).

Safeguards

The following manoeuvres should be applied to every catheter after placement:

1. There should be free aspiration of venous blood into a syringe when gentle suction is applied.

2. After fixation of the catheter and attachment to the administration set, the flow controls on the infusion line should be opened, and the bottle or bag simultaneously lowered below the level of the patient's heart. There should be an easy and free reflux of blood into the first part of the infusion line from the catheter. This should

oscillate in synchrony with the right atrial contractions and with respiration. This is perhaps the simplest and most important safety check to confirm correct central intravenous placement. If no reflux of blood occurs following this manoeuvre, it may, of course, signify that the catheter has been occluded by a small thrombus, is wedged against the wall of the vein or in a tributary. These possibilities should be excluded by gently withdrawing the catheter a centimetre or so and, if necessary, flushing with 1 or 2 ml of sterile heparinized saline. The test should then

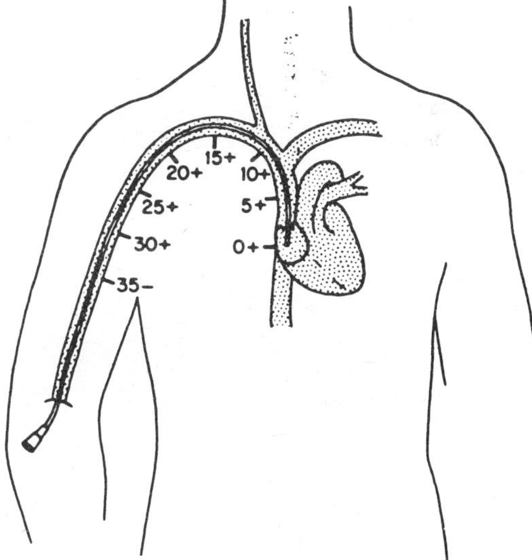

Fig. 5.14. Detection of saline injections through central venous catheters using a praecordial ultrasound Doppler probe. Detectable changes can be heard when the tip is as much as 30 cm from the right atrium. (Reproduced by kind permission of Dr P. S. Colley and the Editor of *Anaesthesiology*.)

be repeated (*Fig.* 5.15), and if there is still no reflux of blood back down the line when the manoeuvre is performed, the line should be considered to have become looped, kinked or even to have perforated out through the vein and into the pleural cavity or mediastinum. No infusions should be passed through the line until the situation has been resolved.

3. Finally, a chest X-ray should be performed, with the arm abducted, to confirm the position of the catheter tip, the absence of knotting, looping or malposition (*Fig.* 5.16). If there is still doubt about the placement because of failure in the manoeuvre described above, a further chest X-ray should be performed whilst 5–10 ml of Conray 280 (May & Baker) are injected down the lumen. When major surgery is to be performed on the abdomen and the decision has been taken to insert a central catheter for parenteral nutrition therapy, it is extremely useful to fit a radiolucent head on to the operating table and the catheter can be accurately positioned using an image intensifier in combination with an injection of Conray 280. When the catheter has been inserted from the antecubital fossa, the check chest X-ray should be taken with the arm abducted at 90° to the trunk in order to obtain an accurate reflection of the catheter tip position.

It is essential that these safeguards are followed because many of the recorded complications have arisen following errors made during the insertion procedure. Knots and loops in the axillary or subclavian vessels predispose to thrombosis. Serious neurological sequelae may result if an arm or subclavian catheter passes in a retrograde fashion high into the jugular vein and is then used for infusion purposes. Coma has been reported following the administration of intravenous lignocaine into the jugular vein via such a misplaced catheter (8). Jugular vein or cerebral venous thrombosis may occur if hypertonic nutrient solutions are infused into the jugular vein in such a retrograde fashion (9).

Balloon flotation catheters are used for short periods with their tips situated in the pulmonary artery. Hickman and Broviac silicone catheters have been used for prolonged periods with their tips sited in the right atrium; however, the majority of central catheters should be placed so that they reach no further than the upper part of the superior vena cava and effectively lie outside the limits of the pericardial sac. Movement of the elbow, arm and shoulder girdle are known to create a to-and-fro piston effect with the result that the catheter tip is able to travel several centimetres, sufficient to allow penetration of the heart in a few instances, with the develop-

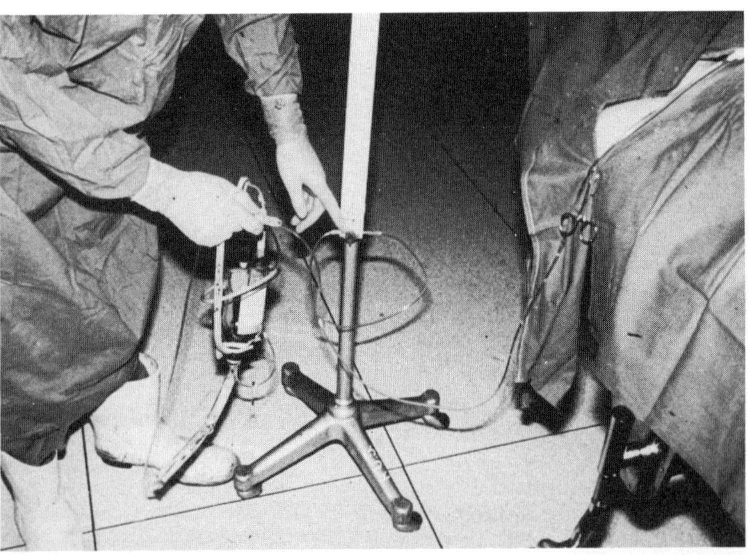

Fig. 5.15. Correct central intravenous placement being checked by lowering the meniscus in the administration set drip chamber below the level of the heart with all flow controls in the 'open position'.

ment of cardiac tamponade from the leakage of blood or the continued infusion of fluid (9).

Since it is unnecessary to place most central catheters into the heart, Defalque has suggested that catheters should remain in the upper segment of the superior vena cava (9). Therefore,

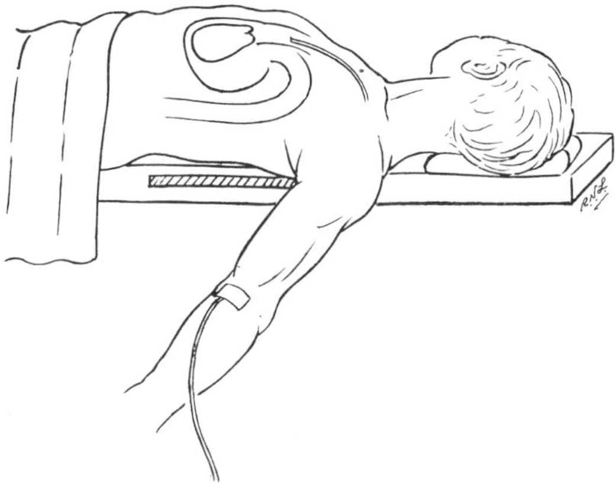

Fig. 5.16. A post-insertion chest X-ray checking correct placement of a long line introduced from a brachial vein. Note that the X-ray is taken with the shoulder in a position of abduction.

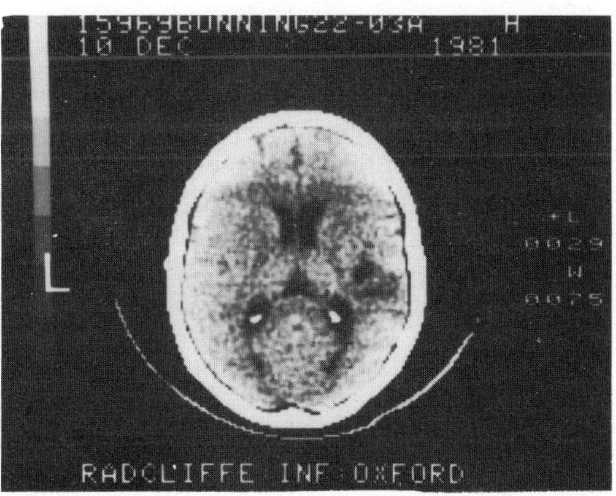

Fig. 5.17. Computed tomogram showing right parietal infarct (low density area enhanced by contrast medium), caused by a spreading cortical venous thrombosis due to the infusion of a hyperosmolar solution into the internal jugular vein. (Reproduced by kind permission of Mr R. G. Souter, Mr A. Mitchell and the Editor of the *British Medical Journal*.)

on reviewing the post-insertion chest X-ray (*see Fig.* 5.16), the catheter tip should be at or just above a plane drawn through the third rib or the T5–T6 vertebral interspace; alternatively, a site 2 cm below the inferior clavicular border or just above the level of the carina may be chosen. When this is confirmed and the dressing completed, it is important to ensure that a record is made concerning the date and time of insertion and the type and length of central catheter used. Precise instructions should be left concerning the regimen for dressing and maintaining the catheter.

References

1. Bozetti F.: Experience at the National Institute of Cancer. Milan. Personal communication, 1978.
2. Howie J. G. R., Cumming R. L. C.: The role of infection in transfusion thrombophlebitis. *Lancet* 1962; **2**: 851–3.
3. Moran J. M., Atwood R. P., Rowe M. I.: A clinical and bacteriologic study of infections associated with venous cutdowns. *N. Engl. J. Med.* 1965; **272**: 554–60.
4. Izaguirre S. F. S.: Surgical venepuncture. *Surg. Gynecol. Obstet.* 1970; **140**: 1095.
5. Simpson K.: Air accidents during transfusion. *Lancet* 1942; **1**: 697.
6. Colley P. S., Pavlin E. G., Groepper J.: Assessment of a saline injection test for location of a right atrial catheter. *Anaesthesiology* 1979; **50**: 258–60.
7. Parkin L., Hopkinson R. B.: Hydrohaemothorax following percutaneous internal jugular cannulation, recognised by intravenous pyelography. *Anaesth. Analges.* 1978; **58**: 507–11.
8. Klein H. O., Di Segni E., Kaplinsky E.: Unsuspected cerebral perfusion; a complication of the use of a central venous pressure catheter. *Chest* 1978; **74**: 109–10.
9. Souter R. G., Mitchell A.: Spreading cortical venous thrombosis due to infusion of hyperosmolar solution into the internal jugular vein. *Br. Med. J.* 1982; **285**: 935–6.
10. Defalque R. J., Campbell C.: Cardiac tamponade from central venous catheters. *Anaesthesiology* 1979; **50**: 249–52.

Chapter 6

Internal Jugular Vein Catheterization

I. C. W. English

Since 1968 the preferred technique for obtaining central venous pressures or infusing intra-operative and postoperative fluids at Brompton Hospital, London, has been by internal jugular vein puncture (1). About two thousand such procedures are now performed annually. During the period when we introduced this technique, Branthwaite and Bradley reported the use of the Seldinger technique to introduce fine-bore cannulas fitted with thermistors via the internal jugular vein, whilst they investigated the measurement of the cardiac output using the thermodilution principle at St Thomas' Hospital, London (2). Other descriptions and variations of surgical technique have also been published (3–6).

Anatomy

After emerging from the base of the skull posterior to the internal carotid artery, the vein descends through the neck behind and deep to the sternomastoid, gradually moving to the lateral side of the common carotid artery and eventually becoming anterolateral. The relationship of the vein to the deep surface of the sternomastoid muscle is the key to understanding the position of the vein in the neck (*Fig.* 6.1). It joins the subclavian vein behind the first rib to form the innominate vein. In practice, surface markings are not a reliable means of locating the internal jugular vein as its position, particularly in a lateral plane, tends to vary considerably.

Advantages

The main advantage of the internal jugular vein as a cannulation site stems from the fact that its blood flow is rapid and never suffers from the periods of stasis that can occur in peripheral veins. Thrombosis is almost never a complication and the same site can be used repeatedly. The right internal jugular vein has been re-cannulated up to five times on a number of occasions.

The neck is a relatively clean area—certainly compared with the femoral region—and infection has not proved to be a major problem. In the case of small children and neonates, internal jugular puncture is probably the only satisfactory percutaneous method of obtaining central venous pressures.

Disadvantages

Experience and a lot of practice are necessary to obtain the best results with the technique, and this applies particularly to neonates. Muscle tone in conscious patients makes cannulation more difficult and one must always be aware of the possibility of air embolism.

Technique for Adults and Large Children (over 25 kg)

It is better, in the first instance, to use the technique on anaesthetized patients placed on an operating table. The right internal jugular vein is better for use with open heart surgery because the left-sided pressures are often artificially raised when the two halves of a divided sternum are separated. This is because the left innominate vein becomes stretched and flattened.

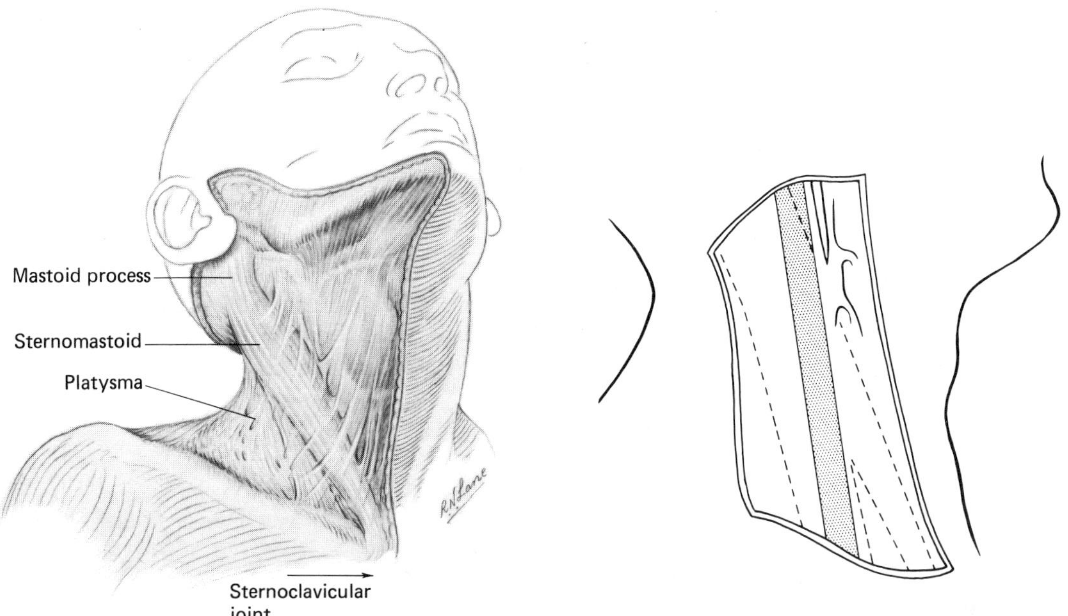

Fig. 6.1. The superficial relations and surface anatomy of the right internal jugular vein. The internal jugular vein normally lies under the sternomastoid muscle throughout its length in the neck.

Assuming the right-sided vein is to be cannulated, the patient's head should be turned to the left and extended. A head-down tilt of about 20° is necessary in most patients to raise the venous pressure in the neck and distend the vessels. Right-sided heart failure or tricuspid valve disease can make the tilt unnecessary. Standing at the head of the patient, the operator should face the patient's feet and try to palpate the internal jugular vein with the fingers of his left hand (*Fig.* 6.2). The best way to achieve this is by a process of ballottement with the fingers

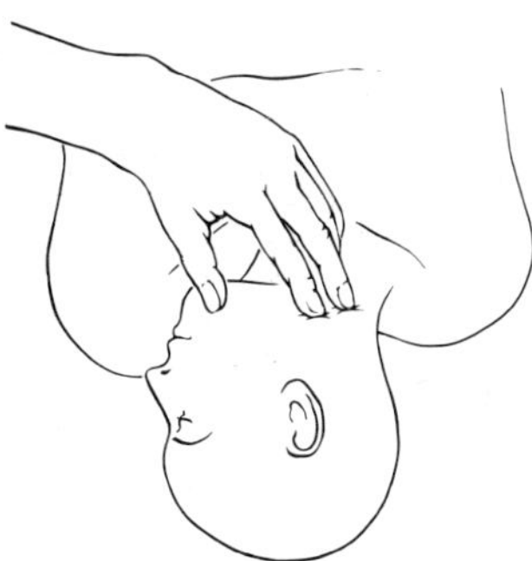

Fig. 6.2. Palpate the internal jugular vein with the fingers of the left hand. The patient has been positioned in a head-down 20° tilt.

exploring the right side of the neck. With a little practice it becomes quite easy to locate the vein, even though it is lying under the sternomastoid muscle. In a variety of conditions it is possible to have a pulsatile pressure in the internal jugular vein and it may be necessary to palpate the common carotid artery separately on its medial side to reassure oneself before attempting cannulation.

Choice of Cannula

Almost any sort of cannula can be used, but ideally it should be about 10 cm long and be introduced over a needle rather than through one. A cannula inserted through a needle has two disadvantages. First, there is a danger of the sharp bevel of the needle cutting segments off the cannula if the latter is removed carelessly with the needle still in place, or if a conscious patient suddenly moves during the insertion procedure. The second disadvantage results from the fact that the needle makes a larger hole in the vein than can be filled by the cannula. If the central venous pressure is high, bleeding will occur around the cannula and in heparinized patients this can be quite serious. For this reason we now use a catheter-over-needle technique on all occasions.

Insertion Technique

Having selected a needle and cannula (14 G for an adult), and after skin preparation, draping and the provision of local anaesthesia in a conscious patient, attach an empty 2 ml syringe to the hub of the needle and puncture the skin over the centre of the palpated internal jugular vein about halfway down the neck, taking care to avoid the external jugular vein where it often crosses superficially. Have the bevel facing anteriorly. Now withdraw the plunger of the syringe to produce a negative pressure and advance the needle and cannula with a jerky motion. The direction to advance is in the line of the vein, i.e. towards the umbilicus and slightly posterior— about 5–20°, depending on the obesity of the patient (*Fig.* 6.3).

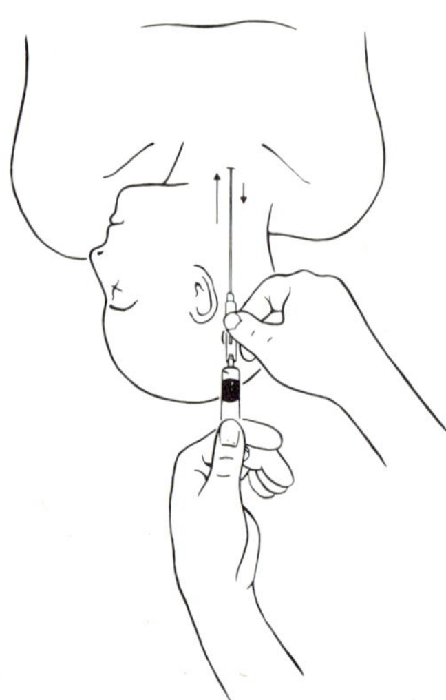

Fig. 6.3. Apply suction with a syringe during venepuncture and approach the vein with a very slight to-and-fro motion of the needle point.

The jerky motion is necessary to prevent the vein being transfixed. In spite of the fact that the table is tipped head-down, the venous pressure is still much lower than that in an arm vein below some sort of tourniquet. It is quite possible to flatten the internal jugular vein with pressure from the needle, and if a steady movement is applied the point will pass through the

anterior and posterior walls simultaneously and no blood will be withdrawn. By advancing the needle say 1 cm and then pulling it back 0·5 cm and so on, it is usually possible to place the whole of the needle bevel within the lumen of the vein. This is immediately obvious because blood appears in the syringe. Although the bevel may be in the lumen, it does not necessarily mean that the tip of the cannula has penetrated the anterior wall of the vein (*Fig.* 6.4). If one attempts to advance the cannula at this stage and slide it off the needle, all that happens is that the vessel is pushed off the needle (*Fig.* 6.5). Both

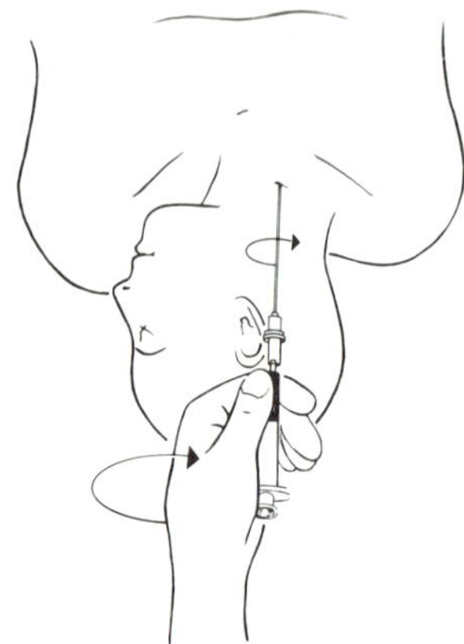

Fig. 6.4. Having aspirated blood, rotate the syringe 180° and advance a further centimetre.

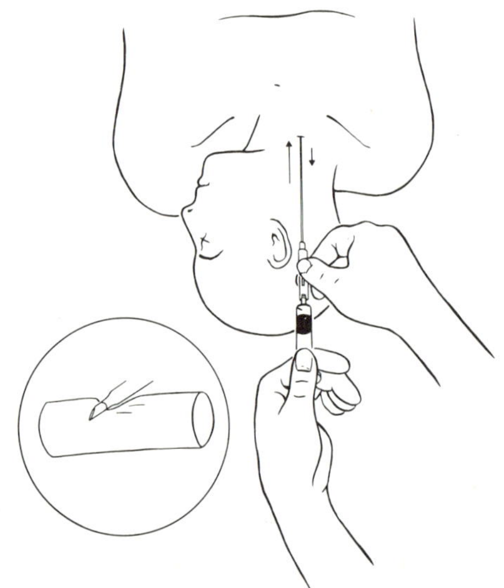

Fig. 6.5. When only the needle point but not the central catheter tip is situated in the vein lumen, further advancement of the central catheter merely pushes the vein off the needle (*see inset*).

the whole of the bevel and the tip of the cannula must be within the lumen before attempting to slide the cannula off the needle. To make sure of this, the syringe should be rotated 180° after blood appears so that the pointed tip of the needle becomes anterior. If the syringe is now advanced about 1 cm, a distinct click can often be felt as the cannula tip passes into the lumen (*Fig.* 6.6). The reason for having the point of the needle anterior at this stage is to prevent it catching on the posterior wall of the vein. Assuming blood can still be withdrawn, the cannula should be pushed fully home and the needle removed (*Fig.* 6.7).

The detail in this explanation may seem unnecessarily tedious, but by paying attention to it

and trying to visualize what is happening under the skin, one's results improve.

As a means of fixation, a sterile adhesive Op-Site sheet without any dressing underneath is satisfactory. It is impervious and does not become stained.

Alternative Technique

It is sometimes impossible to palpate a right internal jugular vein. In such cases it is dangerous to try to cannulate it from surface markings because its position in the neck, particularly in a lateral plane, is variable. If the patient is not going to have open heart surgery, the left internal jugular vein can be used, but it too may be difficult to feel. On these occasions there is an alternative technique for use on the right side. It does depend on surface markings, but as the vein is approached from the medial side, its position in a lateral plane is less important.

It is quite easy to find the centre of the triangle formed by the two heads of the sternomastoid and the clavicle, even in obese subjects or babies (*Fig.* 6.8). The needle and cannula with a 2 ml

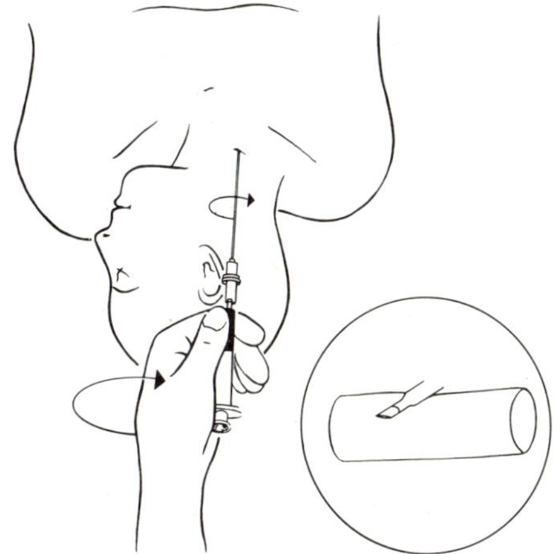

Fig. 6.6. The central catheter has been successfully placed in the internal jugular vein lumen by a 180° rotation of the device (*see inset*).

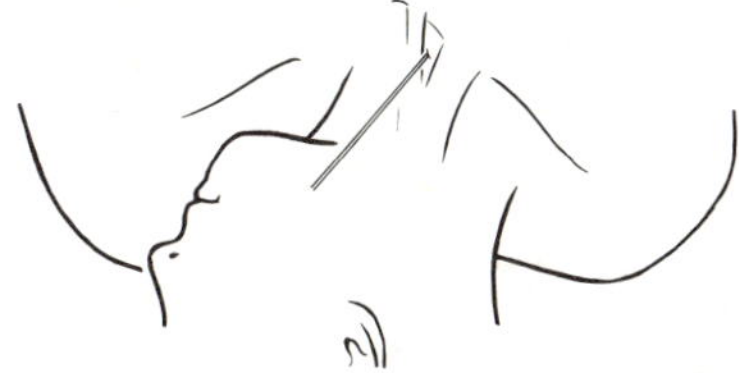

Fig. 6.8. The angle of approach for the alternative technique.

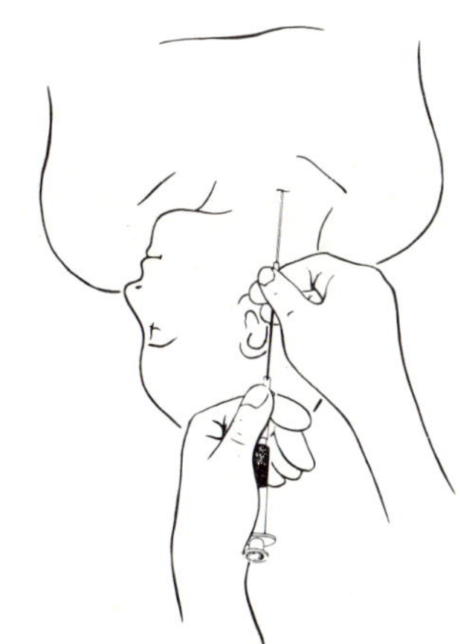

Fig. 6.7. Slide the cannula off the needle.

syringe attached should be inserted through the skin at this point and directed 40° backwards and 20° laterally. Apply suction and advance the needle in the same jerky fashion as has been described already. At the base of the neck the jugular vein lies anterolateral to the common carotid artery and is fairly near the surface. Sometimes the needle enters it immediately under the skin and it is normally unnecessary and undesirable to search any deeper than 2 or 3 cm in this site. Having withdrawn blood and rotated the syringe, the needle and cannula must be aligned with the vein before advancing them both to ensure that the end of the cannula is also in the lumen. The realignment involves a change of direction from 40° back and 20°

laterally to 15° back and 10° medially. Remember that the vein has been approached from the medial side.

This alternative technique is quite useful for conscious patients because tone in the sterno-mastoid muscle makes it difficult to palpate the internal jugular vein higher up the neck. With the lower approach there is no muscle of consequence between the vein and the skin. Conscious patients are normally in bed and a somewhat different method must be used to raise the venous pressure unless the bed can be tipped. The easiest arrangement is to place a pillow under the patient's shoulders to extend the head and to have an assistant hold the legs vertically in the air. Some patients requiring emergency central venous pressure lines are oligaemic and the legs have to be raised for a minute or so before the neck veins become distended.

Left Internal Jugular Vein

It has already been explained that left internal jugular vein cannulation is not recommended for open heart surgery because the left innominate vein becomes stretched and flattened when the sternum is divided. A long cannula that reaches the superior vena cava overcomes the problems of artificially raised pressures but long cannulas increase the resistance to rapid transfusion that may be necessary.

However, if the operator still wishes to use the left side, the technique is the same as for the right-sided elective approach except that the patient's head is turned to the right. The alternative approach on the left is not a very satisfactory one. There is quite an sharp angle where the internal jugular and subclavian veins join and an equally sharp one where the two innominate veins join. Whereas the right innominate and superior vena cava continue in the same line, the left innominate joins at right-angles having crossed the aorta. Moreover, on the left side there is the danger of injuring the thoracic duct.

Neonates and Small Children

It is usually easier and kinder to anaesthetize babies before trying to cannulate their central veins. Crying and wriggling will make the procedure dangerous as well as difficult (*Fig.* 6.9).

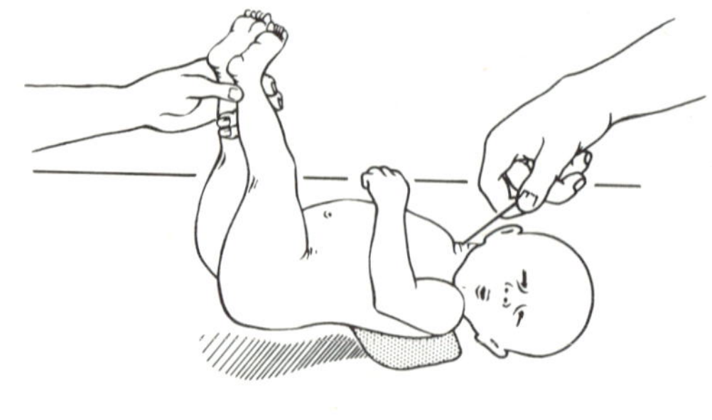

Fig. 6.9. The position for a small child or neonate during jugular venepuncture.

Most small children have short necks relative to the size of their heads and it is impossible to extend the latter sufficiently without an elongated sandbag under the shoulders. Tipping the bed or table serves little useful purpose because the limited length of the child cannot provide a sufficient head of venous pressure. It is better to raise the legs vertically and at the same time lift the buttocks up a few centimetres. As in the case of adults, one should try to palpate the internal jugular vein, but it may be difficult to feel in a plump child. If this is so, the alternative approach is usually successful, although most operators will experience a natural reluctance to insert large cannulas into the base of a baby's neck. The size to use for children under 2 years of age is 18 G.

A crying child will produce large swings of venous pressure which could be the cause of an air embolus if the cannula is disconnected from the drip set at the wrong moment.

The management of an internal jugular line in babies requires a lot of care and experience, but with good nursing it can be kept patent and uninfected for days or even weeks. The main problem is accidental removal when the child is turned.

Complications

A detailed survey of the literature appears in Chapter 12, but in about 14 000 internal jugular punctures at Brompton Hospital there has been a variety of complications related to the insertion procedure. The commonest is a haematoma resulting from accidental arterial punctures. It is normally of no consequence and only becomes more difficult to deal with when the operator does not at first realize his mistake. Even though red blood under pressure has appeared in the syringe, he may still try to introduce the cannula as well as the needle into the vessel and damage the arterial wall further. When this happens, a haematoma will appear rapidly, and may even spread down to the aorta within the vascular sheath. It is better to abandon the attempt and try on the other side of the neck, while firm pressure is applied over the injury. The incidence of haematoma is approximately 1 in 70 when all members of the anaesthetic staff are involved in carrying out internal jugular punctures.

On one occasion, the subclavian artery was transfixed and the pleural cavity entered with the same thrust of the needle. This patient, who was having an open heart operation, developed a haemothorax which had to be drained and the artery did not stop bleeding until after protamine was given.

There have been three cases of accidental pneumothorax following internal jugular cannulation. Two of them followed attempts by inexperienced members of the staff to measure central venous pressures in patients who were in bed, without first making sure that the venous pressure was adequate to distend the vein. At this point, it is again worth emphasizing the fact that it is dangerous to attempt cannulation of the internal jugular vein if the vessel is collapsed as a result of unsuitable posture or oligaemia.

One patient had temporary paralysis of the right vocal cord, presumably as a result of damaging the right recurrent laryngeal nerve where it lies in close proximity to the right innominate vein.

A seriously ill man with pulmonary tuberculosis required central venous pressure measurements when he was admitted to the intensive care unit. A subsequent X-ray showed that the tip of the cannula was lying in a right apical cavity. No permanent harm resulted from this.

An interesting complication in a cyanosed baby having open heart surgery came to light when the pressure transmitted up the cannula was found to be that of the left ventricle. An attempt at venepuncture had failed on the right side of the neck and so it was decided to use the left side with a longer cannula to extend beyond the stretched portion of the left innominate vein. 'Venous' blood was withdrawn and the cannula was easily pushed home. It had entered the left common carotid artery and passed down the aorta and through the aortic valve. Fortunately, the cannula was removed without incident during the operation.

Results

In 1976 one thousand consecutive patients requiring central venous pressure lines at Brompton Hospital were reviewed. All members of the anaesthetic staff took part, and the results are shown in Table 6.1. An overall success rate of 98·5 per cent may seem high, but in some patients the skin may have been punctured twice or more before the cannula could be satisfactorily inserted. Failure has only been registered when all attempts at internal jugular venepuncture at one session were unsuccessful.

New Concepts

In recent months, Gilston of the National Heart Hospital has introduced a catheter-over-needle device fitted with a sterile plastic sleeve which prevents accidental touch contamination of the catheter shaft during the insertion procedure. As the catheter is advanced, the sleeve ruffles up to the hub and may be removed by tearing along the perforations provided by the manufacturer (H. G. Wallace & Co.) (*Fig.* 6.10).

Table 6.1. **The results of attempting 1000 internal jugular vein punctures**

| Age group | No. | Right internal jugular vein | | Left internal jugular vein | Failures | Success (%) |
		Elective	Alternative	Elective		
2 d–2 yr	119	83	17	14	5	95·7
2–14 yr	151	132	13	5	1	99·3
14–84 yr	730	661	39	21	9	98·7
Total	1000	876	69	40	15	98·5

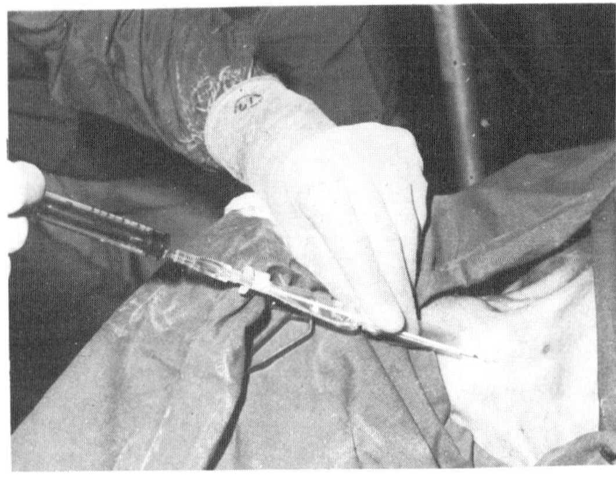

a

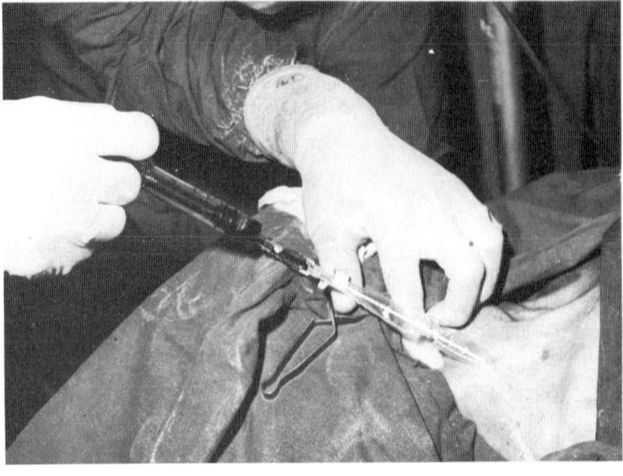

b

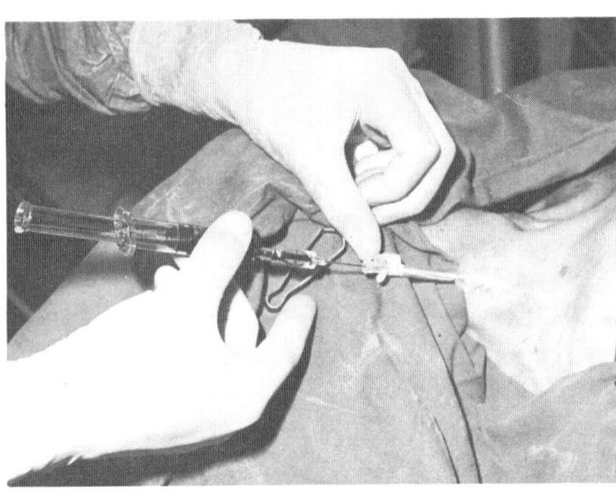

c

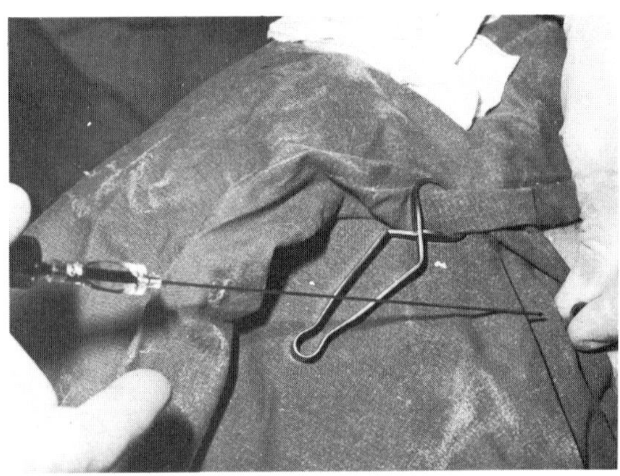

d

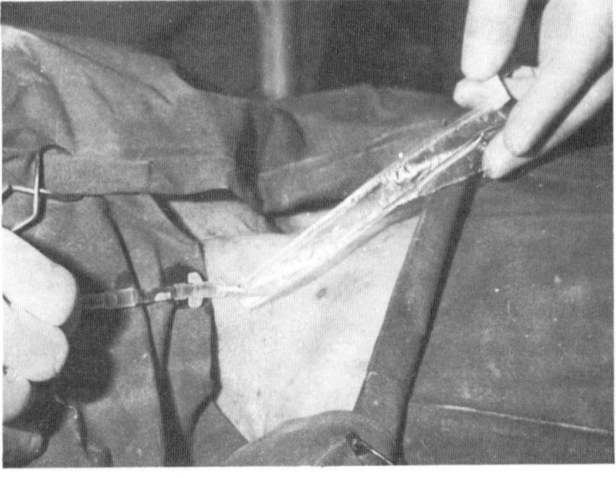

e

Fig. 6.10. Internal jugular cannulation using the Wallace Flexihub cannula fitted with Dr Gilston's protective sleeve. This shows (*a*) the use of a careful no-touch technique whereby the catheter shaft is protected by the sleeve from skin contact; (*b*) successful venepuncture accomplished; (*c*) after cannula advancement, the needle is removed and the flexible hub compressed to prevent air entry or blood egress (*d*); (*e*) the device is linked to an administration set and the sterile protective sleeve removed.

The Gilston cannula also has a compressible hub which allows the clinician to temporarily close off the cannula immediately after the needle is removed and before the administration set or manometer line has been connected. Consequently, air embolism is prevented and the troublesome efflux of blood avoided. This feature is of particular value to the nursing staff during administration set changing procedures, when air embolism is an ever-present risk.

References

1. English I. C. W., Frew R. M., Piggott J. F. et al.: Percutaneous cannulation of the internal jugular vein. *Anaesthesia* 1969; **24**: 521–31.
2. Branthwaite M. A., Bradley R. D.: Measurement of cardiac output by thermal dilution in man. *J. Appl. Physiol.* 1968; **24**: 434–8.
3. Boulanger M., Delva E., Maille J. G. et al.: Internal jugular vein cannulation. *Can. Anaesth. Soc. J.* 1976; **123**: 609–15.
4. Prince S. R., Sullivan R. L., Hackel A.: Percutaneous catheterisation of the internal jugular vein in infants and children. *Anaesthesiology* 1976; **44**: 170–4.
5. Rao T. L. K., Wong A. Y., Salem M. R.: A new approach to percutaneous catheterisation of the internal jugular vein. *Anaesthesiology* 1977; **46**: 362–4.
6. Coté C. J., Jobes D. R., Schwartz A. J. et al.: Two approaches to cannulation of a child's internal jugular vein. *Anaesthesiology* 1979; **50**: 371–3.

Chapter 7

The Supraclavicular Approach to the Subclavian Vein and Temporary Cardiac Pacemaker Electrode Insertion

D. L. H. Patterson

The introduction of cannulas into the subclavian vein by percutaneous techniques is now a commonplace procedure. The ease with which the skilled operator reliably and safely enters the vein is very attractive and may tempt the unskilled to use the technique in preference to a safer puncture of a peripheral vein. The complications of subclavian vein catheterization can be life-threatening. Yoffa, in 1965, introduced the percutaneous supraclavicular approach to the subclavian vein in an effort to minimize the incidence of pneumothorax which had been noted with the infraclavicular approach (1, 2). Argument continues as to whether the supraclavicular or the infraclavicular approach is the safer. It is probably true that the infraclavicular approach is associated with a higher complication rate unless it is performed by doctors experienced in the technique and who are performing it frequently.

The advantages of subclavian vein catheterization are numerous. The vein is always patent and large, often measuring up to 2 cm in diameter in an adult; this renders it particularly useful in the severely shocked patient. Its use often enables both the patient's arms to be kept free. This can be helpful to the patient's morale and comfort and it also leaves the arms free for measurement of other parameters. The site is particularly free from infection and a catheter can often be safely left for weeks without problems. Hypertonic fluids can be infused down the catheter with safety. The central venous pressure can be readily obtained. It is particularly suitable for the introduction of the pacing electrode and obviates the need to bind the patient's arm to his side, as is sometimes necessary if a more peripheral arm vein is used.

Anatomy

The subclavian vein begins at the outer border of the first rib and terminates at the medial margin of the scalenus anterior muscle where it unites with the jugular vein to form the innominate vein. Initially, the subclavian vein arches upwards across the superior surface of the first rib and then inclines medially and downwards across the insertion of the scalenus anterior muscles, to enter the thorax behind the sternoclavicular joint where it unites with the internal jugular vein. Anteriorly the vein is separated from the skin by the clavicle (*Fig.* 7.1). The lateral portion of the vein lies anterior to and below the subclavian artery as both these vessels cross the upper part of the first rib and are

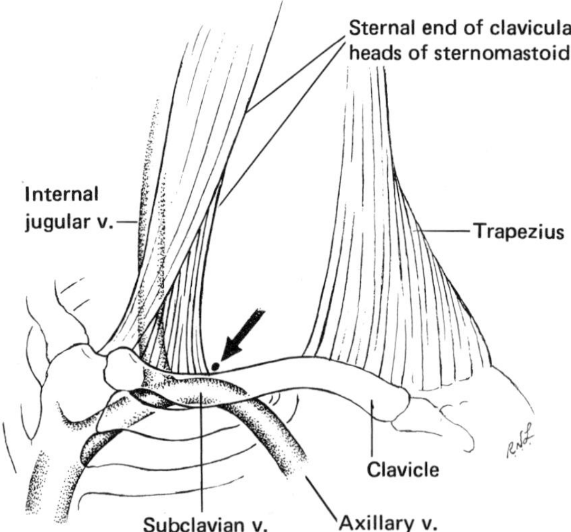

Fig. 7.1. The important musculoskeletal relationships of the left subclavian vein.

separated from one another medially by the scalenus anterior muscle. Behind the artery lies fascia and the cervical pleura (*Fig.* 7.2).

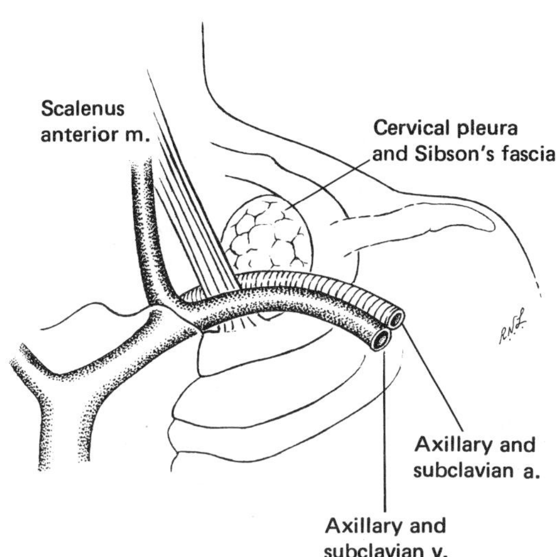

Fig. 7.2. The relationships of the left subclavian vein to the first rib, scalenus anterior muscle, subclavian artery and cervical pleura (the middle and medial thirds of the clavicle are omitted for descriptive purposes).

Technique

There are several techniques of supraclavicular subclavian vein catheterization described. They each use slightly different landmarks and angles. There is also a wide range of central venous catheters. It is important to become familiar and expert with one, although a knowledge of the others is useful. The Wallace Piggy-Back, Argyle Intramedicut and the Vygon long-line Surcath devices are very similar self-contained kits and probably the easiest to use. The E–Z catheter is a useful alternative, although it is more difficult to use in this situation. The size of the catheter to be inserted is an important consideration; in an adult a 14 or 16 G catheter should be used, as anything smaller will produce a much higher resistance to flow and greater damping of pressure recordings. The following description is of the technique preferred by the author.

The procedure must be performed with the patient lying flat and with the legs elevated in order to avoid any possibility of air embolism. If a very low central venous pressure is anticipated,

then it is essential to put the patient in the head-down 20° Trendelenburg position. A right-handed operator will usually find a left subclavian vein easier to enter as there appears to be a natural tendency for the needle to point in the required direction. The identification of the angle between the clavicle and the clavicular insertion of the sternomastoid muscle is vital; the identification will be made easier by getting the patient to raise the head, thus enabling the posterior aspect of the sternomastoid muscle and its clavicular head to be felt and perhaps also to be seen. The patient is then positioned to look directly upwards.

Scrupulous asepsis is mandatory. The operator should 'scrub up' and wear a sterile gown and gloves. The area is thoroughly cleaned and towelled. Local anaesthetic is infiltrated into the site of the identified angle between the clavicle and the clavicular insertion of the sternomastoid muscle (*Fig.* 7.3). The skin should

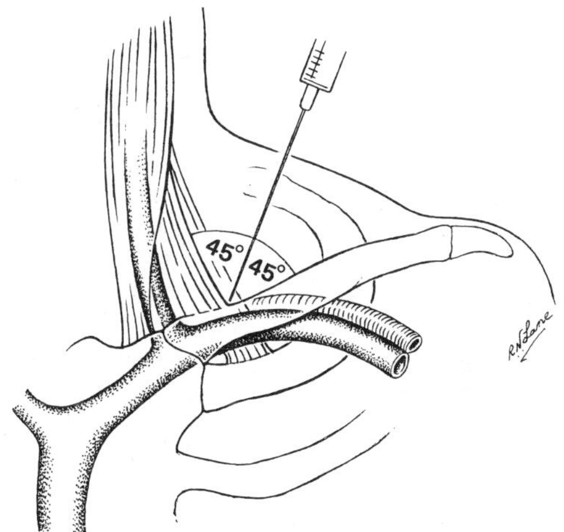

Fig. 7.3. The angle of approach for supraclavicular subclavian vein cannulation.

then be punctured with a scalpel blade. The selected introducing cannula and needle with a firmly fitting syringe attached is introduced through the punctured skin so that it bisects the angle described (*Fig.* 7.3). The needle, cannula and syringe are now raised 15° upwards in the coronal plane. The needle and the cannula should be firmly but gently advanced through the deep cervical fascia maintaining both 15° angulation and the bisection of the described angle. The bevel of the needle should face upwards and the needle will enter the subclavian vein with a slight 'give'. The vein is usually met at a depth of 1–2 cm from the skin. After penetration of the vein, a free flow of blood into the syringe will occur; occasionally, the flow of blood is dependent upon respiration, especially when there is a low central venous pressure. Once the vein is entered, the needle and cannula assembly should be simultaneously rotated and advanced 0·5 cm. The cannula is next advanced slightly over the needle into the lumen of the vein. The syringe and needle are then quickly removed from the cannula, ensuring that the cannula position remains still. The radio-opaque catheter is then threaded down the cannula with a pair of sterile forceps or gently advanced from the sterile plastic protective sheath. It is useful previously to have estimated the length of catheter to be inserted so that, for most purposes, the tip will be in the superior vena cava, approximately 2 cm above the junction with the right atrium. Before connecting up to an infusion, it is mandatory to confirm that the catheter is intravascular by aspirating blood from it. The introducing cannula can then be withdrawn carefully. The catheter is then suitably secured with a purse-string suture and folded across the front of the clavicle and strapped to the anterior chest wall. It is very important to attach the catheter securely, as a restless or confused patient may easily pull it out. Finally, the position of the catheter must be confirmed radiographically before any substantial volume of fluid is infused.

Although the subclavian vein is usually entered easily and safely with this technique, there are occasional difficulties in finding the vein. If the vein is not entered at the first attempt, the needle and cannula should be withdrawn while sucking back on the syringe. The landmarks and angles should be re-assessed and a further attempt made. Minor deviations from the described angles are safe, but it is important not to 'err' too far and accept failure rather than risk a potentially serious complication. Even the most experienced operators have a failure rate. In the elderly patient the anatomical relationships at the base of the neck are slightly altered and the landmarks described above need slight modification. Instead of introducing the needle and cannula at the angle between the sternomastoid and clavicle, it should be introduced approximately 1 cm back from this angle, along the line that bisects it. The other details remain the same.

Occasionally, the subclavian artery is entered. This usually occurs because the angulation of the needle and cannula has been too steep. It is convenient that the anatomy allows suitable prolonged pressure to be exerted on the artery and the bleeding stopped. It is important that at least 5 minutes' pressure is exerted on the artery before proceeding further.

TEMPORARY CARDIAC PACEMAKER ELECTRODE INSERTION

The approach and technique described previously are suitable for the introduction of a temporary transvenous pacemaker electrode. More detailed descriptions of permanent transvenous pacemaker electrode technology are described elsewhere and are beyond the scope of this text.

It is important to have the patient monitored on an oscilloscope during this procedure. A defibrillator should be immediately available and an intravenous line should be present in order to give drug therapy as necessary. A 5 G bipolar electrode may be introduced through a 14 G Argyle Medicut. It is always important to check that the electrode passes through the introducer before starting the procedure. A 6 G bipolar electrode which has more torque than a 5 G can be introduced in an identical manner with a 12 G Medicut. An alternative method is to introduce a guide wire through an appropriate needle which has been first inserted into the subclavian vein. The needle is withdrawn over the guide wire and a 6 G introducing set, comprising a dilator and cannula, is slid over the wire ensuring that there is some projecting wire beyond the end of the introducing set before pushing it on into the vein. Once in the vein, dilator and wire are withdrawn and a 6 G pacing electrode introduced through the cannula.

The electrode is then screened into a position towards the apex of the right ventricle. The right ventricle is often best entered by forming the electrode catheter into a U-shape in the right atrium and then rotating so that the distal end lies adjacent to the tricuspid valve. With a slight withdrawal, the tip usually flicks into the right ventricle and with suitable rotation and advancement, it should be positioned towards the apex of the right ventricle (*Fig.* 7.4). The

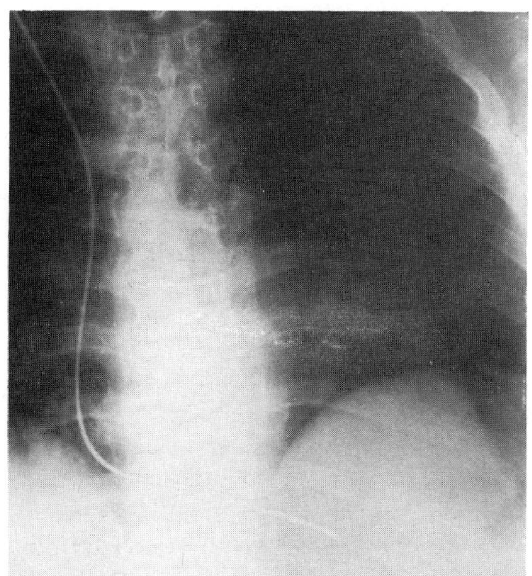

Fig. 7.4. A chest X-ray following the insertion of a temporary transvenous cardiac pacemaking electrode. The tip is shown to be in a satisfactory position near the apex of the right ventricle.

right ventricle is trabeculated and it is usually possible to find a stable and satisfactory electrode position. The final position should allow a smooth curve in the right atrium which is sufficient to prevent dislodgement during deep inspiration; if the curve is too acute, the electrode may loop and become dislodged. Ventricular arrhythmias often occur as the catheter passes through the tricuspid valve, but are usually transient. They are a useful sign that the catheter has passed through the tricuspid valve rather than into the coronary sinus.

When a suitable position has been found, the distal electrode is connected to the cathode of the pacemaker and the proximal electrode to the anode. The threshold is next established. The threshold is the minimum energy required to pace the heart. It should not exceed 1 V or 2 mA with a pulse duration of 1 ms. Higher values may occasionally be accepted in urgent situations or in a patient with a diseased myocardium. It is important that long periods of asystole do not occur when assessing the threshold; it is therefore wise to have one observer watching the

patient's monitor announcing when the first pacemaker artefact fails to capture the ventricle. Meanwhile, the fine voltage adjustment is progressively turned down until the pacing artefact fails to capture the ventricle; whenever this happens the course voltage adjustment is increased, thus ensuring that the heart continues beating. The threshold can then be read at leisure. The threshold should be estimated several times to ensure that it is consistent; if it varies, it can be assumed that the electrode is not in permanent contact with the endocardium and therefore needs repositioning. It is important to wean the patient slowly off the pacemaker before attempting to reposition the catheter. This can be achieved by progressively reducing the rate and the voltage until the patient's own rhythm takes over. The pacemaker should then be switched off and a new position sought.

An electrode position in the coronary sinus or in an hepatic vein can mimic a right ventricular position in the anteroposterior plane (*Fig.* 7.5).

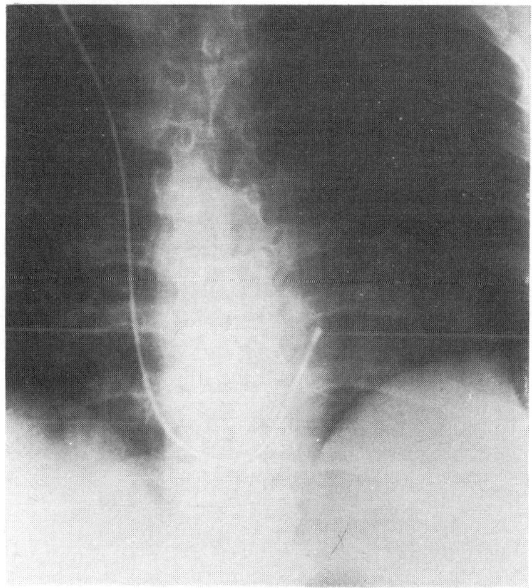

Fig. 7.5. A post-insertion chest X-ray showing undesirable migration of a transvenous cardiac pacing electrode into the coronary sinus.

The threshold, however, will be high, and if the electrode is in the hepatic vein, diaphragmatic stimulation may occur. Lateral screening will help to differentiate between the entry posteriorly to the coronary sinus and the anterior right ventricular position. Intracardiac electrograms may also be useful in distinguishing between a right ventricular and a coronary sinus position; it is important to use an ECG machine that is electrically isolated from the patient, and if there is any doubt about this fact, a battery operated ECG machine should be used. The distal electrode is connected to the chest lead of the ECG machine and the electrograms show marked ST segment elevation if the electrode is in contact with the endocardium. There is no ST segment elevation if the electrode is in the coronary sinus. Any final doubt about the position of the electrode can be resolved by passing it into the pulmonary artery (*Fig.* 7.6), which confirms that it must have been in the right ventricle, and then withdrawing it and manipulating it into its correct position.

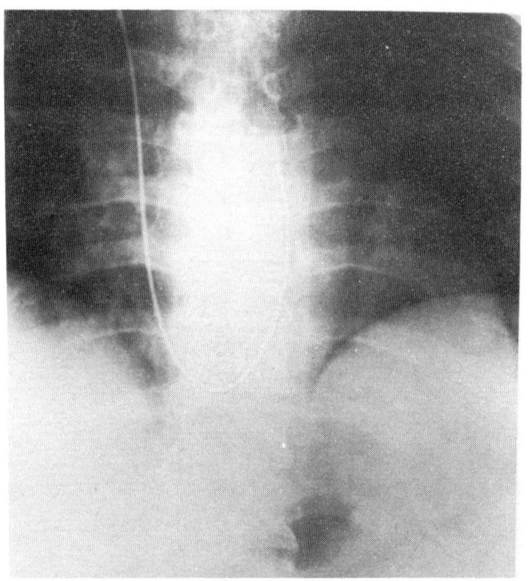

Fig. 7.6. Post-insertion chest X-ray showing the temporary pacing electrode in the pulmonary artery.

Once a satisfactory threshold has been found, the effects of respiration and coughing on the electrical and mechanical stability of the electrode should be tested with the output set at 50 per cent above the threshold. Time spent in ensuring a satisfactory position is worth while and may avoid the necessity of spending further time when the electrode becomes displaced, perhaps in the middle of the night! The introducer can now be withdrawn, ensuring that the electrode does not move. It is wise to check the threshold again at this juncture. The electrode

should next be firmly secured to the skin by at least two sutures and the area covered by sterile gauze and an adhesive dressing (e.g. Op-Site), ensuring that all the exterior part of the electrode is covered; this will avoid the possibility of a restless or confused patient inadvertently pulling it out.

A penetrated chest X-ray and a 12-lead paced ECG should be performed to serve as a base line for the development of any subsequent problems. The electrical connections and threshold should be checked daily and potential complications sought. The threshold will normally rise progressively in the first 2 weeks after insertion but will not usually rise more than two- or threefold above the initial threshold. The pacing rate should be set at an appropriate level, which in most circumstances is between 60 and 90 per minute. The decision about whether to use demand or fixed rate pacing depends on the underlying problems; if the patient's inherent rate is slow at all times, then the fixed rate mode should be used. If the patient's inherent rate is variable, then demand pacing is preferable. The theoretical advantage of demand pacing is that it avoids the possibility of a pacing impulse occurring at the peak of the T wave, which may precipitate ventricular fibrillation.

PROBLEMS ASSOCIATED WITH TEMPORARY PACING

Occasionally serious ventricular arrhythmias occur as the catheter is passed through the tricuspid valve; these will usually disappear if the catheter is moved back into the right atrium, but may occasionally require DC shock or drug therapy. If this problem occurs repeatedly, it may be necessary to start an infusion of lignocaine whilst the electrode catheter is being manipulated into position. An alternative is to try a smaller and therefore softer electrode. Ventricular ectopic beats sometimes occur after pacing has commenced; it is usually possible to eradicate these by altering the pacemaker rate slightly. This is a more satisfactory solution than infusing anti-arrhythmic drugs which inevitably will depress cardiac function.

If the patient's own inherent rate increases, it may approximate that of the pacemaker and, even when this is set on demand, 'competition' may occur; this will result in pacemaker artefacts appearing on the oscilloscope or ECG in spite of preceding QRS complexes. This can sometimes be confused with malfunction of the pacemaker, but in fact can be readily resolved by either increasing or decreasing the pacemaker rate. Occasionally, the pacemaker can stimulate both the heart and the diaphragm. Hiccups at a rate of 70 per minute can be distressing for the patient! This problem is unusual and self-limiting, but occasionally repositioning of the electrode is required.

Should the pacemaker fail to capture the ventricle, then it is important to try to diagnose the problem. This can usually be done quickly. The information required is whether there are pacemaker artefacts on the oscilloscope or ECG and whether the pacemaker box is functioning. If there are pacemaker artefacts present, then this implies that the electrode circuit is intact and that the problem lies at the level of contact with the endocardium. It may be possible to capture the ventricle again by increasing the voltage; if the threshold is consistent although high, it implies that the electrode is still in permanent contact with the endocardium but perhaps has perforated through the myocardium and is lying in the pericardium. It is sometimes possible for the pacemaker to stimulate the left ventricle by this means and this can be confirmed by an ECG, which will show a different pattern of activation or, alternatively, auscultation, which will reveal a change in movement of the second heart sound with respiration. A variable threshold implies intermittent contact with the endocardium and it is likely that the catheter is lying within the right ventricular cavity. In both these instances it is

important to wean the patient off the pacemaker and then to reposition it. The absence of pacemaker artefacts on the oscilloscope or ECG implies that the electrical circuit is not complete. The commonest cause is a loose connection. Other causes include battery failure, a short circuit within the system or a fault in the pacemaker electrode itself.

It is possible for the electrode to perforate the myocardium and cause tamponade. This complication is surprisingly rare but, nevertheless, should be suspected if the patient's condition deteriorates in spite of adequate pacing. There are virtually no problems with infection or with thrombosis; there is therefore no need for either anticoagulation or prophylactic antibiotics. The temporary electrode can, if necessary, be left safely in place for some weeks. It is wise to leave the electrode in place for a few days after return to sinus rhythm following a myocardial infarction complicated by heart block. It is the author's practice to leave the electrode in place but disconnect it from the pacemaker box until the patient is stabilized.

The indications for temporary pacing are outside the scope of this article. Temporary electrical pacing is a very satisfactory therapeutic technique; it is a technique, however, that requires some expertise and should not be embarked upon lightly by the untrained operator.

References

1. Yoffa D.: Supraclavicular subclavian venepuncture catheterisation. *Lancet* 1965; **2**: 614–15.
2. Freeman J.: Subclavian vein catheterisation. *Med. J. Aust.* 1968; **2**: 979–82.

Chapter 8

Percutaneous Infraclavicular Subclavian Vein Catheterization

J. L. Peters and P. A. Belsham

The veins of the arm were used exclusively for central venous cannulation until 1952, when Aubaniac first introduced the concept of using the infraclavicular subclavian vein as a site for venepuncture (1). His technique was adopted by Keeri-Szanto (2), Villafane (3) and Lepp (4) in 1953. Initially, the technique was restricted to venepuncture for obtaining blood samples or giving injections, and central catheterization via the subclavian vein was not performed. In 1954, Aubaniac performed angiocardiography using this approach. A further 8 years elapsed before Wilson in Denver, Colorado, pioneered the introduction of flexible central catheters into the superior vena cava by this route (5). The technique was first described in the United Kingdom by Ashbaugh and Thompson in 1963, while they were working in Edinburgh (6).

The use of this approach for the percutaneous catheterization of the subclavian vein has been the subject of much controversy since those pioneering days. The critics of the technique quite rightly point out that the major drawback of this route of insertion is the frequency with which complications occur, particularly when the procedure is performed by the inexperienced. The creation of new problems for patients already in jeopardy from their original pathology or surgery is to be avoided at all costs. In a review of the literature in 1972, Borja reported complication rates of between 0·4 and 9·9 per cent (7). James and Myers found a 6 per cent complication rate with this technique (8). In 1971, a prospective study by Bernard and Stahl demonstrated that non-infectious complications using the infraclavicular approach correlated with the clinical experience of the operator with

the technique (9). Those clinicians who had performed more than 50 procedures had no complications in their series, whilst an 8·1 per cent complication rate was recorded among personnel who had inserted less than 50 catheters.

The most frequently reported complication, occurring with an incidence of 30 per cent in the literature is pneumothorax. These may be partial, total, under tension and even bilateral (10, 11) (when the inexperienced operator creates one pneumothorax and then immediately attempts to cannulate the contralateral vein). An associated pneumomediastinum may develop, associated with massive subcutaneous emphysema which can obstruct the airway and necessitate a tracheostomy. This is especially likely to occur when the patient is receiving intermittent positive pressure ventilation.

The second most reported mishap occurring during insertion is subclavian artery puncture, which accounts for 20 per cent of all complications. This arises when catheterization attempts have been made too far lateral and posterior with respect to the vein. Usually, no problem arises if adequate pressure is applied; however, this is not always the case, and once an expanding haematoma occurs, serious sequelae can result in the form of a false aneurysm or arteriovenous fistula. Arterial injury associated with simultaneous penetration of the pleura may lead to a major haemopneumothorax. In the light of these and other complications to be described later in this chapter there is sufficient reason for the greatest caution to be exercised when this technique is contemplated.

The major considerations in favour of subclavian vein puncture are practical. The arm, jugular and supraclavicular subclavian routes are all unsatisfactory sites when prolonged catheterization is required. Whereas with the infraclavicular subclavian route the skin puncture site is easy to dress and the patient can move the shoulder girdle, almost without restriction. The jugular insertion site is notoriously difficult to keep clean. In the male it is in the beard area, whilst in both sexes it can be contaminated by oropharyngeal secretions, and movement of the patient's neck is restricted. These latter points of advantage over the other routes are important for patient comfort and safety. Many now suggest that where a subclavian catheter is expected to be necessary for more than 2 or 3 weeks, e.g. for the provision of parenteral nutritional support, the device should be tunnelled away from the clavicular region to a distant site (Chapter 9). This is of particular importance in those patients who require a temporary tracheostomy during the course of their management. It is of paramount importance that junior medical staff do not attempt this procedure for the first time (and indeed, the first ten times) without adequate supervision and revision of the topographical anatomy.

Contraindications

In this particular field of supportive care it is not possible to lay down definitive absolute and relative contraindications. The following guidelines are suggested, although in the bizarre spectrum of cases presenting to surgeons involved with trauma and burns, there may be no alternatives left for the clinician on the spot. The infraclavicular subclavian approach should ideally *not* be used in the following circumstances:

1. Children.
2. Restless and uncooperative patients.
3. Bleeding diatheses.
4. Diminished pulmonary reserve.
5. Apical pulmonary bullae or pathology.
6. Abnormal anatomy, e.g. previous clavicular fractures, thoracoplasty or local radiotherapy.

The technique should be reserved for the controlled insertion of a potential 'life-line' into a well-prepared patient, correctly positioned in a 20–30° head-down tilt and preferably in an operating theatre (*Fig*. 8.1).

Preparation

There is no place for the basic principles introduced by Semmelweiss and Lister, or the elementary foundations of current surgical hygiene, being disregarded. The insertion of a foreign body into the human circulation must be associated with the adoption of a strict aseptic and antiseptic ritual on the part of the surgeon.

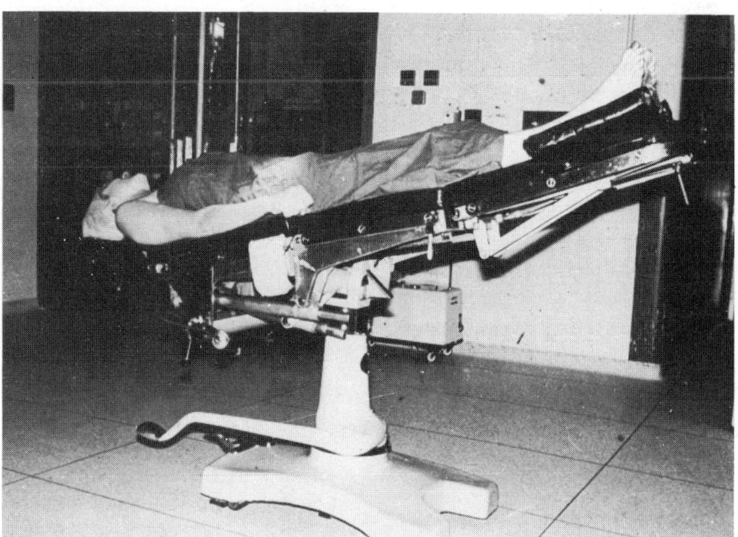

Fig. 8.1. The correct environment and position for the elective percutaneous insertion of infraclavicular subclavian central venous catheters.

Experience gleaned from the 1960s has shown that departure from these principles gives rise to incidences of catheter-related sepsis in excess of 30 per cent, and this should no longer be accepted.

The clinician should liaise with the nursing staff and ensure that all the necessary equipment is to hand and an assistant is available. The appropriate infusion fluids and administration set should be assembled and primed. A good light is essential for this procedure. It is worth while before attempting the procedure to spend some time carrying out the following preliminary activities.

Inspection

Prior to draping the patient, a short time should be spent studying the patient's individual topographical anatomy so that a three-dimensional picture of the subclavian vein's position may be perceived. It is often difficult to cannulate the vein in heavily built subjects with large clavicles and well-developed musculature. Conversely, in many patients of thin or moderate stature, it is sometimes possible to see a venous pulse in the infraclavicular fossa where the subclavian vein passes medially under the clavicle close to the junction of the middle and medial thirds of the bone. It is worth inspecting the anatomy of this region in the cadaver and the course of the vein is easily seen in women who have undergone radical mastectomy in the past. The vein is often prominent in these patients and can be found on a horizontal line drawn from the junction of the mid and medial thirds of the clavicle to the surgical neck of the humerus and the superior aspect of the ipsilateral sternoclavicular joint (*Fig.* 8.2). Whilst the patient is in the Trendelenburg position, palpation of the liver and abdomen may accentuate the venous pulsations in the root of the neck and the infraclavicular subclavian vein. The patient may be returned to the horizontal or head-up position for comfort whilst the necessary further preparations are being made.

Palpation

The next step in the preparatory process is to gently palpate the sternoclavicular joint and the inferior border of the clavicle, noting the re-

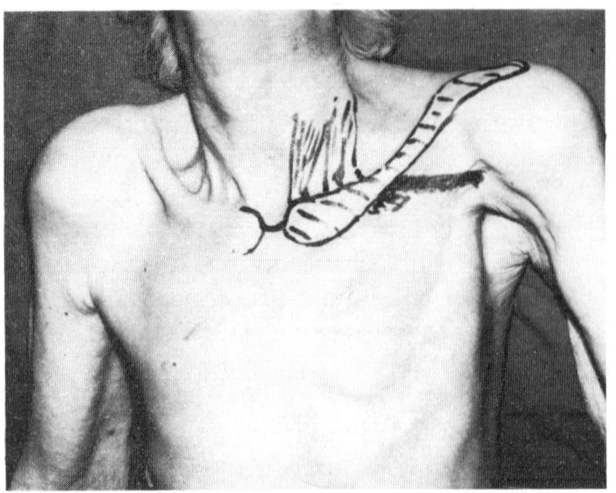

Fig. 8.2. The course of the subclavian vein can be easily seen in patients who have undergone radical breast surgery.

lationship of the external jugular vein to the superior clavicular border. In particular, the point at which the external jugular vein disappears relative to the bone should be marked with an indelible ink fibre-tip pen.

Auscultation

Significant variations in the anatomical relationship of the subclavian vein to the clavicle have been well demonstrated by autopsy studies (12). Contrast radiography studies of the veins have also confirmed these findings (13, 14), leading to the suggestion that television fluoroscopy should be used for accurate localization of the vein prior to the catheterization procedure (15). The slightly different courses of the subclavian vein on the right and left sides, together with positional changes with posture, have also been emphasized by these authors. In patients who have had previous subclavian or long central lines in place, there is a need to check the patency of the vein before further attempts to catheterize the vessel are made. This is normally accomplished by using contrast phlebography (16). The authors have introduced a technique of searching for a more precise localization of the subclavian artery and vein before commencing the procedure (17). This involves the use of a Doppler ultrasound probe (Model BV 102R, Sonicaid Ltd); using this instrument the vessels can be accurately located and, moreover, the patency of the vein investigated. The skin of the infraclavicular fossa is lubricated with Aquasonic Transmission Gel and the Sonicaid probe placed just below the junction of the medial and middle thirds of the clavicle. The probe is moved until the position of the artery is determined by listening for the pulsatile flow sounds and this point is marked with an indelible fibre-tip ink pen, after the skin has been cleared of jelly at that point with a tissue or gauze. The probe is next moved more medially and the characteristic venous hum detected by trial and error. This is made easier by giving the ipsilateral arm a firm, rapid, squeeze and hence the patency of the vein can be established. This point should also be marked and the remaining jelly cleaned from the skin (*Fig.* 8.3). This

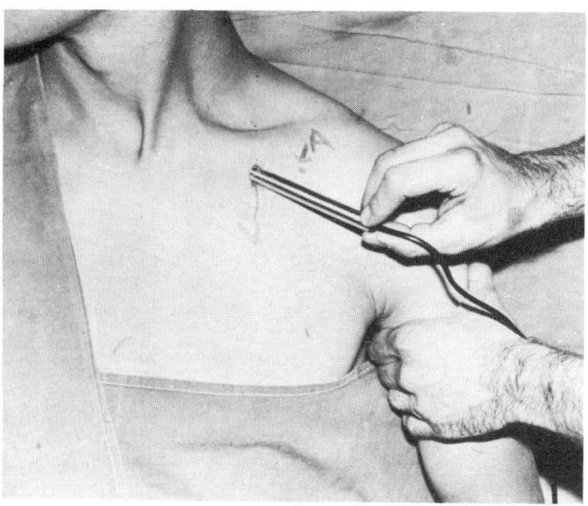

Fig. 8.3. The use of the Sonicaid Doppler ultrasound probe to detect the position of the subclavian artery and vein prior to percutaneous puncture. Note the firm squeeze being applied to the ipsilateral arm.

technique has now been used in 35 patients and the vessels have been effectively localized. The artery has not been punctured and the brachial plexus cords lying close to the artery have not been injured. Sometimes more than one attempt has been required to cannulate the vein, and this has been achieved without creating a pneumothorax. The subcutaneous position of the vein is known with greater confidence. Although the technique will not eradicate pneumothorax if other safeguards are neglected by the clinician, it is hoped that the incidence of pleural, arterial and neurological injury will be substantially reduced, especially when the percutaneous infraclavicular approach to the subclavian vein is being attempted by those new to the technique.

The application of this inspection, palpation and auscultation routine prior to draping should be associated whenever possible with examination of a recent chest X-ray. The upper zones of each hemithorax should be scrutinized in order to detect bullae or other abnormalities which may deter the clinician from using this approach. With practice, these extra steps take less than 5 minutes to perform and can be done whilst the nurse is collecting the trolley and other equipment.

Requirements

Trolley
Cleaning sponges, antiseptic skin disinfectant, e.g. povidone-iodine, chlorhexidine in 70 per cent spirit
Drapes and towels
Towel clips
Instrument pack with sterile scissors
Op-Site incise drape (Smith & Nephew) (28 × 45 cm)
Lignocaine 1 per cent w/v 5–10 ml
Sterile disposable syringes: 5–10 ml
Hypodermic needles: 21 G, 23 G and 25 G
Sterile gauzes
Central venous catheter: 28–33 cm, 14–16 G
Heparinized saline (Hepsal: 10 i.u./ml, Weddell Pharmaceuticals)
3/0 silk suture on a cutting atraumatic needle
Op-Site I.V. dressing (28 × 45 cm, 10 × 14 cm or 6 × 8·5 cm)
Povidone-iodine spray (Disadine, Stuart Pharmaceuticals)

There are now complete kits commercially available and these are based upon a sequential tray principle (Abbott Laboratories, *Fig.* 8.4). Such products are of considerable benefit since they save appreciable amounts of time on behalf of the nurse and the clinician.

The procedure may be performed under local anaesthesia or concurrently with other surgery being performed under general anaesthetic. In view of the risks of pneumothorax, the procedure is best performed at the end of a surgical operation under general anaesthesia. This diminishes the risk of the patient developing a pneumothorax whilst being ventilated. If the procedure is to be performed under local an-

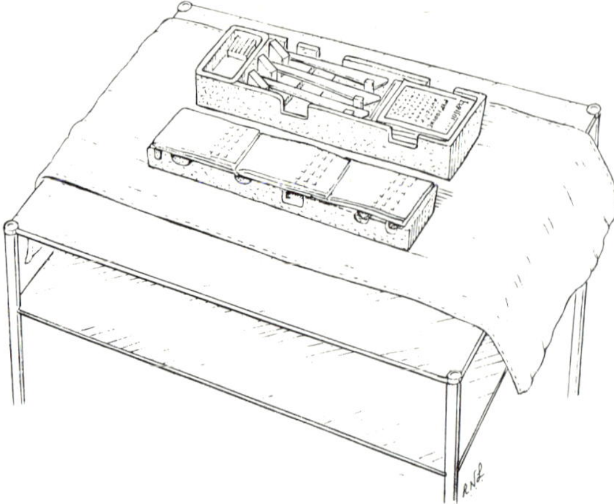

Fig. 8.4. Pre-sterilized two-layer subclavian catheter kit (Abbott Laboratories).

aesthesia, it is kinder to give some form of premedication, e.g. an appropriate dose of pethidine and/or diazepam. If the patient already possesses a peripheral infusion, then a small dose (in adults, 5–10 mg) of diazepam can be given intravenously just prior to the event.

The correct position has been depicted in *Fig.* 8.1, and it is useful to tilt the table slightly towards the chosen side. Many surgeons advocate placing a rolled towel or small sandbag between the patient's shoulder blades so that the clavicles and shoulder girdles are slightly extended during the procedure. The head of the patient should be rotated to face away from the site of insertion. In some units the patient is also fitted with a mask during the procedure. If the operation has to be performed on the patient's bed in a ward, the foot of the bed must be elevated and adequate space made available. It is therefore useful to detach the head of the bed. Right-handed surgeons will find the procedure easier to perform on the left subclavian vein and vice versa. The skin should be shaved when necessary over a wide area so that the subsequent dressings can be applied and removed without discomfort.

The operator should next 'scrub up', donning a mask, gown and gloves. The chosen operation site should be generously cleaned for at least 3 minutes with povidone-iodine, iodine in 70 per cent w/v spirit or chlorhexidine in 70 per cent w/v spirit. The area cleaned should extend up on to the posterior triangle of the neck, over the suprasternal notch of Burns and on to the

contralateral side of the anterior chest wall (*Fig.* 8.5). This enables the various landmarks to be easily seen and palpated during the procedure. All the excess fluid should be dried off with a sterile towel. When a commercial kit is not being used, surgical linen or paper drapes should be arranged as depicted in *Fig.* 8.6. It is important to be able to see the external jugular vein and the superior aspect of the sternoclavicular joint. The towel covering the patient's face should naturally be lifted clear by a nurse during the procedure. Paper drapes invariably fall on the floor or dislodge and they rarely maintain a satisfactory sterile field. It is useful, therefore, to fix the drapes in place using a transparent incise drape (*Fig.* 8.7), e.g. Op-Site. The nurse and clinician should explain the procedure prior to each manoeuvre in order to reassure the patient. This is of particular importance, because when the actual puncture takes place, it is extremely helpful if the patient can remain relaxed and immobile and either hold his breath or perform a Valsalva manoeuvre.

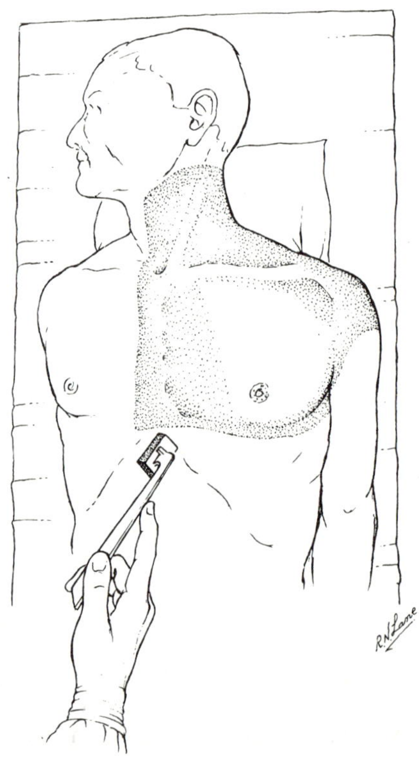

Fig. 8.5. Area of skin preparation for subclavian vein catheterization.

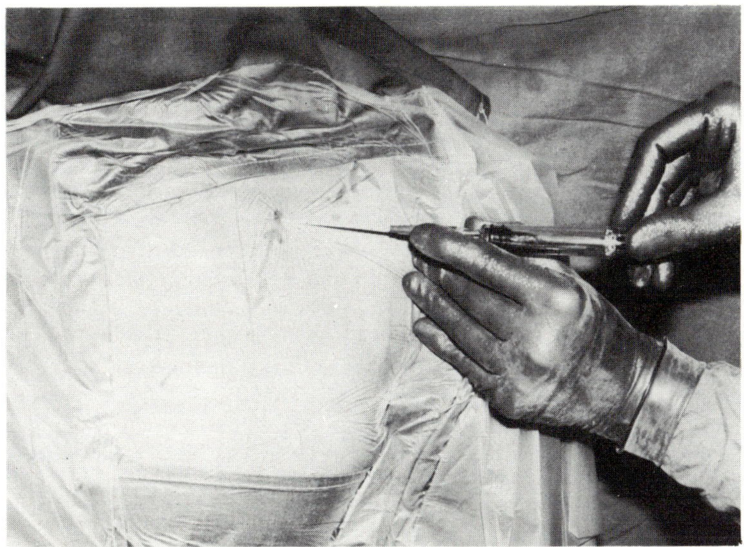

Fig. 8.6. The surgical drapes must be carefully placed to allow further inspection and palpation.

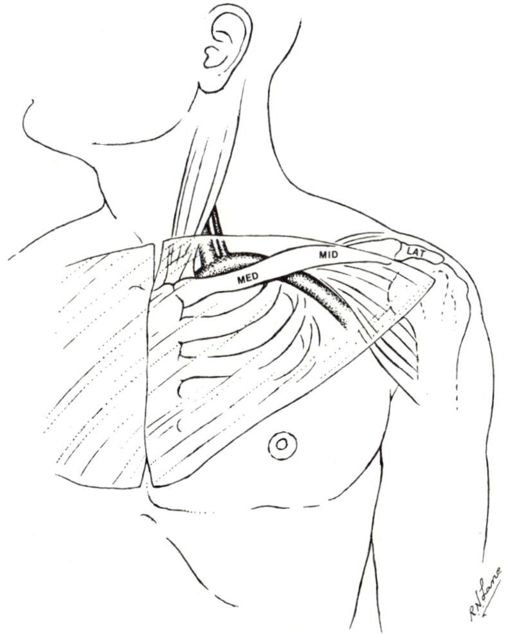

Fig. 8.7. To show the relationship of the draped area, the clavicle, subclavian vein and first rib.

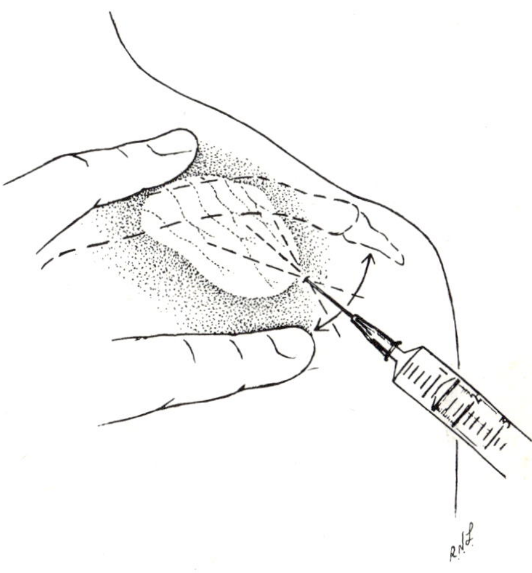

Fig. 8.8. The skin overlying and below the junction of the middle and medial thirds of the clavicle should be carefully infiltrated with local anaesthesia. The relevant cervical nerves pass over the anterior aspect of the clavicle. The anaesthetic agent must also be introduced into the deeper layers around the vein.

Local Anaesthesia

The infraclavicular fossa should be anaesthetized by infiltrating lignocaine 1 per cent w/v into the subcutaneous tissues as shown in *Fig.* 8.8, using first a 25 G needle and then a 21 G needle. The innervation of the skin in this region is from small supraclavicular branches which cross the anterior aspect of the clavicle. It is important to allow the lignocaine time to act. With experience, a small amount of the anaesthetic solution can be gently infiltrated into the subclavius muscle and around the vein without puncturing the vessel. The anaesthetic solution may be dispersed into the tissues by gently pressing the area with a swab.

Insertion Technique

A through-needle technique should never be used because of the risk of catheter embolism. Even if the clinician has the steadiest of hands, the patient may suddenly move or cough and the catheter can be transected on the needle bevel. The same risk exists with splitting needles. Goy has described a Seldinger wire technique and this is a safe way of avoiding the necessity of passing a cannula through the needle if the equipment described below is not available (18).

A through-cannula technique will be described, and this is generally provided for by manufacturers at the present time. The kit shown in *Fig.* 8.4 contains the introducing cannula and syringe together with all the other equipment required. If such an arrangement is not available, the catheter assembly selected by the clinician, e.g. a Wallace Piggy-Back, No. 33816, should be carefully delivered from its package on to the sterile trolley area by the assistant using a no-touch aseptic technique. The introducing cannula, needle and syringe should be assembled and the syringe pushed firmly home. Some may prefer to half-fill the syringe with heparinized saline (e.g. Hepsal, 10 i.u./ml). Individuals may prefer holding different-sized syringes for comfort, and this aspect is important if a smooth and atraumatic procedure is to be performed. The central catheter in its plastic dispensing sheath should be arranged in a convenient position and it is wise to gently free the sheath because the catheter is often adherent to the PVC.

Once all these preparations are completed, the following points concerning the patient should be re-checked:

1. The patient is relaxed.
2. There is a 20–30° head-down Trendelenburg tilt.
3. The shoulders are extended over a towel or sandbag (e.g. *Fig.* 8.9).
4. The head is turned towards the contralateral side.
5. The arms lie alongside the thorax.

With the patient in this position, the introducing cannula held by its attached syringe should be introduced through the skin approximately 2–3 cm below the junction of the mid and medial thirds of the anterior clavicular border. The clinician should then palpate the surgical neck of the humerus, the anterior border of the clavicle and the ipsilateral sternoclavicular joint and, finally, make a mental note of the position of the

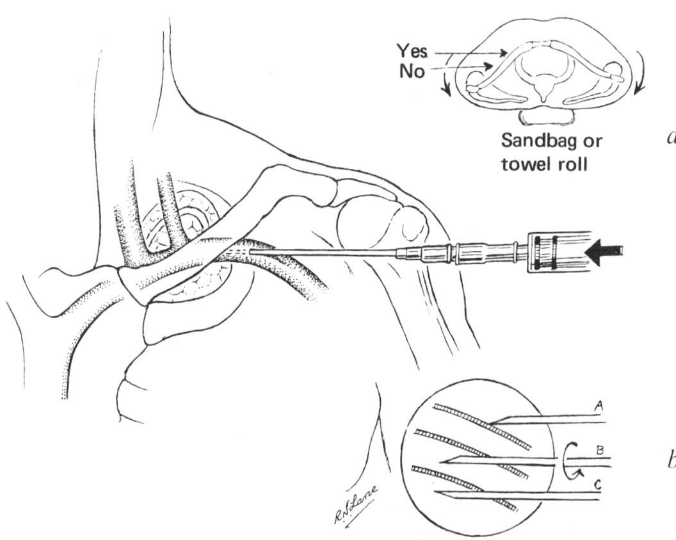

Fig. 8.9. The correct angle of approach of the insertion cannula and needle (*see also inset a*). A sandbag or towel roll should be placed between the shoulder blades so that the scapulae may be retracted. *Inset b*, the importance of rotating the needle during the entry manoeuvre (A, B, C).

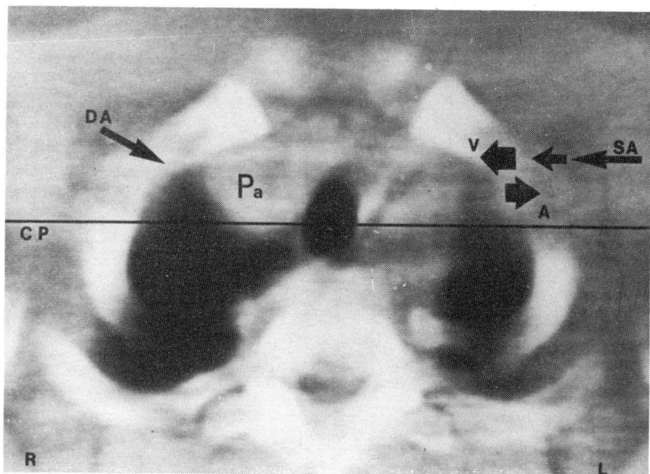

Fig. 8.10. A CAT scan at the level of the thoracic inlet and clavicles illustrates important features. Note the occult apical pulmonary pathology on the right side of the neck. The dangerous angle of approach (DA) shows how easily a pneumothorax can be created. The safe angle of approach (SA) to the subclavian vein (V) is shown together with the subclavian artery (A). Note how the line of approach should be parallel to the coronal plane (CP).

external jugular vein. When Doppler ultrasound has been used, the skin can be penetrated as marked (*see Fig.* 8.3). A safe procedure can only be accomplished if the clinician has a comprehensive knowledge of the topographical anatomy of this region and has a three-dimensional concept in respect of the structures adjacent to the vein. A CAT scan, which depicts the relationships of the first rib, subclavian vessels and apical pleura (*Fig.* 8.10), is shown here to assist those attempting the procedure (under supervision) for the first time. The value of inspecting a preliminary chest X-ray is apparent here, where abnormal apical pathology (Pa) would possibly distort the subclavian venous anatomy. The dangerous angle of approach (DA) is shown, and it can be seen that in order to avoid injury to the pleura, the safe angle (SA) of approach is on a plane parallel to the coronal plane of the body (CP) in the line of the vein (V) and just anterior to the line of the artery (A). This angle of approach lies horizontal to the floor and bed when the patient has been placed in the position previously described. The anatomy of this region involved in a percutaneous infraclavicular subclavian vein puncture, as seen in a sagittal section of the relevant area, is highlighted in *Fig.* 8.11.

Once the introducing needle and cannula have been pushed through the skin into the subcuta-

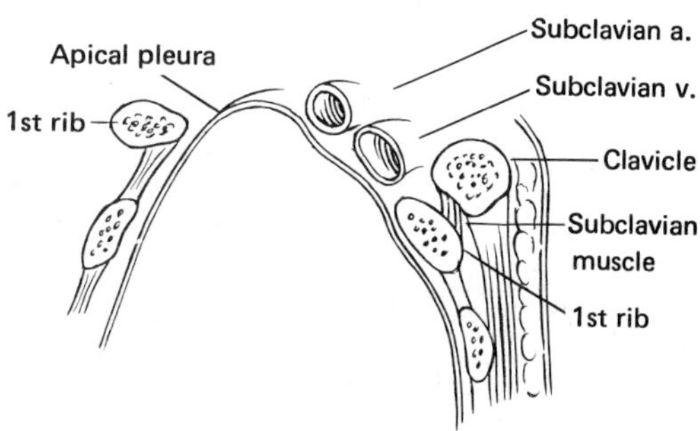

Fig. 8.11. A sagittal section through the junction of the upper thorax and clavicle, illustrating the relationship of the subclavian artery, vein, pleura and clavicle.

neous fat, this assembly should be advanced towards the inferior border of the clavicle with a gentle negative suction being applied to the syringe using only one finger on the plunger. The bevel of the needle should face upwards and it is useful intermittently to rotate the cannula and needle through 90° as the vein is approached. By the time the pectoral muscles are reached, the cannula should have been positioned so that the 'safe angle (SA)' of approach has been achieved. Useful coordinates to follow are that the cannula should be parallel to the coronal plane (CP), as shown in *Fig.* 8.10, and also the cannula should be advanced slowly and carefully along an imaginary line extending from the surgical neck of the humerus, through the junction of the medial and middle thirds of the clavicle, to the top of the ipsilateral sterno-clavicular joint. This 'line' is shown well in the post-insertion chest X-ray (*Fig.* 8.12), where unfortunately malposition into the jugular vein has occurred! The needle should travel in a plane 0·5–1 cm posterior to the clavicle and the vein will be entered at the outer border of the first rib (*see Fig.* 8.9). The introducing cannula should be simultaneously rotated through 180° and advanced a further half-centimetre. Venous blood should aspirate freely into the syringe before the needle and syringe are withdrawn. It is useful to place a sterile gauze beneath the hub to catch any escaping blood (*Fig.* 8.13).

Recently, an introducing cannula has been developed which possesses a compressible hub, and this design enables the clinician to prevent unnecessary haemorrhage or air entrainment (*see* Chapter 6). If this form of plastic introducing cannula is not available, the patient should be instructed to stop breathing momentarily whilst the syringe and needle are quickly removed. Speed is essential at this point and the introducing cannula with its tip in the sub-clavian vein must be held with a steady hand.

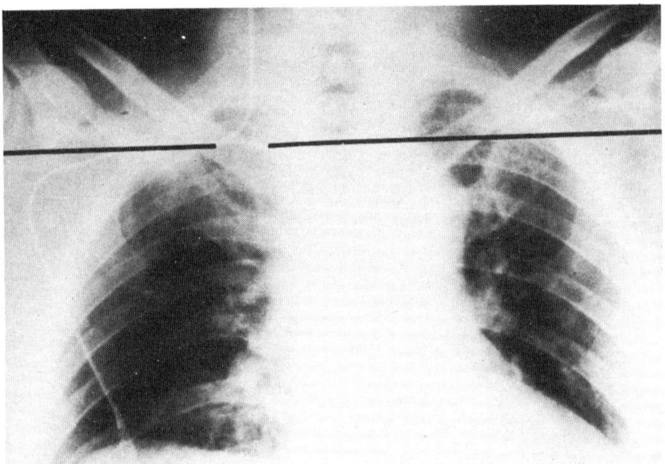

Fig. 8.12. Chest X-ray illustrating the horizontal 'line' of approach extending from the anatomical neck of the humerus through the junction of the middle and medial thirds of the clavicle to the superior aspect of the sterno-manubrial joint. The X-ray also shows how the catheter has been malpositioned into the internal jugular vein and this would not have occurred if on-table screening had been performed.

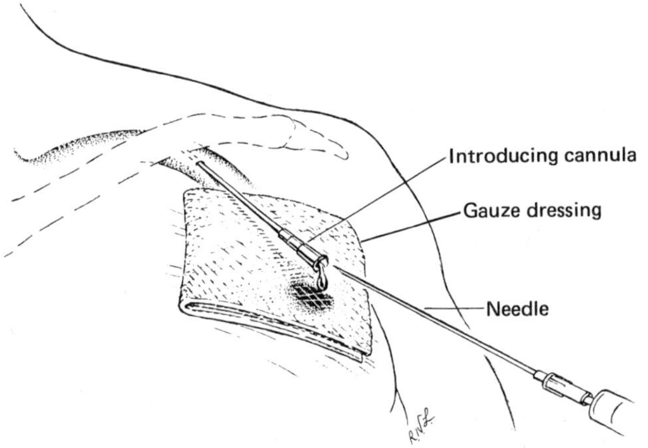

Fig. 8.13. A sterile swab placed beneath the introducing cannula hub absorbs any escaping blood.

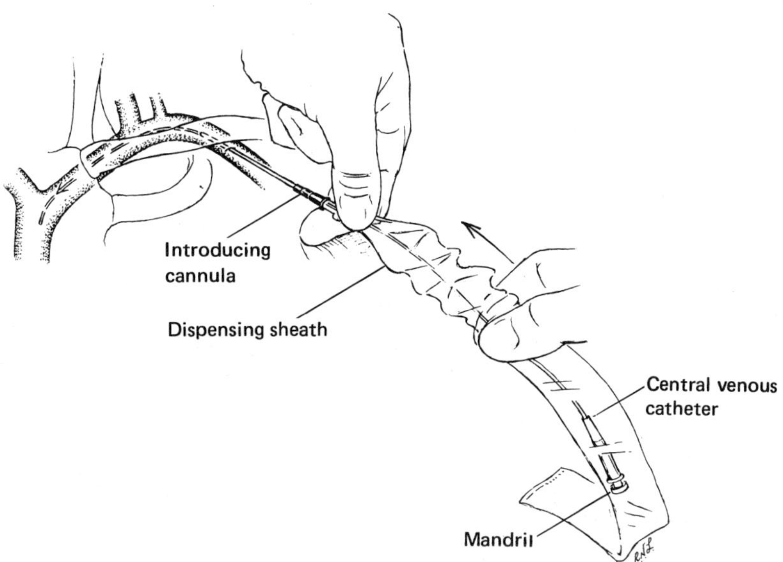

Fig. 8.14. No-touch introduction of a central venous catheter and mandril into the superior vena cava.

The definitive central catheter and its protective sheath should be fitted on to the hub and the central catheter gently passed through the introducing cannula by a 'tweaking' action of the index finger and thumb through the plastic dispensing purse (*Figs.* 8.14, 8.15). The catheter should enter the vein without difficulty. Some may prefer to remove the central line completely from the sheath in order to improve their dexterity at this critical point in the procedure.

Subclavian central catheters stiffened with mandrils in their lumen are less likely to pass in a retrograde fashion up the jugular vein, but they must be handled very carefully lest they perforate the innominate vein or superior vena cava as they are advanced. Any difficulty experienced in passing the catheter should be taken seriously, since the tip may be impacting in a tributary; loop formation may have occurred or the catheter may have started to dissect the endothelium of the vein; the catheter may even have passed through into the perivenous space, pleura or mediastinum. If difficulty does occur, the catheter should be withdrawn slightly, rotated through 90° and the angle of the introducing cannula altered a fraction, before a further attempt is made to advance the central line. If this also fails, then the clinician should establish whether or not the introducing cannula is still in the vein, since dislocation may have occurred

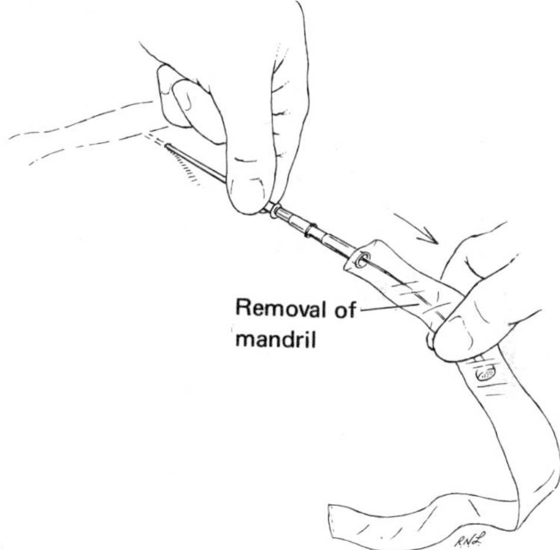

Fig. 8.15. After insertion, the central mandril should be removed, the introducing cannula and central venous catheter hubs firmly engaged and adjustments made to the final position of the device.

with a slight movement of the hand or of the patient's chest wall. The cannula can be completely withdrawn, pressure applied and the assembly cleared out with sterile heparinized saline before a further attempt is made. It is worth while to try to position the patient in a steeper degree of head-down Trendelenburg tilt. The temptation to change the *angle* of approach should be resisted; although the path chosen may be a few millimetres away, the direction of approach should still be one which is parallel to the coronal plane.

Once a successful cannulation and subsequent passage of the central catheter has been achieved, care must be taken not to insert the device too far into the superior vena cava. When the central catheter has been sited, the plastic introducing sleeve may be removed and the mandril or terminal Luer plug removed from the central catheter hub. The authors prefer to occlude the catheter hub with a 2 or 5 ml syringe of heparinized saline (e.g. Hepsal 10 i.u./ml) whilst the final positional and dressing arrangements are being completed. Small aliquots (0·5 ml) of heparinized saline can be used intermittently to flush the central line. Next, the introducing cannula should be withdrawn out of the vein over the shaft of the central line and clear of the original puncture site. The central catheter should be carefully held to avoid accidental dislodgement during this manoeuvre. The introducing cannula should then be threaded further back over the catheter and the hub of the central line locked into the hub of the introducing cannula. This is an important point since death from air embolism has occurred when the introducing cannula has remained in the vein and the central venous catheter has been accidentally pulled out leaving a patent and unprotected portal for air entry into the circulation (19). New devices are now to be made so that the introducing cannula locks on to the central line with the aid of a plastic screw thread. The catheter may be fixed to the skin with a 3/0 silk suture, and if this is performed it should be done carefully in case the lumen of the catheter is obliterated or a stress fracture induced in the catheter shaft. The puncture site should be sprayed with povidone-iodine powder (Disadine) before applying a small square of gauze and an Op-Site dressing. The shaft of the catheter should be fixed separately to the anterior chest wall in a gentle curve using a sheet of Op-Site so that the hub is left free for administration set changes. Finally, the syringe containing the heparinized saline can be removed and the catheter linked to an intravenous administration or manometer set. Attention to detail in the fixation of the catheter is extremely important in order to prevent the device from 'telescoping' in and out of the wound or kinking

under the influence of the infusion tubing. The junction between the catheter and administration set should be sprayed with povidone-iodine and enclosed in an envelope made with a sterile gauze swab.

Correct Placement Checks

During the course of the procedure it is important to ensure that the catheter is placed into the lumen of the vein and the tip of the catheter is situated in the upper half of the superior vena cava as described in Chapter 5 (*Fig.* 8.16). Moreover, there should be no looping or malposition of the catheter shaft.

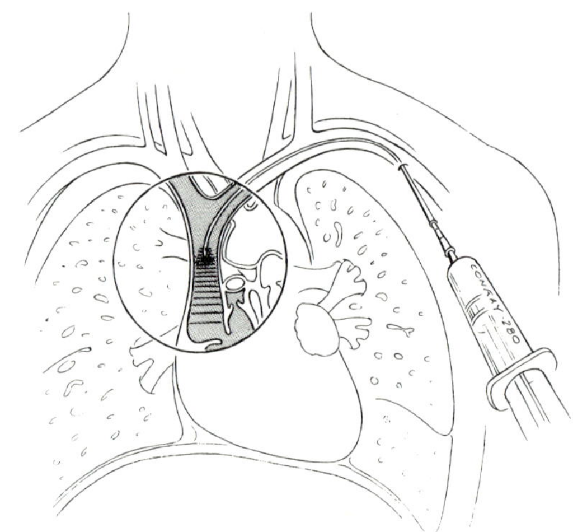

Fig. 8.16. Accurate placement should always be confirmed by performing an immediate post-insertion X-ray using contrast medium (Conray or Hexabrix). This is best performed using on-table screening with an image intensifier.

There should, therefore, be free aspiration of blood down the introducing cannula after the initial puncture of the vein; the definitive central catheter should have entered the vein without difficulty; it should be possible to aspirate blood down the central catheter using a syringe. The most important criteria which must be applied in order to confirm the correct placement are:

1. After the central catheter has been connected to the primed administration set, and with all the control taps etc. open, the bottle or bag of fluid should then be slowly lowered to a level below the patient's heart and venous blood should reflux easily and oscillate in synchrony

with atrial contraction and respiratory excursions. If this test fails, it suggests that the central catheter has become blocked by a thrombus, looped, kinked or has passed outside of the vein. It is wise not to use the catheter until one has taken the necessary steps to discover the problem.

2. A plain chest X-ray should be performed. It is useful to inject a small quantity of Conray 280 or Hexabrix 320 into the catheter in order to enhance the X-ray view. It is preferable to visualize the catheter using these contrast media and an image intensifier.

3. If there is any doubt as to the correct placement, a chest X-ray should be performed after the injection of 5–10 ml of sterile contrast medium down the lumen of the catheter.

Once these checks have confirmed a satisfactory placement of the catheter, the prescribed infusion can be commenced with confidence or else the line used as a manometer. A record should be made of the time and date of insertion together with the length and type of catheter used. Clear instructions should be issued to the nursing staff concerning the care of the catheter and dressing change routine.

Complications

A comprehensive discussion of the complications related to central venous catheterization procedures is provided in Chapters 12, 13 and 14. The following list illustrates the problems that have been related to the infraclavicular subclavian vein insertion procedure.

Embolism
  Air embolism
  Catheter embolism
Vascular
  Pneumothorax
  Haemothorax
  Subclavian artery puncture
  Arteriovenous fistula formation
  Carotid artery puncture
  Pulmonary artery laceration (apical branch)
  Internal mammary artery laceration
Nerve
  Brachial plexus injury
  Phrenic nerve palsy
  Left recurrent laryngeal nerve injury

Bone
  Osteomyelitis of the clavicle
  Tracheal perforation and endotracheal tube cuff perforation
Miscellaneous
  Malposition
  Knotting and loop formation

Such complications have been documented intermittently throughout the medical and surgical literature since 1952. It is to be hoped that the application of careful technique and an appropriate degree of caution on behalf of the clinician will in the future eliminate many of these problems. Once a catheter has been safely inserted, the patient must be subjected to a careful and regular examination with respect to the potential complications and the nursing staff must be encouraged to maintain the central catheter using a scrupulously aseptic technique. Once a catheter is safely inserted, the complications which are to be feared most are: air embolism from disconnection of the catheter and the infusion system, catheter sepsis, septicaemia and secondary bacterial or fungal endocarditis; subclavian vein thrombosis or suppurative thrombophlebitis; superior vena cava perforation with the development of hydromediastinum; a cardiac tamponade as a consequence of the endocardium being eroded by hypertonic solutions or mechanical perforation by the tip of the central catheter. Catheter embolism can also occur at a late stage because of fractures which develop in the catheter shaft due to the rigours of clinical practice.

References

1. Aubaniac R.: L'injection intraveneuse sous claviculaire. *Presse Méd.* 1952; **60**: 1456.
2. Keeri-Szanto M.: The subclavian vein, a constant and convenient intravenous injection site. *Arch. Surg.* 1956; **72**: 179.
3. Villafane E. P.: Technica de la transfusion por via subclavicular. *Prensa Med. Argent.* 1953; **40**: 2379.
4. Lepp H.: Über eine neue Intravenuse Injektions und Punktionsmethode. *Deutsch. Zahnarztl. Z.* 1953; **8**: 511.
5. Wilson J. N., Grown J. B., Demong C. V. et al.: Central venous pressure in optimal blood volume maintenance. *Arch. Surg.* 1962; **85**: 563.
6. Ashbaugh D., Thompson J. W. W.: Subclavian vein infusion. *Lancet* 1963; **2**: 1138.
7. Borja A. R.: Current status of infraclavicular subclavian vein catheterisation. *Ann. Thorac. Surg.* 1972; **13**: 615–24.

8. James P. M., Myers R. T.: Central venous pressure monitoring; complication and a new technique. *Am. Surg.* 1973; **39**: 75–81.

9. Bernard R. W., Stahl W. M.: Subclavian vein catheterisation; a prospective study. (i) Non-infectious complication. *Ann. Surg.* 1971; **173**: 182–90.

10. Matz R.: Complications of determining central venous pressure. *N. Engl. J. Med.* 1965; **273**: 703.

11. Maggs P. R., Schwaber J. R.: Fatal bilateral pneumothoraces complicating subclavian vein catheterisation. *Chest* 1977; **71**: 532–3.

12. Borja A. R., Henshaw J. R.: A safe way to perform infraclavicular subclavian vein catheterisation. *Surg. Gynecol. Obstet.* 1970; **130**: 673.

13. Land R. F.: Anatomic relationships of the right subclavian vein. A radiologic study pertinent to percutaneous subclavian venous catheterisation. *Arch. Surg.* 1971; **102**: 178.

14. Land R. F.: The relationship of the left subclavian vein to the clavicle. Practical considerations pertinent to the percutaneous catheterisation of the subclavian vein. *J. Thorac. Cardiovasc. Surg.* 1972; **63**: 564.

15. Lane R. F., Garrett J. C., Hedberg S. E.: Television fluoroscopy and specification of the subclavian vein. *Arch Surg.* 1970; **101**: 429–30.

16. Axelsson C. K., Efsen F.: Phlebography in long-term catheterisation of the subclavian vein. *Scand J. Gastroenterol.* 1978; **13**: 933.

17. Peters J. L., Belsham P., Garrett C. P. O. et al.: Doppler ultrasound, an aid to percutaneous infraclavicular subclavian vein catheterisation. *Am. J. Surg.* 1982; **143** (3): 391–3.

18. Goy J. E.: Guide wire technique for central vein cannulation. *Br. Med. J.* 1976; **2**: 21.

19. Ross S. M., Freedman P. S., Farrer J. V.: Air embolism after accidental removal of intravenous catheter. *Br. Med. J.* 1979; **1**: 987.

Chapter 9

Tunnelling Techniques

J. L. Peters and P. A. Belsham

During the late 1960s, at the University of Pennsylvania in Philadelphia, Dudrick and his colleagues, during their earliest survival experiments concerned with providing total parenteral nutrition in dogs, were faced with the technical problem of finding a method of gaining continuous and safe access to the circulation in free ranging laboratory animals (1–3). No greater test could have been devised, and history has vindicated their technical expertise. They used PVC catheters introduced by a cut-down procedure and the catheters were tunnelled to a point between the scapulae on the animal's back. Using this technique, the catheters could be kept functioning for periods extending up to several hundred days.

Perhaps the effectiveness of these procedures should have been predicted, for the aphorism of Sir Alexander Fleming points out that: 'The greatest of all antiseptics is living tissue'. The creation of a long skin tunnel for a catheter entering a major tributary of the great veins effectively provides a skin dressing for the portion of the catheter adjacent to the endothelial puncture site. The subcutaneous tunnel is much longer than the 1 or 2 cm track, lined by granulation tissue, which surrounds a catheter inserted by the conventional percutaneous technique; furthermore, the catheter which has been tunnelled is not subjected to the same 'piston or telescoping' effect. Such movement at the catheter insertion site is likely to result in the progression of skin bacteria into the granulation tissue lining the wound, and ultimately infection of the fibrin sheath known to surround the intravascular portion of the catheter (4). The greater length of subcutaneous tissue which envelops the catheter shaft presumably allows a more effective control of nosocomial bacterial penetration around the catheter by the immune defence mechanisms of the patient. The catheter exit site is removed away from obvious sources of contamination, such as saliva, spillage from nasogastric, endotracheal and tracheostomy tubes and the perspiration that accumulates in the 'beard' area. The reduced incidence of catheter-related sepsis found in patients where catheters were tunnelled over a distance of 20–30 cm was initially an empirical observation made upon a few patients requiring total parenteral nutrition. More recently, reports of controlled trials are validating the technique (5). In the United Kingdom, Moghissi reported a zero incidence of complications in his series of thoracic surgical patients who were given parenteral nutrition in the perioperative period (6). Another major advantage of tunnelled catheters is that they are more secure and less prone to the problem of gradual or accidental withdrawal. The Broviac–Hickman type of catheter has been fitted with a Dacron cuff on the subcutaneous portion to fortify the security of the catheter when prolonged placement is required (*Fig* 9.1).

These twin advantages of increased catheter security relative to the body surface and a reduced incidence of catheter-related sepsis are significant benefits. The problem of sepsis occurring early in the course of intravenous nutritional therapy was recognized in 1969 by Altemeier and subsequently called 'third day fever' (7). Since sepsis following conventional cannulation of veins can be established so early, surgeons are now tending to create some form of subcutaneous tunnel from the outset, when a

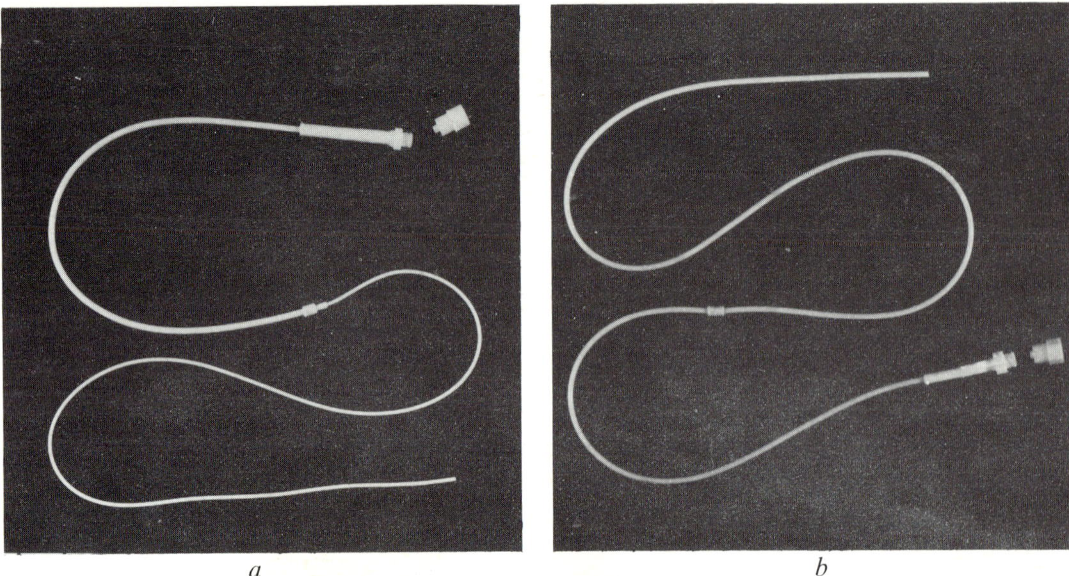

a　　　　　　　　　　　　　　*b*

Fig. 9.1. *a*, The Broviac silicone right atrial catheter. This possesses an intravascular portion, a subcutaneous segment carrying a Dacron felt collar. The sterile cap used for the heparin-lock technique is also shown. *b*, The Hickman catheter, which has a slightly larger intravascular portion and also possesses a Dacron felt collar.

period of prolonged parenteral nutrition is envisaged (8, 9). The advances in technique which have derived from patients requiring prolonged home total parenteral nutrition can be applied to good effect for the safer management of patients who may require intravenous nutritional support for shorter periods. A further beneficial feature of the current generation of catheters designed for tunnelling and prolonged placement in the great veins or right atrium is often overlooked, namely the importance of the increased strength of the devices, e.g. Hickman and Broviac catheters. It is generally acknowledged that infusion systems should be closed and contain the minimum number of connections which can be accidentally separated (allowing air entrainment) or contaminated by pathogenic micro-organisms. The maintenance of sterility and the integrity of the infusion system achieves supreme importance in the management of prolonged fluid or drug therapy, to malnourished patients or those with an attenuated immune response. Professor H. A. Lee, Professor of Medicine at Southampton University, has pointed out that 'angio-access obsession leads to perfection and not infection'. In selected cases the provision of a resilient and inert central venous catheter, carefully tunnelled and sub-

sequently well maintained, should achieve the objectives sought by Professor Lee and should last for many weeks without causing harm to the patient.

During the past 10 years a variety of techniques has been suggested for the creation of subcutaneous tunnels. The Broviac catheter, which has found favour for prolonged parenteral nutrition, requires the surgical exposure of a cephalic, external jugular or internal jugular vein (10, 11). The tunnel is usually created by passing a long artery or biopsy forceps away from the cut-down wound for 10 cm and pulling the catheter through until correctly sited, before performing a venotomy and inserting the intravascular portion of the device into the superior vena cava or right atrium (11, 12). Solassol and Joyeux in Montpellier developed a technique of exposing a tributary of the axillary vein and inserting a silicone catheter with a Teflon tip so that this lay flush with the internal lumen of the main vein. The silicone catheter was then mounted upon a trocar and tunnelled for 20 cm to an exit site on the anterior thoracic wall (13). In between infusions, this 'Scurasil' catheter was capped with a small plug. In New York, Parsa and Ferrer described a tunnelling technique for PVC catheters in which the hub was cut off and re-attached after the catheter had been tunnelled 10 cm (14). In 1978, Benotti, whilst working with Blackburn in Boston, reported a tunnelling technique whereby the hub was pulled through the tunnel after percutaneous guide-wire placement into the internal jugular vein (15). Whilst the aim to maintain the integrity of the parenteral nutrition feeding line is achieved, the technical drawbacks created by this particular technique are important (*Fig.* 9.2), namely (*a*) the risk of hub fracture; (*b*) impaction of fat into the hub and catheter lumen; (*c*) air embolism during the procedure.

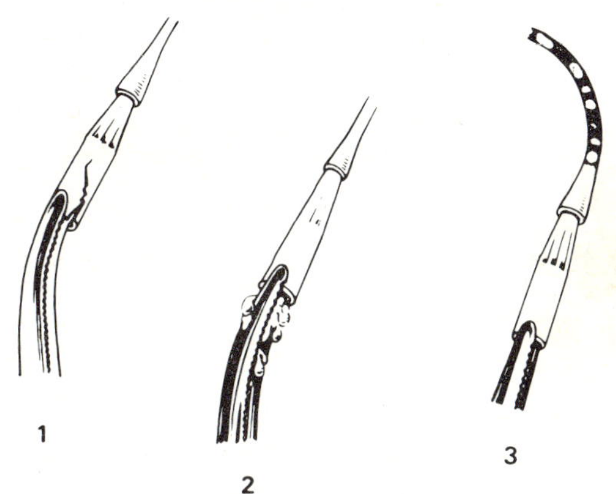

Fig. 9.2. The technical problem of tunnelling a central catheter hub through the subcutaneous tissues. *a*, Fracture of the hub may occur; *b*, impaction of fat in the hub lumen; *c*, there is a risk of air entrainment.

In the United Kingdom Powell-Tuck reported a modification of the technique described by Dudrick (1), Parsa (14) and Titone (16) whilst working at St Mark's Hospital (17). This entailed the percutaneous through-cannula insertion of a subclavian catheter, detachment of the hub and withdrawal of the introductory cannula from over the silicone central catheter, which is then clipped with an artery forceps in order to prevent air entry. Next, the introductory cannula and needle are re-introduced via a skin puncture site situated 8–10 cm away from the initial venepuncture wound; the cannula and needle assembly is guided subcutaneously towards the small stab incision through which the percutaneous insertion was performed. The artery forceps must then be removed and the needle removed from the cannula before the central catheter can be threaded back through the introducing cannula lumen. The original catheter hub is then reconnected and the subclavian wound closed with a suture; the catheter is also made secure by using part of the introducing cannula as a splint. There have been several similar techniques described in which a variety of hollow needles (e.g. Vim-Silverman) have been used to tunnel catheters (18–22). The tunnels so created are usually short, and the integrity of the junction between the catheter shaft and hub is destroyed. Keilly has noted, in a small neonatal series, that the only episodes of septicaemia that occurred were associated with separation of the catheter shaft from the hub adaptor (21). In 1979, Moghissi described a technique for pre- and postoperative parenteral nutrition in patients who were undergoing thoracic surgical procedures (6). This involved exposure of the external jugular vein under local anaesthesia and insertion of the central catheter through a venotomy. A subcutaneous tunnel being created using blunt dissection with a long artery forceps (e.g. Roberts) for a distance of 20 cm. A piece of urinary catheter or suction tubing was then pulled through the subcutaneous tunnel up into the neck wound and the central catheter hub inserted into the lumen of this tubing. The urinary catheter tubing is subsequently withdrawn, carrying with it the central line to its new exit site.

The introduction in 1975 of the Hickman Silastic catheter, which possesses a 1·6 mm lumen and a Dacron cuff, for prolonged intravenous therapy in patients with leukaemia and allied disorders, has proved to be a valuable innovation for the comfort and care of patients with such severe diseases. The incidence of septicaemia, in patients having both their blood samples removed and receiving their intravenous fluids, chemotherapy and haematological support by the solitary Hickman catheter, was less than in a control group of patients being managed with conventional peripheral intravenous therapy (23). A similar experience has also been reported from the Royal Marsden Hospital, London, by Thomas (24), and Blacklock and colleagues, working in Auckland, New Zealand (25).

The advent of skin tunnelling techniques has considerably simplified the problem of gaining and maintaining a portal into the circulation where prolonged venous access is required. The insertion procedures naturally take a little longer to perform, however, when an 'artificial gut' is being created for the patient; it is necessary that this synthetic venous tributary should be fashioned very carefully from the outset. In view of the dissection involved with the tunnelling process, it is important that the catheter tip correctly placed into the superior vena cava and confirmation obtained by peroperative contrast radiology studies. The ideal operative sequence is as follows:

1. The catheter is placed either by a percutaneous through-cannula technique or by surgical exposure of a proximal tributary of the superior vena cava.

2. X-ray confirmation of the correct position is obtained.

3. The catheter hub is then tunnelled away from the venepuncture wound to a distant exit site.

Sites of Insertion for Tunnelled Catheters

These may be listed in order of preference, in respect of the patient's comfort, technical difficulty and intravenous infusion line maintenance problems as follows:

1. Cephalic vein
2. External jugular vein (26)
3. Subclavian vein
4. Axillary vein tributaries
5. Internal jugular vein
6. Anterior or common facial vein
7. Long saphenous vein or tributaries

All these approaches are straightforward, the techniques are essentially simple to perform and should lie within the capability of junior surgical staff in training. Indeed, in 1954, Gordon, Grant and Grigor in Glasgow's Royal Victoria Infirmary first published a report on the technique of resuscitating bleeding patients by catheterizing the cephalic vein using PVC tubing (27). In their paper, Gordon et al. quote Antia as being the originator of the technique. Shortly afterwards, Antia published his data accumulated whilst working as a surgical registrar in Preston, Lancashire (28). The value of this route for massive blood transfusion in thoracic surgery was confirmed by Dolton of Wolverhampton in 1955 (29). The obvious advantage of direct surgical exposure techniques for tributaries

such as the cephalic vein is that the risk of pneumothorax is avoided.

Contraindications

There are no absolute contraindications to performing these tunnelling procedures and, indeed, many of the patients with acute leukaemia are in such a parlous state that the prompt commencement of their therapy represents the only chance of achieving remission. It is preferable that an attempt should be made to correct any haematological deficits by platelet, blood, granulocyte and fresh frozen plasma infusions.

Premedication

It is preferable to give some form of analgesia prior to the procedure. This is of particular relevance if it is planned to carry out the operation under local anaesthesia, and an appropriate dose of pethidine combined with diazepam is effective. In addition, some units provide prophylactic antibiotic cover before and for 3 days after the operation (e.g. a cephalosporin) (30).

The clinician should also be aware that some Hickman and Broviac catheters sold in the United Kingdom are *not sterile* and advice should be taken from the microbiology department and CSSD staff concerning the most appropriate technique for preparing the catheter for insertion (*see* Chapter 17).

The patient should be reassured and the operation about to be performed should be explained and informed consent obtained.

Preparation

These procedures must be performed in the operating theatre, where there are adequate lighting facilities, suction pumps, diathermy apparatus and, preferably, the facility to screen the position of the catheter using an image intensifier. The operating table should therefore be fitted with a radiolucent extension. If no X-ray image intensifier is available, the patient should be placed upon the bridges used for operative cholangiography and the appropriate size of film plates ordered. Both the operating theatre and X-ray department staff need to be informed in advance, and the contrast medium (meglumine iothalamate injection BP 60 per cent w/v; Conray 280) should be ready and at hand for injection.

Anaesthesia

These procedures can be performed under a local or general anaesthetic. In the series recently reported by Thomas 75 per cent of catheters were inserted under local anaesthesia (30). If it is intended to perform the procedure under general anaesthesia (e.g. in children or very anxious adults), it is advisable to insert an endotracheal tube, because once the procedure has commenced, the operation should not be disturbed by manipulations on the part of the anaesthetist trying to maintain the airway.

Position

The patient should be made comfortable in the supine position. Since the vein is opened under direct vision and ligature control, the risk of air embolism must be eliminated. It is useful to have the patient in a slight head-down Trendelenburg tilt during the period of perivenous dissection and then alter the table to the horizontal position when the vein is about to be cannulated.

Requirements

For an expeditious procedure to be performed in sick patients, it is imperative to have adequate assistance. An intravenous administration set (e.g. Continu-Flo, Travenol Laboratories) should be primed with the appropriate solution and the dressings required at the end of the procedure should be made readily available. These small points, if remembered and passed on to the nursing staff, can save a great deal of time.

The following items should be available:

Trolley

Minor general or plastic surgical instrument set

Galley pot, sponges and forceps for skin preparation

Povidone-iodine skin preparation lotion in 10 per cent alcohol

Surgical drapes and 6 towel clips

Sterile towel for drying the skin

Op-Site incise drape (28 × 45 cm)

Disposable syringes: 3 × 20 ml, 2 × 10 ml

Hypodermic needles: 21 G, 23 G and 25 G

Spinal needle: 18 G—15 cm (Steriseal Ltd)

Local anaesthetic: bupivacaine hydrochloride BP 0·25 per cent w/v (Marcain, Duncan, Flockhart)

Heparinized saline, 20 ml (Hepsal, 10 i.u./ml, Weddell Pharmaceuticals)

X-ray contrast medium, meglumine iothalamate 60 per cent, 5–10 ml (Conray 280 or Hexabrix 320, May and Baker Ltd.)

Instruments

Scalpel and No. 10 or 20 blade

Cutting diathermy point attachment

Fine diathermy coagulation forceps

Gillies' fine-tooth forceps

Fine non-tooth forceps

West's self-retaining retractor

Langenbeck retractor

Fine curve scissors

Fine straight scissors

McIndoe's scissors

Lepine's fine right-angled curved artery forceps or aneurysm needle

Mosquito artery forceps × 6

Tunnelling stylet

Central venous silicone catheter

Venotomy sucker/retractor

Angled catheter introducing forceps

Coronary artery probes or dilators

4/0 silk ligatures

4/0 Dexon sutures on an atraumatic needle

3/0–6/0 silk or Prolene on a cutting atraumatic needle

Procedure

Prior to cleaning the skin, the chosen forequarter of the body should be carefully and completely shaved. This shaved area should extend across the midline to the opposite side, thus ensuring that at the end of the procedure the adhesive dressings can be neatly applied. The area of the vein selected for catheterization should then be studied and some may prefer to mark the skin surface with an indelible fibre-tip pen. The deltopectoral groove can be first gently palpated with the patient relaxed, and then after the patient has been asked to protract the arm against a resistance (*Fig.* 9.3). This will highlight the plane of subsequent dissection and is especially valuable in the obese patient. Similarly, the external jugular vein can be filled by transiently

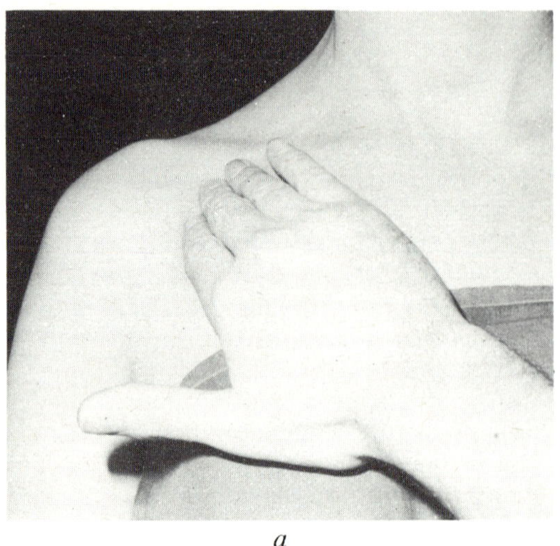
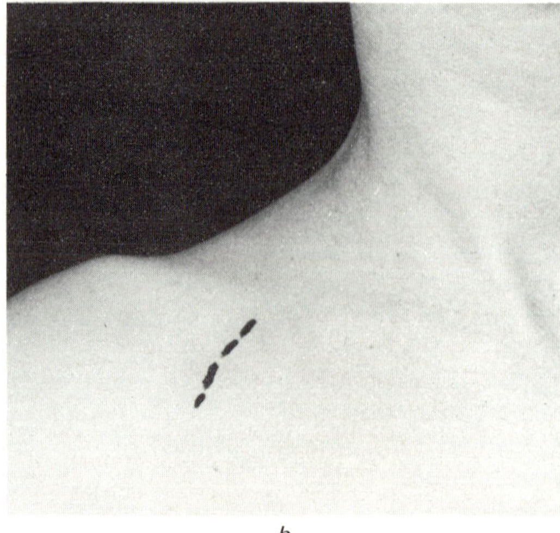

a   b

Fig. 9.3. *a*, Preliminary palpation of the deltopectoral groove. *b*, Marking the intermuscular fissure.

tilting the patient into a head-down position whilst the supraclavicular course of the vein is marked on the skin. The patient should be fitted with a face mask, at least during the initial draping procedure. Once the towels are in position, they can then be arranged so that the mask can be discarded if necessary.

Once these preliminary activities have been completed, the surgeon should put on a protective lead-lined radiologist's jacket; then scrub up and don a gown and gloves before cleaning the skin over a generous area. The axilla, insertion wound and the tunnel skin exit site must be adequately prepared with povidone-iodine solution in alcohol, chlorhexidine in 70 per cent spirit or iodine in 70 per cent spirit. The essential feature is that this procedure should be carried out for a full 3-minute period. Any excess fluid can be removed by using a dry sterile drape, which is then carefully discarded. The draping towels should be arranged so that the skin over the relevant vein and intended tunnel track (extending 30 cm or more) is clearly exposed. The axilla should be excluded by the drapes, which should extend the full length of the patient to prevent the catheter or other items of equipment becoming contaminated during the procedure (*Fig.* 9.4). The patient's face can be kept free of the towels by organizing a screen. The whole area of exposed skin can then be covered by an incise drape (e.g. Op-Site 28 × 45 cm).

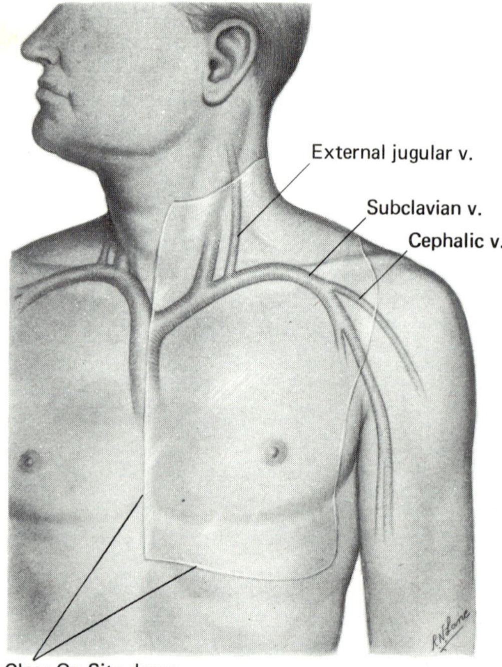

Fig. 9.4. A wide area of exposure can be achieved by using a transparent Op-Site incise drape. The wound should be draped so that more than one vessel can be approached if necessary.

When the procedure is performed using local anaesthesia, an adequate diamond-shaped zone over the relevant vein and towards the relevant cutaneous nerves should be infiltrated with bupivacaine 0·25 per cent w/v (Marcain). The proposed exit site of the tunnel should then be infiltrated with 1–2 ml of bupivacaine and finally the intervening tunnel track can be slowly and gently infiltrated with local anaesthetic solution introduced through a 15 cm long 18 G spinal needle (Steriseal). Thus, in essence, an anaesthetized fluid 'tunnel' is created across the anterior chest wall. This can be led in any direction from the intended site of cannulation, according to the site and nature of any pre-existing wounds or stomas. The anaesthetized zone can be gently pressed using a large sterile swab in order to disperse the fluid. The local anaesthetic agent must be given time to take effect. Occasionally, it will be necessary to inject further small aliquots around the vein and the deepest layers of the wound.

INSERTION TECHNIQUE

Exposure of the Cephalic Vein in the Deltopectoral Groove

The radiographer should be informed at the commencement of the dissection so that the image intensifier and television screen can be manoeuvred into position in good time. It is wise to mark the deltopectoral groove prior to the operation by asking the patient to protract the arm against resistance when the anatomical defect between the muscles is easily identified. A curved 2·5–5 cm incision should be made, commencing 1–2 cm below the clavicle and extended in the direction of the groove through the skin. This must be carefully deepened, and the authors prefer to use cutting diathermy. It is particularly important to maintain meticulous haemostasis in patients with leukaemia, most of whom have a bleeding diathesis. The tissues can be stretched slightly by inserting a self-retaining retractor or applying Alliss forceps. The superficial fat should be divided and the clavicular fibres of the deltoid and pectoralis major muscles displayed. A band of deltopectoral fascia covers the muscle edges forming the groove and this must be divided before these muscles are gently retracted. The vein usually appears at this point in the dissection, although it may be absent or too small for cannulation in about 9 per cent of individuals. There is often a

small branch of the acromio-thoracic artery superficial to, or accompanying the vein; in addition, the lateral pectoral nerve branch of the brachial plexus often runs across the floor of the deltopectoral groove adjacent to the vein. If this small artery is injured, it should be identified with the sucker and carefully controlled, using diathermy or a ligature without causing injury to the cephalic vein. The periadventitial fascia ensheathing the vessel should be incised and the vein cleaned before a fine right-angled curved Lepine forceps is slipped under the vessel in order to carry back a 4/0 silk ligature. A single throw should be put on the ligature and slid down to within 1 cm of the vein before being clipped to the drape with a mosquito artery forceps. Any tributaries draining into the cephalic vein are best ligated in continuity using 4/0 silk. These can then be used to secure the vein during the insertion procedure. If they are not tied, very occasionally, the silicone catheter will find its way to a subscapular or pectoral vein. Once the tributaries have been ligated, the main trunk of the vessel should be encircled with a ligature and a mosquito forceps applied. It is wise to loop another strand of 4/0 silk around the vessel just proximal to the subclavian vein, so that the assistant will be in perfect control of this relatively fragile vein when the central catheter requires to be introduced. Once this phase of the dissection has been completed and haemostasis established, the retractors can be removed and the ligatures arranged in an orderly fashion.

Tunnelling Procedure

The Hickman, Broviac or similar central catheter should be delivered from its outer sterile wrappings on the scrub nurse's table and the sterile screw caps which are supplied with the device (for use when a heparin-lock technique is required) should be preserved in a sterile container. The catheter should be primed with Hepsal and kept covered carefully on the towels because of the static attraction of particles to the silicone. It should always be handled using instruments rather than gloved hands. If the procedure is being performed under local anaesthesia, at this stage an assistant may administer an intravenous injection of pethidine and/or diazepam in the appropriate dosage through a peripheral vein. The tunnelling stylet should then be passed through the wound in a cephalad to caudal direction. Initially the spatulated point of the instrument (*Fig.* 9.5) should be passed

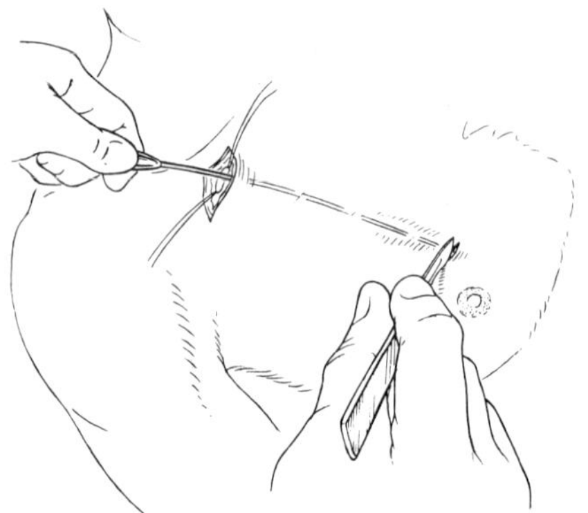

Fig. 9.5. The tunnelling stylet is passed in a caudad direction through the cephalic vein exposure wound via the subcutaneous tissue to the anterior chest wall, where an exit incision is created.

through the fat close to the pectoralis muscle and then quickly guided into a subcutaneous plane before the chest wall is traversed just superficial to and around the periphery of the breast, and along the anaesthetized track to the exit site, which is best placed adjacent to the xiphisternum, or in the anterior axillary line. The catheter should not emerge through skin in the submammary fold where a fungal intertrigo can develop. An incision is next made with a No. 10 blade on to the stylet. This should be withdrawn 7 cm back into the wound and the skin of the tunnel adjacent to the exit site undermined for a few centimetres using McIndoe's scissors, so that the Dacron cuff of the Hickman variety of catheter will pass without difficulty. The stylet should then be pushed through this wound and the free end of the Hickman catheter slipped over the shaft of the instrument (*Figs.* 9.6, 9.7). This stylet is next withdrawn through the tunnel to the infraclavicular wound exposing the cephalic vein. The Dacron cuff of the catheter should be directed under the skin by gently applying traction (*Fig.* 9.8) so that it rests in an intercostal space. It is wise to fix the catheter at the skin exit site with a 3/0 silk suture before proceeding to the subsequent stages.

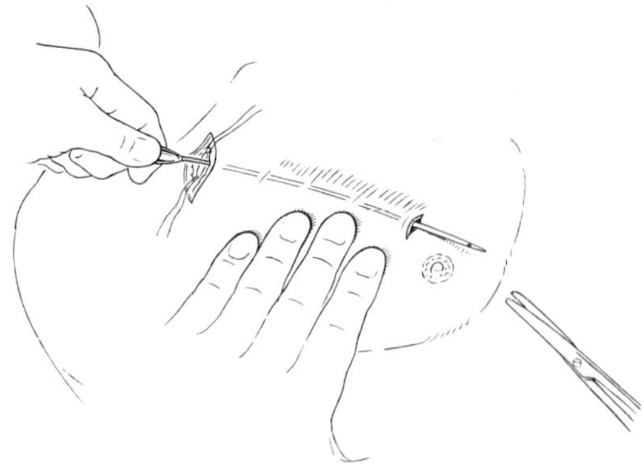

Fig. 9.6. The spatulated end of the stylet has been passed through the tunnel.

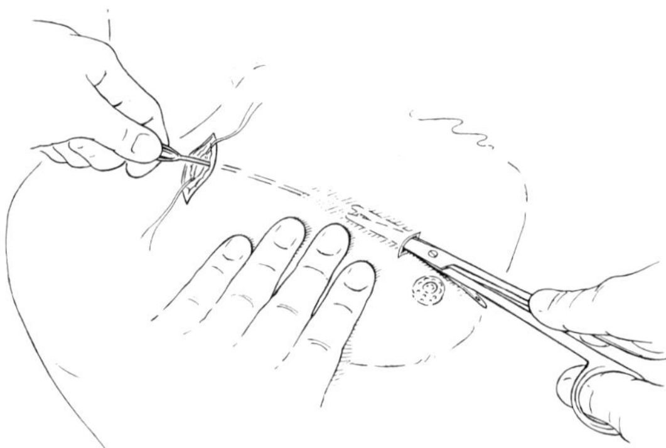

Fig. 9.7. The subcutaneous track is gently widened using McIndoe's scissors to allow the passage of the Dacron cuff.

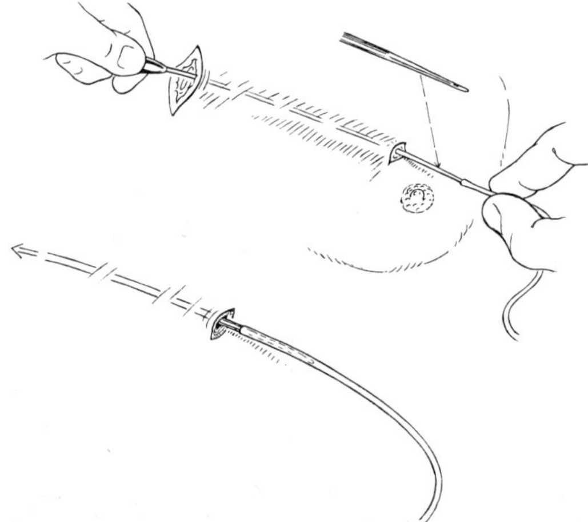

Fig. 9.8. The silicone catheter is mounted on the specially shaped spatulated tip and drawn back through to the venotomy exposure wound.

Venotomy and Insertion of the Catheter

After the catheter has been brought through to the wound, the self-retaining retractor should be inserted and the controlling ligatures rearranged. The distal ligature on the cephalic vein can be tied off and used for retraction; the ligatures holding tributaries should be utilized to stabilize the vein in a statisfactory position for cannulation. The free end of the catheter, held by instruments, should be laid on the towels along the line of the subclavian and innominate veins before being cut cleanly with scissors at the level of the superior vena cava. The catheter should then be placed in a convenient position on a sterile gauze swab whilst the assistant gently retracts the proximal controlling ligatures around the cephalic vein in order to prevent the efflux of venous blood from the subclavian vein.

A small venotomy should be made adjacent to the distal ligature using fine scissors. The vein may require slight dilatation with a curved mosquito forceps or coronary artery dilators. Alternatively, the venotomy cannulation sucker shown in *Fig.* 9.9 can perform this function and be used to open up the vein whilst gentle suction is intermittently applied by the finger control vent on the shaft of the sucker. Next, the catheter should be grasped 1 or 2 cm from its tip using forceps (specially angulated and grooved to facilitate this manoeuvre, *Fig.* 9.9) and gently introduced under the grooved venotomy cannulation sucker into the lumen of the vein. The assistant should control the vein by releasing the traction on the first ligature and then on the most proximal ligature as the catheter is advanced by the surgeon. The process may be assisted by the nurse gently flushing small aliquots of heparinized saline through the line from a syringe which must guard the catheter hub at all times in order to prevent air embolism.

Once the first 2 cm of the catheter have been introduced, it can be assumed to have entered the subclavian vein. If any resistance to advancement of the catheter is encountered, this invariably means entrapment by a valve, or that the catheter is passing into an unrecognized tributary. It is best to gently withdraw the catheter a half-centimetre, rotate it through 90° and try advancing it again in synchrony with a Hepsal flush. The central catheter may then be advanced very slowly so that it is carried by the

blood flow into the superior vena cava. It is useful if an assistant passes a hand beneath the drapes and presses gently on the root of the neck over the line of the jugular vein in order to prevent malposition into this vessel. After the catheter is fully advanced, the ligature encircling the vein should be slipped down and tied. The patency of the catheter lumen should be further confirmed by another injection of heparinized saline.

Correct Placement Check

There should always be free aspiration of venous blood obtained at this stage. The head of the image intensifier or X-ray camera should be manoeuvred into place and the position of the catheter confirmed by injecting 2–5 ml of Conray 280 or Hexabrix 320 whilst the mediastinum is screened. It is a useful ploy to place a steel forceps or scissors on the surface of the body overlying the mediastinum in the region of the superior vena cava so that this is easily picked up on the X-ray. Once the catheter position is acceptable, the silk ligatures can be cut short, almost on the knots.

Wound Closure and Dressing Technique

It is vital to achieve careful haemostasis in this operation. The deltoid and pectoralis major muscles can be approximated around the catheter using 4/0 interrupted absorbable sutures (e.g. Dexon) and the deltopectoral fascia can also be reconstituted. Extreme care must be taken not to puncture the catheter inadvertently. The superficial layers of fascia should also be approximated and the subcutaneous space obliterated. The skin is best closed with interrupted 3/0–5/0 silk or Prolene sutures. The wound and catheter exit site should be carefully cleaned with hydrogen peroxide, dried and treated with sterile mastic (Mastic Paint Compound BPC, J. M. Loveridge Ltd), dressed with sterile gauze and covered with Op-Site (10 × 14 cm and 6 × 8·5 cm. The catheter should be arranged on the chest wall in a gentle curve and further fixation with Op-Site performed. The syringe can then be discarded and the hub connected to an administration set (e.g. Continu-Flo, Travenol). This assembly should also be sprayed with povidone-iodine before being enveloped in a

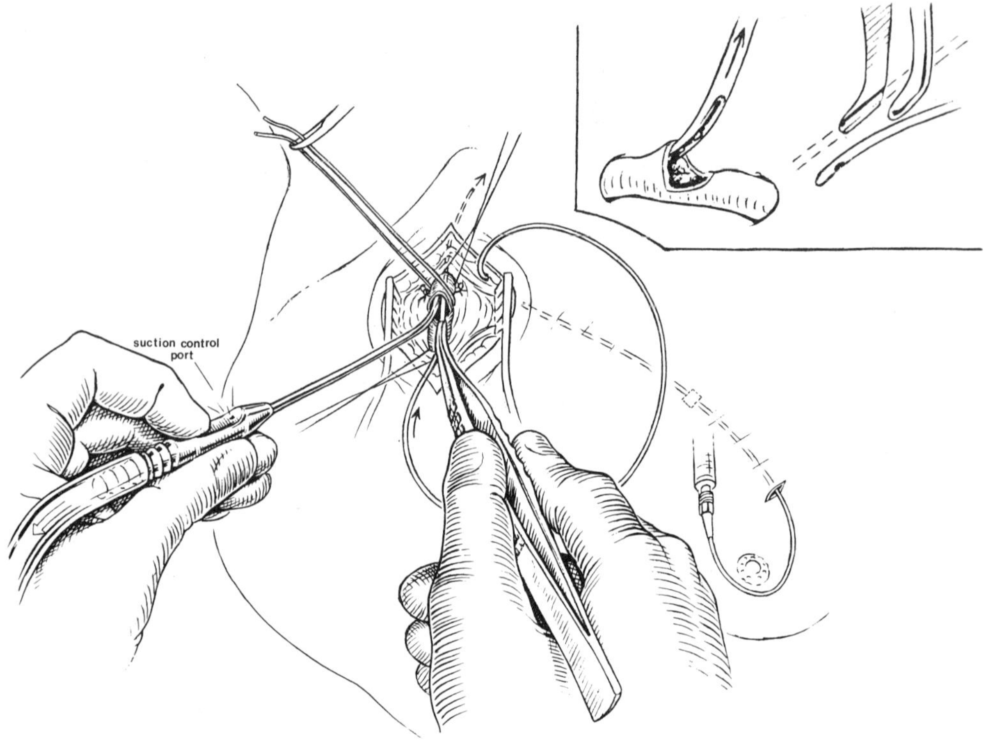

a

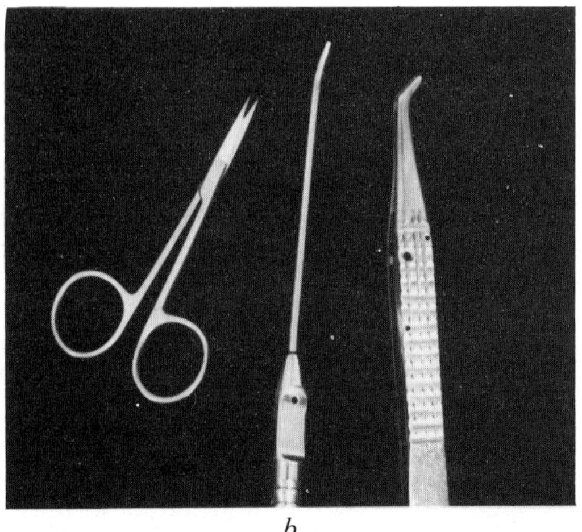

b

Fig. 9.9. *a*, A venotomy in progress with proximal control of the vein using a silicone sling and silk ligature; the venotomy flap is being elevated gently by the sucker whilst the catheter is introduced using angled forceps as the assistant releases the proximal ligatures (*see inset*). The catheter has already been passed through the tunnel to the wound. *b*, Instruments for performing central venous catheter venotomy: *left to right*, fine scissors, a grooved angled vein elevator and venotomy sucker, grooved and angled catheter introducing forceps.

rolled sterile gauze swab and fixed to the chest wall using another sheet of Op-Site.

In patients with a bleeding diathesis associated with leukaemia, there is sometimes a slow, constant ooze of blood from capillaries. In such circumstances, successful control and prevention of haematoma formation may be achieved by applying hydraulic pressure for several hours. This is simply achieved by laying a sterile 1-litre plastic sachet or bag of intravenous fluid over the dressed wound and along the line of the tunnel. This may be fixed in place by applying a shoulder spica, using 150 mm (6-in) wide sterile crêpe bandages (*Fig.* 9.10).

Exposure of the External Jugular Vein

This vein provides an easy and convenient route of access to the central veins. Moghissi has demonstrated that catheters introduced by this route can remain sterile and patent for the duration of the patient's intravenous therapy when they are tunnelled to the anterior chest wall. The dissection for exposure of the vessel is easier than for the cephalic vein. There is a slight

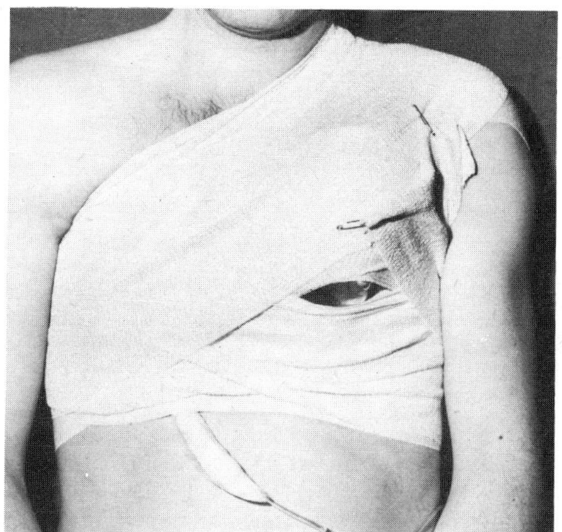

Fig. 9.10. The use of a 1-litre or 500 ml bag of intravenous fluid to provide a temporary 'hydraulic' shoulder spica.

drawback, however, in that the tunnelled catheter must cross the anterior aspect of the clavicle, and the angulation of the catheter during neck movements can occlude the lumen and impede the flow of fluid (*Fig.* 9.11). This approach is of particular value in children, where the cephalic vein may be too small for successful cannulation; in obese patients, where dissection of the cephalic vein can be a tedious

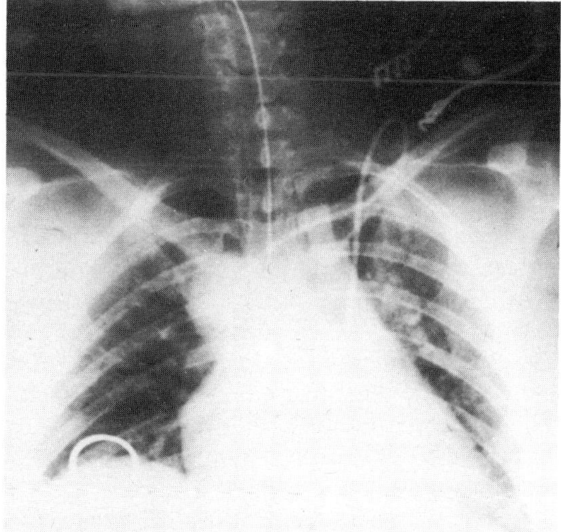

Fig. 9.11. A peroperative post-insertion X-ray showing the angulation and tortuous course of a catheter inserted via the external jugular vein after being tunnelled in front of the clavicle.

procedure; and where the other routes of insertion have already been sacrificed.

The skin preparation, draping, anaesthesia and position remain the same as described earlier in this chapter. Naturally, the superior drape should be taken further up the neck so that the posterior triangle is adequately exposed. As mentioned, it is useful to mark the course of the vein with indelible ink before cleaning the skin. A transverse incision (2 cm) should be made over the vein and continued through the superficial fascia, platysma and deep cervical fascia until the vein is exposed. Using fine dissection scissors, the periadventitial tissues must be incised and the vein cleaned before a fine right-angled Lepine forceps can be slipped under the vessel and used to place a 4/0 silk ligature around the vein. Particular care should be taken to avoid a small supraclavicular nerve branch which often accompanies the vessel. It is wise to continue the dissection and expose and ligate in continuity tributaries close to the subclavian vein. The ligatures should be left long at this stage so that they may be used for retraction purposes and enable the valves in this region to be opened. Sometimes there is a sizeable vein which enters the lateral aspect of the external jugular vein close to the subclavian vein (transverse cervical) and this tributary can be cannulated allowing the principal vessel to remain patent on occasions. After the tributaries have been controlled, the proximal part of the vein should always be encircled by two 4/0 silk ligatures. Some surgeons prefer to use fine silicone slings for vascular control. Many prefer to allow the vein to remain patent and function after cannulation. If this is to be the case, the ligatures and a fine purse-string vascular suture at the proposed site of venotomy should be arranged as shown in *Fig.* 9.12.

The subcutaneous tunnel should then be created using a stylet as described for the cephalic vein. The tunnelling instrument can be easily guided over the clavicle onto the anterior chest wall by picking up a fold in the skin before passing it through the subcutaneous fat to the chosen exit site. An incision (0·5 cm) should be made onto the spatulated point of the stylet, which is subsequently pushed out of the wound, and the first 7 cm of the tunnel track adjacent to the exit site should be undermined using McIndoe's scissors. The silicone catheter may

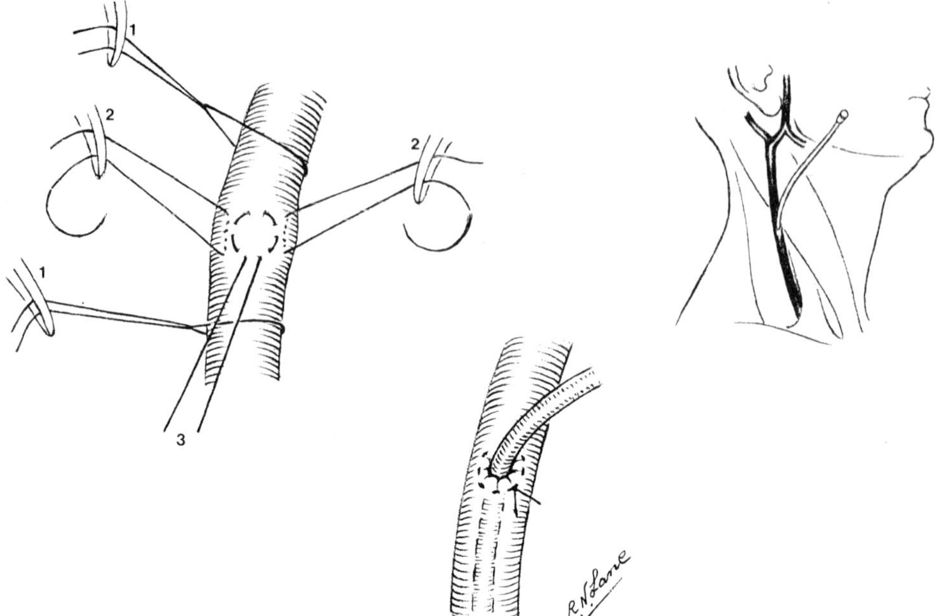

Fig. 9.12. Techniques for controlling veins and performing a venotomy with larger vessels.

then be delivered from its package as previously described and primed with heparinized saline before the free end is slipped over the tunnelling stylet point and pulled slowly back through to the neck wound. The Dacron cuff must then be snugged into the subcutaneous track by gently pulling the catheter through, and this should be secured to the exit site using 3/0 silk or Prolene. The length of the intravenous segment should be gauged and the catheter cut cleanly with scissors at the appropriate point. The segment of the catheter removed should be preserved so that, in the future, the length can be re-checked if there is any doubt about accidental breakage and embolism when the catheter is finally removed.

The ligatures and silicone slings should then be arranged, and the position of the table adjusted so that the patient is in a slight head-up tilt. The venotomy should be fashioned using fine scissors and any efflux of venous blood can be prevented by gentle traction on the proximal ligatures. The venotomy cannulation sucker and grooved forceps will allow the slippery silicone catheter to be passed into the vein with ease. The ligatures should be released sequentially by the assistant and the catheter moved slowly towards the subclavian vein. If any difficulty is experienced, the catheter must be withdrawn slightly, the

traction on ligatures occluding the tributaries altered, and the angle of the venotomy cannulation sucker may be changed slightly. Usually, these manoeuvres are successful and the catheter may be floated into the superior vena cava by advancing the device very slowly using grooved cannulation forceps. The ligatures or purse-string sutures may then be tied in order to provide further fixation of the catheter.

Once the catheter has been advanced fully into the vein, careful attention should be paid to the way in which the catheter lies in the perivenous space and the patency of the lumen checked by aspirating blood and gently syringing with heparinized saline. The placement must then be checked as previously described using contrast medium and an image intensifier or chest X-ray. The wound should be closed in layers of 4/0 Dexon over the catheter and the skin approximated with interrupted 3/0–6/0 silk or Prolene. The dressing procedure and subsequent catheter fixation are the same as described for the cephalic vein technique.

Surgical Exposure of the Internal Jugular Vein

This procedure is rarely indicated in order to establish venous access. It should not be attempted by clinicians with limited surgical experience in view of the depth and complexity of the dissection required. It is unwise to attempt the procedure on patients with a bleeding diathesis. This approach has been recommended for the insertion of tunnelled LeVeen peritoneovenous Silastic shunts. The technique may also be required by patients needing prolonged intravenous feeding in whom the external jugular and cephalic veins have already been sacrificed.

After the previously described preparatory steps have been taken, an incision of 5–10 cm may be made either transversely or obliquely over the lateral border of the lower third of the sternomastoid muscle. This must be continued through the platysma and investing cervical fascia which envelops the sternomastoid muscle. The muscle should then be retracted medially. The exposure of the internal jugular vein is occasionally simplified by dividing the lateral aspect of the muscle and by grasping the muscle edges with Alliss or similar forceps so that the sternocleidomastoid can be lifted off the carotid sheath and jugular vein. In children and neonates, it is easy to gently split the muscle in the direction of its fibres (22). Once the internal jugular vein has been located, it must be carefully dissected and controlled by encircling with proximal and distal silk ligatures or silicone slings. There have been reports of the vein being safely ligated during the procedure with only transient unilateral facial oedema being noted. Alternatively, a venotomy can be made into the vessel carefully controlled in the manner illustrated in *Fig.* 9.12.

The Hickman, Broviac or similar catheter should be tunnelled through to the neck wound according to the technique already described in the previous sections and the hub protected at all times with a syringe primed with heparinized saline in order to prevent accidental air embolism. The length of the intravascular segment required should be measured and the excess catheter cut off cleanly with scissors and this segment preserved for the reasons previously mentioned. Once the venotomy has been performed, any efflux of blood from the wound in the vein before the purse-string suture is secured can be prevented by gentle digital pressure and traction on the appropriate slings. The central catheter, having been introduced into the lumen

of the jugular vein, should be advanced gently and slowly so that it 'floats' in the bloodstream towards the heart. The final placement should be checked with the image intensifier or a chest X-ray using contrast medium as described. The muscle and fascia can then be approximated in layers with interrupted 3/0 Dexon and the skin closed with interrupted 3/0–6/0 silk or Prolene sutures, before the dressing detailed in the previous descriptions is applied.

SUBCUTANEOUS TUNNELLING AFTER PERCUTANEOUS INFRACLAVICULAR SUBCLAVIAN VEIN PUNCTURE

In all the aforementioned techniques, the catheter has to be pulled through from the distant skin site and then inserted through the venotomy wound to its ultimate position in the central veins. To date, tunnelling techniques performed after percutaneous central venous cannulation have been based upon a technique described by Titone in 1974 (16). These have involved the insertion of the catheter through a cannula or needle, removal of the hub and tunnelling of the catheter shaft to a distant site, either by using forceps (14) or the introducing cannula as a conduit through which the hub-less catheter shaft can be threaded and then reconnected to the hub following the withdrawal of the introducing cannula from beneath the skin (8, 9, 14, 16, 31). This creates an extra and superfluous defect in the infusion system. Benotti and Blackburn described their manoeuvre for pulling the hub through the subcutaneous tissue with forceps, and Moghissi utilized a Foley catheter to obtain the same objective (6). A technique is described below which is a further progression in this field and has been developed in order to provide:

1. The ability to tunnel with ease the central catheter, integral hub and introducing cannula assembly as a unit.

2. Safe protection of the plastic central catheter and introducing cannula assembly during its subcutaneous passage.

3. A facility for occluding the Luer female hub of the central catheter in order to prevent the entry of air or subcutaneous fat during the tunnelling procedure.

In addition, this technique establishes a more logical sequence of operative steps by which the patient is spared an unnecessary tunnelling procedure if malposition occurs as aberrant locations of the catheter tip are actively sought and corrected before the tunnel is completed. A recent review of this problem has once again revealed how frequently malposition and the aberrant location of catheter tips do occur when the position is reviewed with plain chest X-ray examination minutes or even hours after the insertion procedure (32). This study reinforces the need for the correct catheter position to be confirmed by screening during the operation. The correct operative sequence, therefore, is:

1. Central catheter placement.
2. Confirmation of correct position by contrast X-ray and screening studies.
3. Creation of the subcutaneous tunnel.

The principal advantages obtained are that the venotomy is achieved neatly using a conventional through-cannula manoeuvre; and once the definitive central catheter has been placed, the complete introducing cannula and central catheter hub assembly can be tunnelled out through to a distant wound over a considerably greater distance than feasible by previous techniques. A special tunnelling stylet has been developed in conjunction with H. G. Wallace Ltd. The way in which this device encapsulates the central catheter is illustrated in *Figs*. 9.13 and 9.14. The most important point to realize before using the instrument is that the subcutaneous tunnel is gently created using McIndoe's or Nelson's scissors; the tunnelling stylet simply provides a safety capsule to transport the hub mechanism and catheter shaft without difficulty through the track beneath the skin. A tunnelling procedure should be considered for those patients in whom it is expected that a central venous nutrition catheter will be required for more than 2 or 3 weeks. This particular technique is not suitable in the presence of a bleeding diathesis; in such circumstances, the same stylet can be used in an alternative fashion, as previously described.

Technique

Meticulous attention must be paid to aseptic technique and therefore the procedure must be

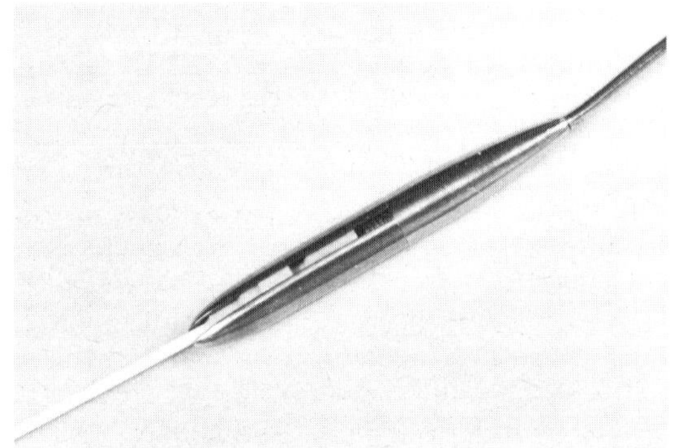

Fig. 9.13. A central venous catheter hub and introducing cannula mounted on the tunnelling stylet.

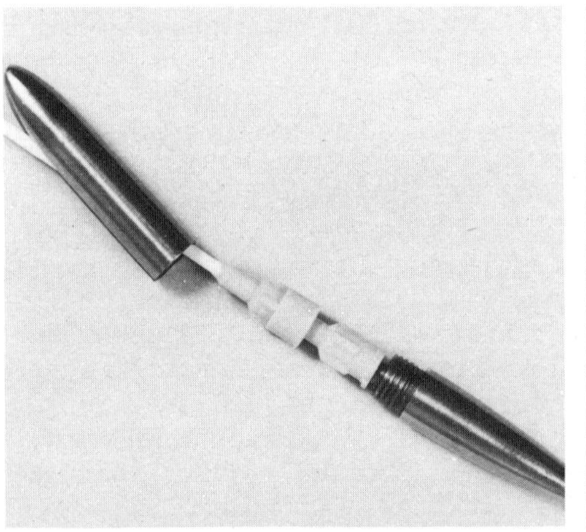

a

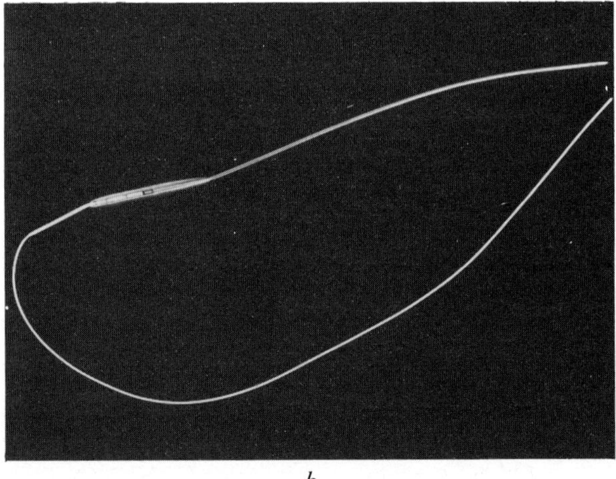

b

Fig. 9.14. The design features of the tunnelling stylet include a Luer plug, on to which the central venous catheter hub is inserted, and a protective shell, which encapsulates the hub mechanism as shown (*a*). The complete arrangement is shown in *b*.

carried out in an operating theatre, preferably as part of an elective operating list. The authors have found it useful to perform emergency surgery with the operating table fitted with a radiolucent image intensifier attachment. This allows a decision to be made towards the end of the procedure whether or not to insert a central feeding catheter. The surgeon requires to scrub-up, don a protective lead radiologist's jacket and wear a sterile gown together with gloves. The staff of the radiology department need to be informed of the time and venue for the procedure well in advance, and called to the theatre at the appropriate hour. They will need to be informed of the intention to perform either screening using an image intensifier and contrast medium (e.g. Conray 280 or Hexabrix 320) or a chest X-ray once the catheter has been inserted. Accordingly, the operating table must be equipped with a radiolucent extension or bridges to allow an expeditious screening procedure to be performed. The theatre staff should be aware of the precise central venous catheter, instruments and drapes required, according to the surgical approach intended. The procedures depicted concern the use of a Wallace Two-Stage central venous catheter (66 cm, 16 G, Teflon FEP) introduced using a 57 mm 13 G introducing cannula (Code No. 6616 or 66816). The preliminary preparations are the same as described for the percutaneous puncture technique described in Chapter 8 with the added provision of ensuring that a greater area of the anterior chest wall is prepared and left exposed through the incise drapes as illustrated in *Fig. 9.4*.

Requirements

The following items will be required for the skin preparation, draping and operative procedure, in order:

Skin preparation sponges and forceps
Povidone-iodine, chlorhexidine or iodine in 70% alcohol
Sterile towel for drying the skin
Sterile drapes, sufficient to cover the whole patient
Towel clips
Incise drape; Op-Site (28 × 45 cm) (Smith & Nephew)
Disposable plastic syringes (3 × 20 ml, 2 × 10 ml)
Local anaesthetic solution (e.g. bupivacaine injection BP 0·25% w/v; Marcain, Duncan, Flockhart)
Hypodermic needles: 21 G, 23 G and 25 G
A spinal needle: 18 G × 15 cm (Steriseal)
Sterile gauze swabs
Scalpel and No. 10 blade
Gillies' or similar fine-tooth forceps
Central venous catheter (Wallace Two-Stage: 6616 or 66816)
Heparinized saline, 20 ml 10 i.u./ml (Hepsal, Weddell Pharmaceuticals)
Meglumine iothalamate injection BP 60% w/v (Conray 280, May & Baker)
Tunnelling stylet (H. G. Wallace)
McIndoe's or Nelson's scissors
3/0–6/0 silk or Prolene on a curved cutting or straight-hand needle
Hydrogen peroxide
Mastic paint Compound BPC (J. M. Loveridge)
Op-Site (6 × 8·5 cm and 10 × 14 cm) (Smith & Nephew)

After the infiltration and dispersal of a small volume of local anaesthetic solution (bupivacaine 0·25 per cent), an oblique transverse skin incision (1·5 cm) should be made approximately 2·5 cm below the mid-point of the clavicle (*Figs. 9.15* and *9.16*). Through this wound the introducing cannula needle mounted upon a syringe should be slowly introduced following the coordinates for percutaneous subclavian puncture described in Chapter 8. As previously mentioned, the author also highlights the position of the vessels by using an ultrasound auscultation technique. The needle should therefore be parallel to the coronal plane or operating table and travel along an imaginary line extending from the surgical neck of the humerus, through a point just below the junction of the middle and medial thirds of the clavicle to the postero-superior aspect of the ipsilateral sternoclavicular joint. Once the subclavian vein has been penetrated, and free aspiration of blood from the vein confirmed, the needle and cannula assembly should be rotated through 180° and advanced a further half-centimetre before the needle is withdrawn. The conscious patient should be instructed to stop breathing momentarily or perform a Valsalva manoeuvre at this stage, as the definitive central catheter is gently inserted via the introducing cannula. The authors prefer to

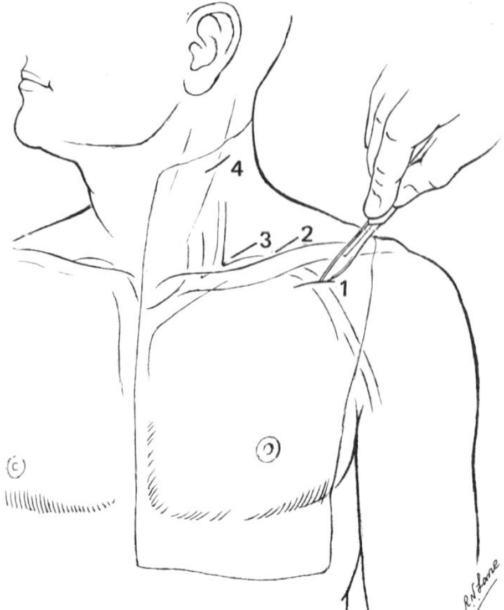

Fig. 9.15. The area of skin prepared and draped is shown together with alternative sites for percutaneous insertion of catheters into the infraclavicular subclavian vein (**1**), the external jugular vein (**2**), the supraclavicular subclavian vein (**3**) and the internal jugular vein (**4**).

remove the central catheter from its PVC sheath and place it on to the sterile drapes so that this manoeuvre can be completed quickly. Once this has been achieved (and with the introducing cannula still situated in the subclavian vein), the central catheter should be flushed through with sterile heparinized saline solution (10 i.u./ml, Hepsal) whilst the image intensifier or X-ray camera are being manoeuvred into place (*Fig.* 9.17). The correct position of the catheter tip in the upper superior vena cava must be confirmed on screening before the tunnel is created (*Fig.* 9.18). It is a useful ploy to have infiltrated the proposed tunnel track with local anaesthetic solution so that this can take effect during the X-ray procedure and hence as little time as possible is wasted. After the confirmatory X-ray has been completed, the catheter should be cleared of the contrast medium using heparinized saline and the introducing cannula removed and backed-off along the central catheter shaft until both hubs are united and fitted snugly together. Extreme care should be taken at this stage in the procedure to ensure that the central catheter does not accidentally fall out of the vein. Prior to the creation of the tunnel, it is a kindness to the patient if an appropriate dose of diazepam is

injected intravenously through the central catheter using a sterile syringe.

Creation of the Tunnel

The exit site for the tunnelled catheter should be carefully selected and placed away from stomas, flexural and submammary skin creases. It can be made as much as 30 cm away from the subclavian vein using one pass of the tunnelling stylet. In the conscious patient (and very emaciated patients under general anaesthesia), a fluid track should be created by injecting local anaesthetic solution diluted with normal saline through a long spinal needle in the subcutaneous plane (*Fig.* 9.19). When this has taken effect, a 1·5 cm skin incision should be made at the exit site selected and, using McIndoe's scissors, a tunnel should be created in the subcutaneous plane by opening the blades 1 cm, closing them and advancing the scissors a further 5 cm. This procedure should be carried out gently, and the surgeon can ensure that the scissors remain in the correct plane by palpation with his free hand (*Fig.* 9.20). This procedure can also be performed down the proposed tunnel from the insertion site wound. Once the 'tunnel' has been created in this manner, the stylet should be slipped through until the tip protrudes from the exit site, whilst the protective capsule for carrying the combined catheter hub assembly beneath the skin remains at the insertion wound (*Fig.* 9.21). It is then a simple task to unscrew the protective shell, expose the male Luer plug and fit the central catheter hub. The protective shell should then be slipped over the central catheter shaft using the radial groove and screwed on to the stylet (*Fig.* 9.21). Finally, the surgeon should place the palm of one hand on the chest wall along the line of the tunnel and between the wounds, whilst the stylet is gently pulled through beneath the skin. As the protective capsule containing the hubs emerges from the tunnel, the surgeon's attention should focus upon ensuring that the catheter unfolds slowly, that the proximal portion of the catheter does not kink or dislodge from the vein and that it comes to rest in the floor of the insertion wound. The catheter exit site wound should then be closed and the catheter secured with 3/0 silk using an atraumatic needle and neat vertical

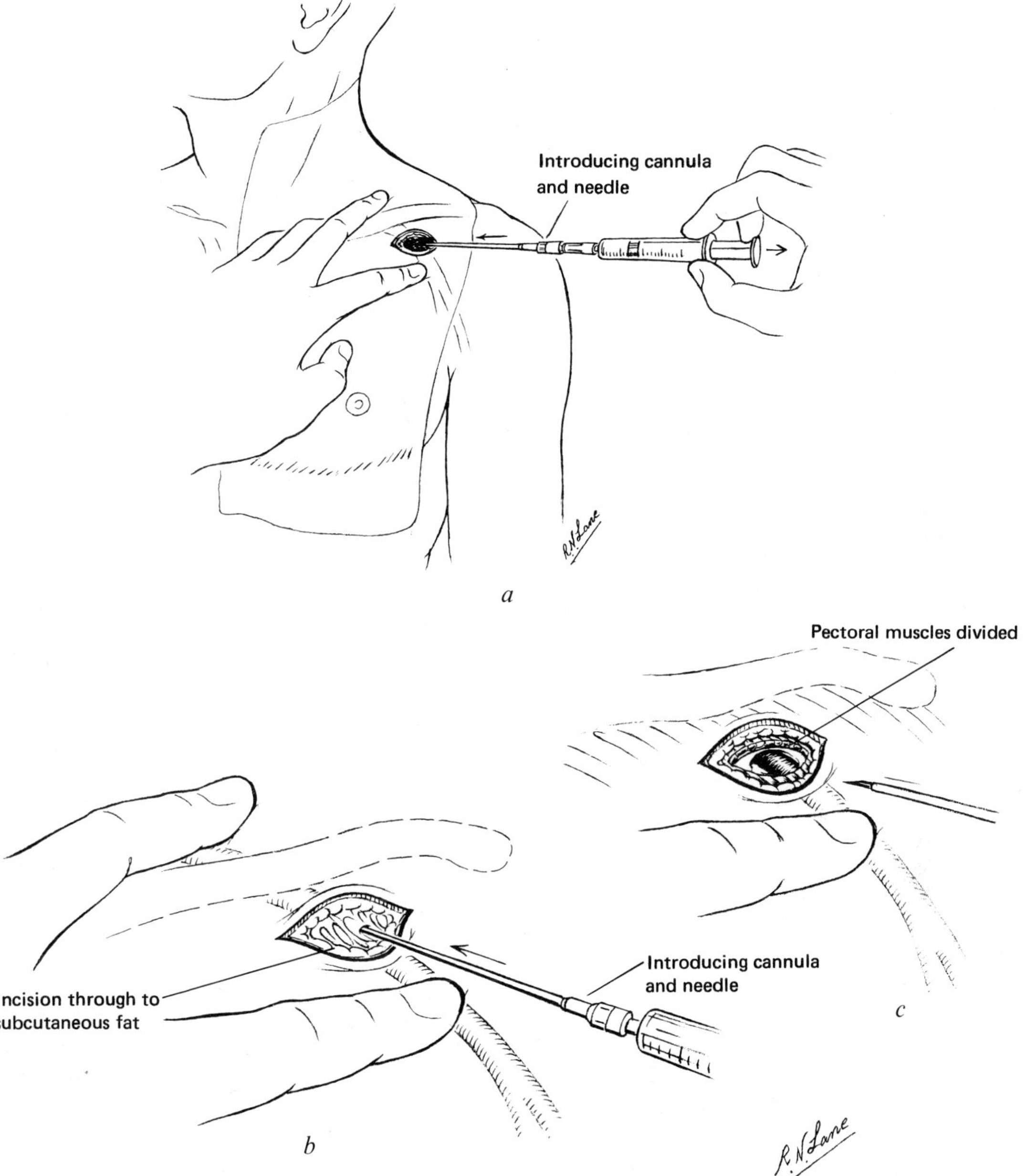

Fig. 9.16. *a*, After making an incision through to the subcutaneous fat (the subclavian vein is illustrated for purposes of clarity), percutaneous through-cannula puncture of the infraclavicular vein is performed. *b*, This situation is highlighted in greater detail, and in *c*, the technique of Osterlee and Dudley is illustrated. The junction of the subclavian and axillary vein has been exposed by dividing the pectoral muscles. NB: The incisions depicted in these subsequent drawings have been enlarged for the sake of clarity. In reality, they are approximately 1·5 cm in length.

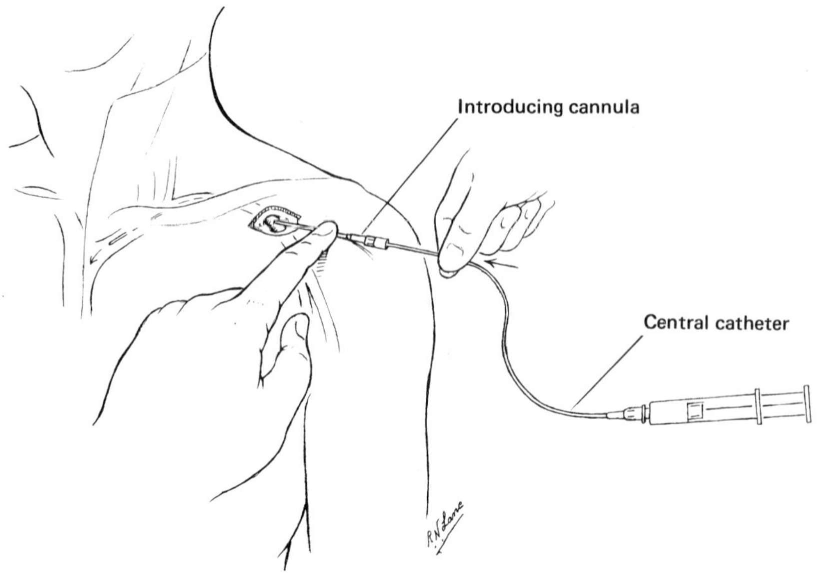

Fig. 9.17. After successful percutaneous cannulation, the central catheter is introduced into the superior vena cava with its hub protected by a syringe containing heparinized saline. (Gloves and drapes omitted for illustration purposes.)

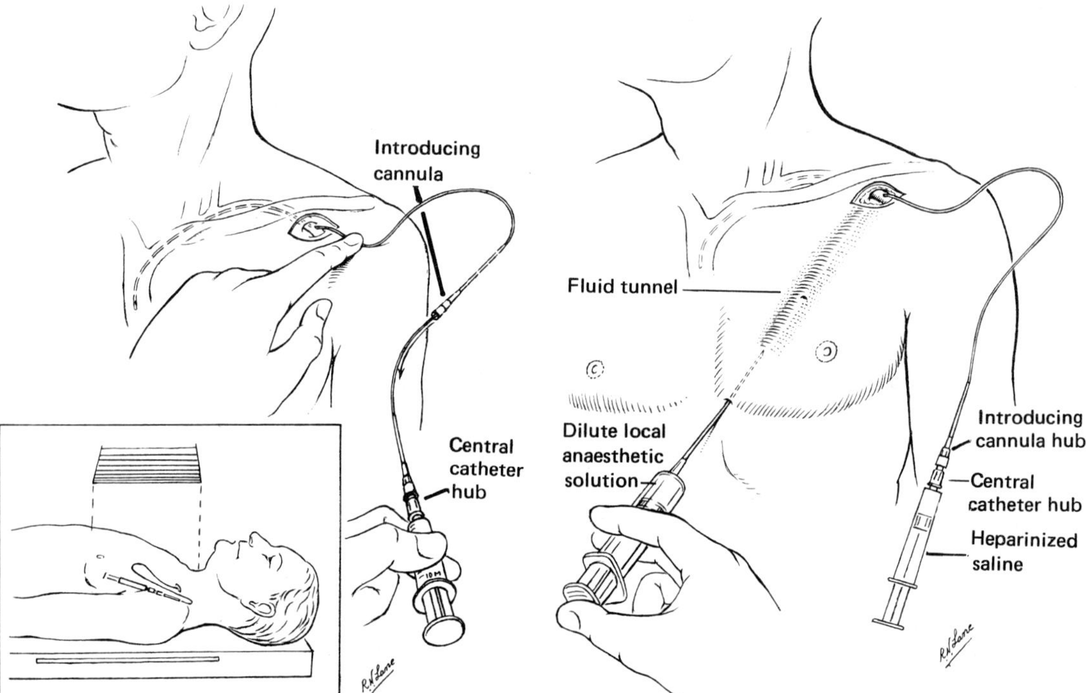

Fig. 9.18. After placement, the correct position of the catheter tip is checked using an image intensifier and an injection of Conray 280 (*see inset*). Once this position is confirmed, the introducing cannula is then withdrawn back over the central catheter shaft and fixed to the central catheter hub (arrow).

Fig. 9.19. Creation of a local anaesthetic fluid tunnel whilst the central venous catheter hub is protected by a syringe of heparinized saline.

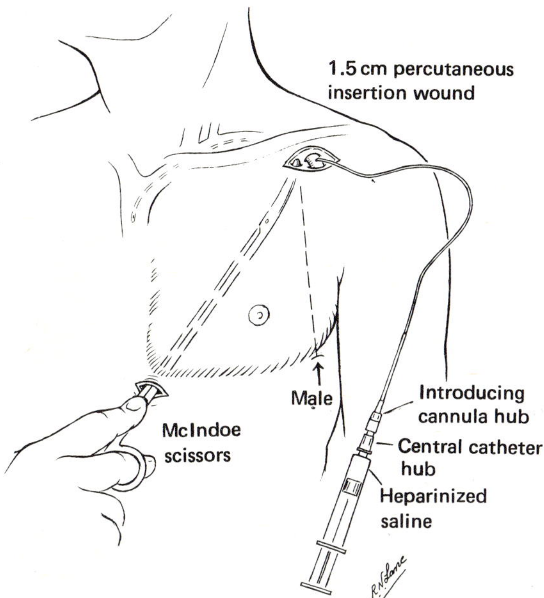

Fig. 9.20. Creation of the subcutaneous tunnel on the anterior chest wall using McIndoe's scissors. In the male, the tunnel can be taken down to the anterior axillary line. (The subclavian vein has been exposed for clarity: gloves and drapes have been omitted.)

mattress sutures. The stylet can then be completely removed and the catheter hub protected with a syringe filled with heparinized saline whilst the insertion wound is also closed with 3/0–6/0 silk of Prolene mattress sutures (*Fig. 9.22*).

Dressing

The catheter wound sites should be cleaned with hydrogen peroxide solution, dried and treated with mastic before a thin ribbon of gauze dressing is applied to the wound and covered with an Op-Site I.V. dressing ($6 \times 8 \cdot 5$ cm). The catheter should then be laid carefully along a gentle curve on the body surface, and fixed with a separate and larger sheet of Op-Site (10×14 cm) (*Fig. 9.23*). It is important to note that this dressing is to prevent dislodgement of the line and should not cover the hub assembly or the exit site dressing. Finally, the catheter can be connected to an administration set fitted with a Luer-locked short extension tube (12 cm: Wallace) and primed with intravenous fluid. The hubs should be sprayed generously with povidone-iodine powder spray (Disadine) and wrapped

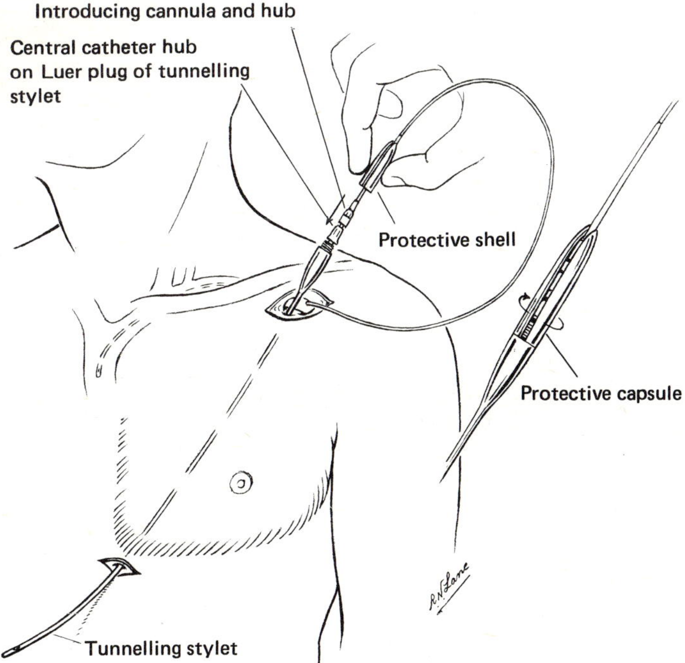

Fig. 9.21. The tunnelling stylet has been passed through the track created by scissor dissection and the combined assembly of central catheter hub and introducing cannula mounted on the Luer plug of the stylet. The protective capsule shell with its radial groove is then slipped over the central catheter shaft and screwed into place (*see inset*).

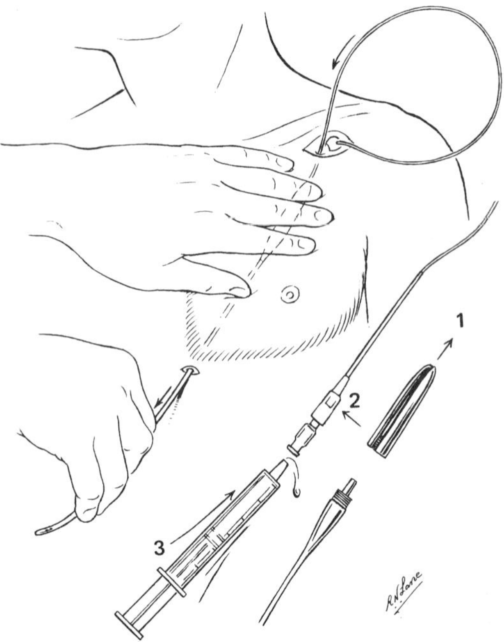

Fig. 9.22. Illustrates the passage of the tunnelling stylet, protective capsule and the combined assembly of the central catheter hub and introducing cannula through the subcutaneous tissues. Note how the surgeon's hand should be placed firmly on the anterior chest wall as the device is pulled through. The protective capsular shell mechanism can then be unscrewed and removed from the central catheter shaft (*insets* 1 and 2). A syringe containing heparinized saline should then be immediately placed into the central catheter hub to prevent air entry (*inset* 3).

carefully in a sterile gauze envelope. This should also be fixed to the body using a sheet of Op-Site.

ALTERNATIVE CANNULATION TECHNIQUES

Osterlee and Dudley in 1979 (31) described a technique by which the junction between the infraclavicular axillary vein and subclavian vein could be exposed by partially dividing the pectoral muscles and inserting a central catheter, through a plastic introducing cannula, into the subclavian vein under direct vision. They pointed out the important advantage of avoiding the risk of pneumothorax when the vein was thus exposed. The technique of using a through-cannula insertion of the central venous catheter, X-ray screening for the confirmation of correct placement and finally tunnelling the integral hub assembly to a distant site, can also be adopted

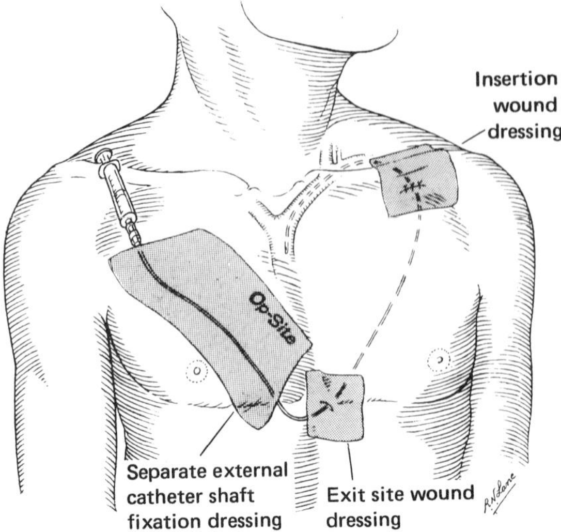

Fig. 9.23. Op-Site and sterile gauze dressings have been arranged to cover separately the insertion wound and catheter exit site; a separate sheet of the material is used to provide external catheter shaft fixation on the chest wall. Note the syringe containing heparinized saline protecting the catheter hub until this is connected to a primed administration set and extension tube.

for the cephalic and external jugular vein. Both veins require surgical exposure as previously described in this chapter, followed by the through-cannula insertion of the central catheter. Once in the correct place, the introducing cannula can be withdrawn over the shaft of the central line, the hub assembly and the tunnelling procedure can then be completed using the stylet as described (*see Figs.* 9.15–23).

The creation of subcutaneous tunnels also allows the use of the femoral vein or one of its tributaries to be contemplated in those rare cases where the more conventional routes have been destroyed or sacrificed.

COMPLICATIONS

There have been no complications related to the tunnelling procedures performed as described to date, except for occasional transient linear bruising along the track of the tunnel. Hickman and Broviac catheters have been reported to have snapped during removal, and this is due to the Dacron cuff being firmly encased by granulation tissue and inappropriate force being applied (33). The removal procedure techniques are described later in Chapter 15.

The effectiveness of tunnelled catheters in providing safe and prolonged venous access continues to be emphasized together with the relatively low incidence of catheter-related complications. With regard to Broviac and Hickman catheters, Thomas et al., in 1980, noted an incidence of eight episodes of catheter-related sepsis per 6308 catheter days (30), whilst Broviac (10) reported 2 per 2599 catheter days and Byrne, 2 per 1139 catheter days (34). Catheter failure necessitating removal of the device has also been reported to occur because of dislodgement, thrombotic catheter occlusion and axillary vein thrombosis. At the present time, the evidence accumulating suggests that the creation of a long skin tunnel for central venous catheters is not only beneficial, but provides the patient with a comfortable portal for venous access. This convenience, in order to be safe for patients, must be rigorously protected and maintained by vigilant nursing and medical staff trained in the art of intravenous therapy and using faultless aseptic techniques at all times.

NEW DEVELOPMENTS

Recently, at University College Hospital, London, a new silicone central venous catheter has been developed. This device possesses a titanium hub in order to prevent the problem of fracture which occurs with current devices when their hubs are made of plastic. These catheters are designed for prolonged placement and tunnelling subcutaneously; they may also be obtained with or without a dacron cuff on the catheter shaft. The devices have been produced with the kind cooperation of Mr H. G. Wallace (H. G. Wallace & Co. Ltd., Essex).

References

1. Dudrick S. J., Vars H. M., Rhoads J. E.: Growth of puppies receiving all nutritional requirements by vein. *Fortschr. Parenteral. Ernahrung.* 1966; **2**: 16–18.
2. Dudrick S. J., Wilmore D. W., Vars H. M.: Long term total parenteral nutrition with growth in puppies and positive nitrogen balance in patients. *Surg. Forum* 1967; **18**: 356–7.
3. Dudrick S. J., Steiger E., Wilmore D. W. et al.: Continuous long term intravenous infusion in unrestrained animals. *Lab. Anim. Care* 1970; **20**: 521–9.
4. Hoshal V. L., Ause R. G., Hoskins P. A.: Fibrin sleeve formation in indwelling subclavian central venous catheters. *Arch. Surg.* 1971; **102**: 253.
5. Bos L. P., Berbee G. M., Scherder M. et al.: The importance of subcutaneous tunnelling of central venous catheters in the prevention of catheter related septicaemia. In: *Proceedings of the First European Congress on Parenteral and Enteral Nutrition.* Stockholm, September 1979: 62.
6. Moghissi K.: A technique of superior vena caval catheterisation for prolonged intravenous feeding. *J. R. Coll. Surg. Edinb.* 1979; **66**: 673–4.
7. Altemeier W. A., Culbertson R., Fullen W. D. et al.: Serratia marcescens septicaemia—a new threat in surgery. *Arch. Surg.* 1969; **99**: 232–7.
8. Ross A. H. M., Anderson J. R., Walls A. D. F.: Central venous catheterisation. *Ann. R. Coll. Surg. Engl.* 1980; **62**: 454–8.
9. Mitchell A., Draper C., Lee D. R. et al.: A simple system of parenteral nutrition. *Ann. R. Coll. Surg.* 1981; **63**: 173–6.
10. Broviac J. W., Cole B. S., Scribner B. H.: A silicone rubber atrial catheter for prolonged parenteral nutrition at home. *Surg. Gynecol. Obstet.* 1973; **136**: 602.
11. Heimbach D. M., Ivey T. D.: A technique for placement of a permanent home hyperalimentation catheter. *Surg. Gynecol. Obstet.* 1976; **143**: 635.
12. Riella M. C., Scribner B. H.: Five years' experience with a right atrial indwelling catheter for prolonged parenteral nutrition at home. *Surg. Gynecol. Obstet.* 1976; **143**: 205.
13. Solassol C., Joyeux H., Etco L. et al.: New techniques for long-term intravenous feeding: An artificial gut in 75 patients. *Ann. Surg.* 1974; **179**: 519–22.
14. Parsa M., Ferrer J. (ed.): *Safe Central Venous Nutrition; Guidelines for the Prevention and Management of Complications.* Springfield, Ill.: Thomas, 1974.
15. Benotti P. N., Bothe A., Blackburn G.: Safe cannulation of the internal jugular vein for long-term hyperalimentation. *Surg. Gynecol. Obstet.* 1977; **144**: 574.
16. Titone C., Lefton C., Sakwa S.: A technique for chronic subclavian vein catheterisation. *Surg. Gynecol. Obstet.* 1973; **137**: 489–90.
17. Powell-Tuck J.: A skin tunnel for central venous catheter: non-operative technique. *Br. Med. J.* 1978; **1**: 625.
18. Feliciano D. V., Telander R. L.: Total parenteral nutrition in infants and children. *Mayo Clin. Proc.* 1976; **51**: 647.
19. Filler R. M., Coran A. G.: Total parenteral nutrition in infants and children. *Surg. Clin. North Am.* 1976; **56**: 395.
20. Zumbro G., Mullin M., Neilson T.: Catheter placement in infants needing parenteral nutrition using common facial vein. *Ann. Surg.* 1971; **102**: 71.
21. Keilly E.: Placement of central feeding catheters. *Br. Med. J.* 1978; **2**: 1123.
22. Pereyra R., Andrassy R. J., Mahour G. H.: Central venous cannulation in neonates. *Surg. Gynecol. Obstet.* 1980; **151**: 253–4.
23. Hickman R. O., Buckner C. D., Clift R. A. et al.: A modified right atrial catheter for access to the venous system in marrow transplant recipients. *Surg. Gynecol. Obstet.* 1979; **148**: 871–5.
24. Thomas M.: The use of the Hickman catheter in the management of patients with leukaemia and other malignancies. *Br. J. Surg.* 1979; **66**: 673–4.

25. Blacklock H. A., Hill R. S., Clarke A. G. et al.: Use of a modified subcutaneous right atrial catheter for venous access in leukaemic patients. *Lancet* 1980; **1**: 993.

26. Blitt L. O., Wright W. A., Petty C. et al.: Central venous catheterisation via the external jugular vein. A technique employing the J-wire. *JAMA* 1974; **229**: 817–18.

27. Gordon I., Grant J. C., Greigor K. C.: Operation on the exsanguinated patient; reduction of risk. *Lancet* 1954; **2**: 899.

28. Antia N. H.: Use of the cephalic vein in intravenous therapy. *Br. Med. J.* 1955; **1**: 652.

29. Dolton E. G.: Massive blood transfusion through the cephalic vein. *Lancet* 1955; **1**: 1052.

30. Thomas J. H., McCarthur R. I., Pierce G. E. et al.: Hickman–Broviac catheters, indications and results. *Am. J. Surg.* 1980; **140**: 791–6.

31. Osterlee J., Dudley H. A. F.: Central catheter placement by puncture of exposed subclavian vein. *Lancet* 1980; **1**: 19–20.

32. Dunbar R., Mitchell R., Lavine M.: Aberrant locations of central venous catheters. *Lancet* 1981; **1**: 711–14.

33. Fleming C. R., Witzke D. J., Beart R. W.: Catheter related complications in patients receiving home parenteral nutrition. *Ann. Surg.* 1980; **192**: 593–9.

34. Byrne W. J., Halpin T. C., Asch M. J. et al.: Home total parenteral nutrition: an alternative approach to the management of children with severe chronic small bowel disease. *J. Paediatr. Surg.* 1977; **12**: 359.

Chapter 10

Intracardiac Oxygen Measurement

R. F. Armstrong and J. Moxham

Adolph Fick, professor of physiology at the Hochschule of Wurzburg, laid the foundations for the current continuing interest in cardiac output measurement when he presented a brief note in 1870 entitled, 'On the measurement of blood flow in the heart' (1). Fick never personally reported any animal experiments describing simultaneous determination of arteriovenous gas differences and pulmonary gaseous exchange. His principle was first applied in 1886 by Grehant and Quinquaud (2). These workers inserted cannulas into the jugular veins, right heart and carotid arteries of dogs. More exhaustive validation of this principle was provided by Zuntz and Hagemann, who performed experiments upon horses during 1886 to 1894; their work culminated in the publication of a monograph in 1898 (3).

In man, the first controlled catheterization of the right atrium was performed by Forssmann in 1929 (4); in the following year, Diaz and Cuenca described their catheterization of the right atrium with a ureteric catheter in a moribund patient, and location of the tip in the right atrium with a radiograph. They suggested many possible developments of the procedure, including the sampling of mixed venous respiratory gases (5). They also reported studies performed upon a few patients with cardiorespiratory insufficiency in which they compared the oxygen content in peripheral veins and atrial blood, and the arteriovenous difference was estimated in one case. Cournand and Ranges reported their initial experience in 1941 (6), and subsequently they, together with Richards and others, performed an exhaustive series of experiments using right atrial catheters (7). McMicheal and

Sharpey-Schafer were responsible for introducing these techniques and cardiac output estimations into England and were the first to study the effects of intravenous digoxin in cardiac failure (8). During the past 40 years, it has been recognized that the oxygen content of blood leaving the right side of the heart is one of several useful measurements that can be made during right heart catheterization. The value of this measurement lies in the relationship of venous oxygen content to cardiac output and arterial oxygen content, as illustrated in the rearranged Fick equation:

$$C v o_2 = C a o_2 - V o_2 / Q_t$$

$C v o_2$ = mixed venous oxygen content; $C a o_2$ = arterial oxygen content; $V o_2$ = oxygen consumption; Q_t = cardiac output.

From this equation it is clear that changes in $C v o_2$ will follow alterations in arterial oxygen content—as, for example, in respiratory failure or anaemia—changes in cardiac output and changes in oxygen consumption. Therefore, mixed venous oxygen content falls when oxygen delivery (arterial oxygen content × cardiac output) fails to meet the oxygen demand of the tissues. In this way, a knowledge of $C v o_2$ may offer advantages to the clinician when compared with arterial oxygen measurements or cardiac output estimations which provide information about oxygen supply in isolation from tissue requirements.

Although the value of measuring mixed venous oxygen content is based on sound theory, in practice there are several substantial problems. The measurement of true mixed venous oxygen requires catheterization of the pulmonary artery. With more proximal placement, in the right atrium, is the possibility that streaming of the venous blood returning from the venae cavae could give variable and misleading results. Pulmonary artery placement imposes technical limitations if facilities for catheter flow guidance are not available. In some patients, for example, following acute myocardial infarction, the risk of arrhythmias may make pulmonary artery placement unacceptable. An additional problem concerns the question of how well Cvo_2 reflects whole body oxygenation. A study of the contribution of different organs to venous blood, in terms of oxygen tension and blood flow (Table 10.1),

Table 10.1. **Distribution of cardiac output at rest**

	Blood flow (ml/min)	$\% O_2$ delivered	Pvo_2 (mmHg)	$C(a-v)o_2$ (vol %)
Splanchnic	1400	25	43	4·1
Muscle	1200	30	34	8·4
Kidney	1100	7	56	1·3
Brain	750	20	33	6·3
Skin	500	2	60	1·0
Heart	250	11	23	11·4
Other	600	5		
	5800	100	40	5·0

Reproduced from Sykes M. K., McNicol M. W. and Campbell E. J. M.: *Respiratory Failure*, by kind permission of the authors and Blackwell Scientific Publications Ltd, Oxford.

illustrates that, as perfusion patterns alter during regional vasoconstriction, it is possible that several organs could provide a reduced proportion of the total venous effluent. As a consequence, hypoxia of particular tissues may not be apparent from a study of mixed venous oxygen. How important this problem is in practice is hard to assess. Certainly, from the point of view of routine measurements of mixed venous oxygen tension (Pvo_2) in a large number of sick patients, we have observed no marked disparity between the clinical course of the subjects and Pvo_2 readings. Only in septicaemia have relatively normal Pvo_2 levels been seen in patients with obvious shock states. Presumably this is due to the impaired oxygen utilization described in these disorders. To be set against these objections there is good evidence that measurement of mixed venous oxygen is a useful guide to cardiorespiratory function and oxygen utilization. Several studies have sought to establish the importance of central venous oxygen measurement.

Relationship of Cardiac Output to Mixed Venous Oxygen Content

As early as 1950, Boyd and co-workers compared mixed venous oxygen saturation (Svo_2) with cardiac output during postoperative recovery from open heart surgery (9). Of a total of 34 patients, 19 maintained Svo_2 levels above 60 per cent and a cardiac output greater than $2·4 \, \mathrm{l \, min^{-1} \, m^{-2}}$: all survived. The remainder developed levels below 60 per cent and cardiac outputs less than $2·0 \, \mathrm{l \, min^{-1} \, m^{-2}}$. Of this group 10 died. The authors concluded that Svo_2 was the most important denominator of cardiac output. Later workers (10) arrived at similar conclusions and, although unable to demonstrate a linear correlation with cardiac index, noted that serious complications following cardiothoracic surgery were observed much less frequently when the Svo_2 remained above 65 per cent. They concluded that for clinical purposes Svo_2 provided a reliable first approximation of cardiac output, and that its determination should reduce the need for frequent cardiac output measurement.

Other workers, notably Kirklin (11) and Parr (12), demonstrated variability in the relationship between cardiac output and mixed venous oxygen tension, but both workers considered it to be an important measurement in postoperative surgical care. Presumably, mixed venous oxygen and cardiac output will only show a close correlation when arterial oxygen content and oxygen consumption remain stable—an unlikely event in postoperative patients who have changing haemoglobin levels and metabolic rates.

Mixed Venous Oxygen Content as an Index of Tissue Perfusion

If tissue perfusion is sluggish, increased oxygen extraction will lower Cvo_2. In 1974, Stanley used this relationship to determine flow rates during cardiopulmonary bypass (13). Using bicarbonate needs to restore normal pH values, and urine output as an index of adequate tissue perfusion, he showed that better results were obtained when flow was regulated to keep venous oxygen tensions within normal limits than when flow rates were based on the patient's weight.

Mixed Venous Oxygen Content as an Index of Tissue Oxygenation

In 1974 Tenney (14) made a theoretical analysis of the relationship between mixed venous oxygen tension and tissue oxygen tension using a mathematical model (15). He concluded that whilst venous oxygen levels can be misleading, they are nevertheless a surprisingly good approximation of mean tissue oxygen tension under normal conditions.

Support for this view has emerged in several papers describing relationships between venous oxygen levels and lactate measurements. Kasnitz (16) studied 20 patients with serious cardiac and pulmonary disease and reported that all patients (10) with hyperlactataemia (>2 mmol/l) died. Values below 2 mmol occurred in 11 survivors, suggesting that lactate measurement as an index of anaerobiosis was a good predictor of survival. These workers then compared lactate levels with cardiac output, arterial oxygen tension and mixed venous oxygen tension (Pv_{O_2}) and demonstrated that Pv_{O_2} correlated most closely with lactate. Below a Pv_{O_2} of 28 mmHg, 8 patients had elevated lactate concentrations and all died. In an experimental study of dogs, Simmons produced hyperlactataemia by severe hypoxaemia and by reductions of cardiac output (17). He showed that Pv_{O_2} was the best predictor of hyperlactataemia as compared with arterial oxygen tension (Pa_{O_2}), cardiac output (Q_t) or oxygen delivery ($Ca_{O_2} \times Q_t$) and also described a threshold value for Pv_{O_2} of 27 mmHg, below which hyperlactataemia always occurred.

Finally, Hiller studied tissue oxygen tensions directly using intramuscular electrodes and demonstrated a good correlation between tissue P_{O_2} and Pv_{O_2} (18).

Although results of this sort make it tempting to consider Pv_{O_2} and tissue oxygenation as synonymous, further work by Cain introduced an element of doubt (19). He showed that in dogs with hypoxic hypoxia, oxygen uptake did not decrease until Pv_{O_2} values of approximately 17 mmHg were reached. When anaemic hypoxia was produced, significant reductions in oxygen uptake occurred at Pv_{O_2} levels of 44 mmHg.

Using Pv_{O_2} as a measure of tissue oxygenation in these dogs would have been misleading and suggests that dissociation curve movements or re-direction of blood flow may obscure changes in Pv_{O_2}. By monitoring Pv_{O_2} continuously in over 100 patients we have, nevertheless, found Pv_{O_2} to accord well with the patient's clinical condition. In 26 patients studied following myocardial infarction, sustained right atrial oxygen tensions ($RaPv_{O_2}$) below 34 mmHg (11 patients) were associated with a mortality of 70 per cent. Of 15 patients whose $RaPv_{O_2}$ was above this figure, all survived. Examples of 3 patients with differing degrees of cardiac dysfunction are shown in *Fig.* 10.1.

Clinical Applications of Central Venous Oxygen Measurement

1. The arteriovenous oxygen difference ($A-V_{O_2}$) is a commonly used index of cardiac function. If oxygen consumption remains steady, then the arteriovenous difference in oxygen content (normally 5 ml/100 ml) will bear an inverse relationship to cardiac output. When greater than 6 ml/100 ml, the cardiac output is falling (<4.0 l/min). Below 3 ml/100 ml, cardiac output is high.

2. In the evaluation of respiratory function it is customary to consider arterial oxygen tension or the alveolar arterial oxygen tension difference ($A-aP_{O_2}$). At high inspired oxygen concentrations the alveolar–arterial difference bears a close relationship to the proportion of cardiac output perfusing non-ventilated alveoli (shunt fraction). However, the value of this measurement is limited by the influence that cardiac output has on arterial oxygen tension. In the presence of intrapulmonary shunting, a proportion of the mixed venous blood will traverse the pulmonary capillary bed without becoming oxygenated and will modify the arterial oxygen tension accordingly.

When cardiac output is low, the reduction in mixed venous oxygen content which occurs will thus result in a lower Pa_{O_2} even though respiratory function and shunt fraction have not changed. Similarly, a high cardiac output will improve Pa_{O_2} (*Fig.* 10.2).

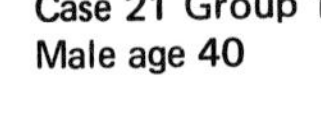

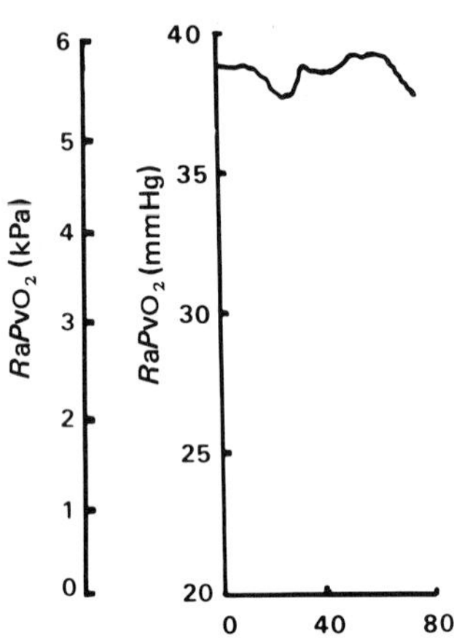
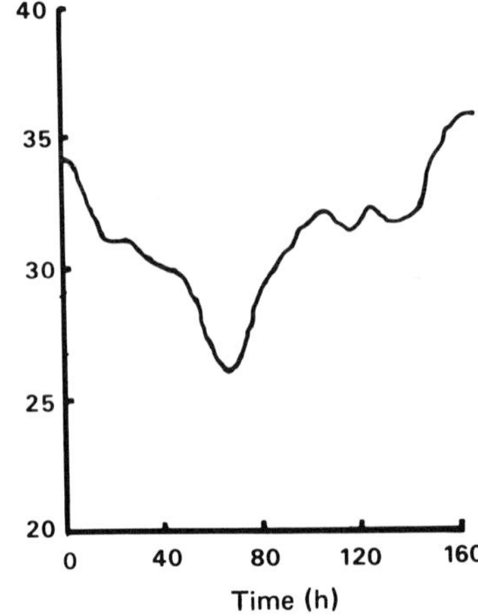
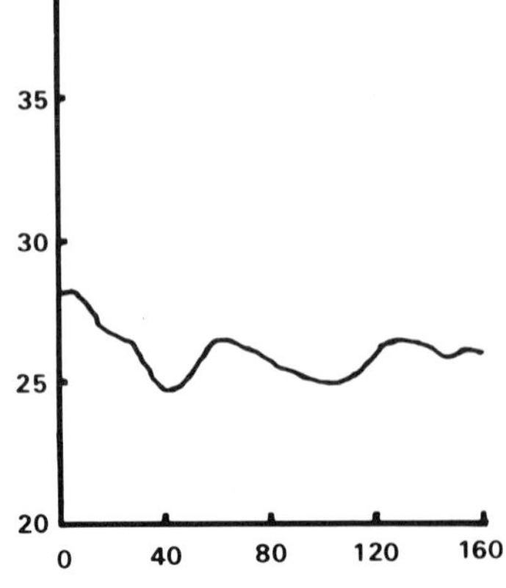

Fig. 10.1. Continuous measurement of $RaPvo_2$ in 3 patients with different levels of cardiopulmonary dysfunction. (Case 21 was a patient with a completely uncomplicated infarction. Case 5 was well on admission but then developed complete heart block, his clinical condition and $RaPvo_2$ improved with transvenous pacing. Case 20 was admitted with cardiogenic shock and eventually died.) (Reproduced from Moxham J. and Armstrong R. F. (23) by kind permission of the Editor of *Intensive Care Medicine.*)

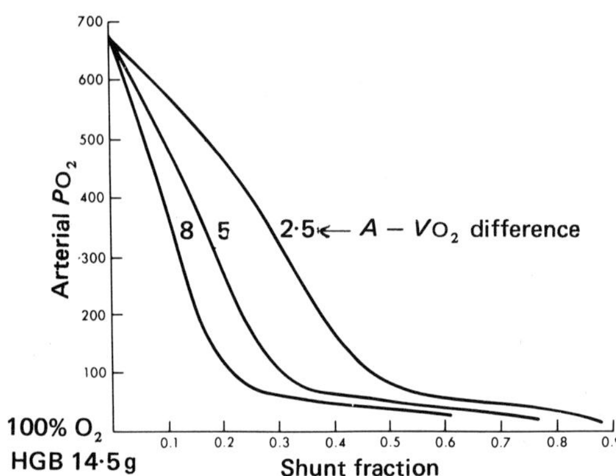

Fig. 10.2. The influence of variation in cardiac output on Pao_2 at different shunt fractions. (Reproduced from Blaisdell F. W. and Lewis F. R.: *Respiratory Distress Syndrome of Shock and Trauma* (*Major Problems in Clinical Surgery*, Vol. XXI) by kind permission of W. B. Saunders Co.)

To exclude this cardiac effect, calculation of the shunt can be made by the shunt equation:

$$\frac{Q_s}{Q_t} = \frac{Cco_2 - Cao_2}{Cco_2 - Cvo_2}$$

which will involve sampling both arterial and mixed venous blood. Q_s = flow through shunt; Q_t = cardiac output; Cco_2 = pulmonary capillary oxygen content; Cao_2 = arterial oxygen content; Cvo_2 = mixed venous oxygen content.

Sampling Sites

Because venous inflow into the right atrium is to some extent in separate streams, sampling of mixed venous blood should be from the right ventricle or pulmonary artery. However, as right atrial catheterization is more commonly employed in clinical practice, it is tempting to use blood from this source as a mixed venous sample. Several workers have compared this site with pulmonary artery sampling and have reached different conclusions. Suter and co-workers (20), consider right atrial and distal pulmonary artery sampling to be inaccurate measures of MVo_2, but other workers, notably Lee (21), demonstrated good correlation between right atrial (RA) and pulmonary artery (PA) samples in patients with and without shock (correlation coefficient 0·95). In 2 patients with oxygen electrodes recording simultaneously in both PA and RA, the authors have noted almost identical traces over many hours of monitoring (*Fig.* 10.3).

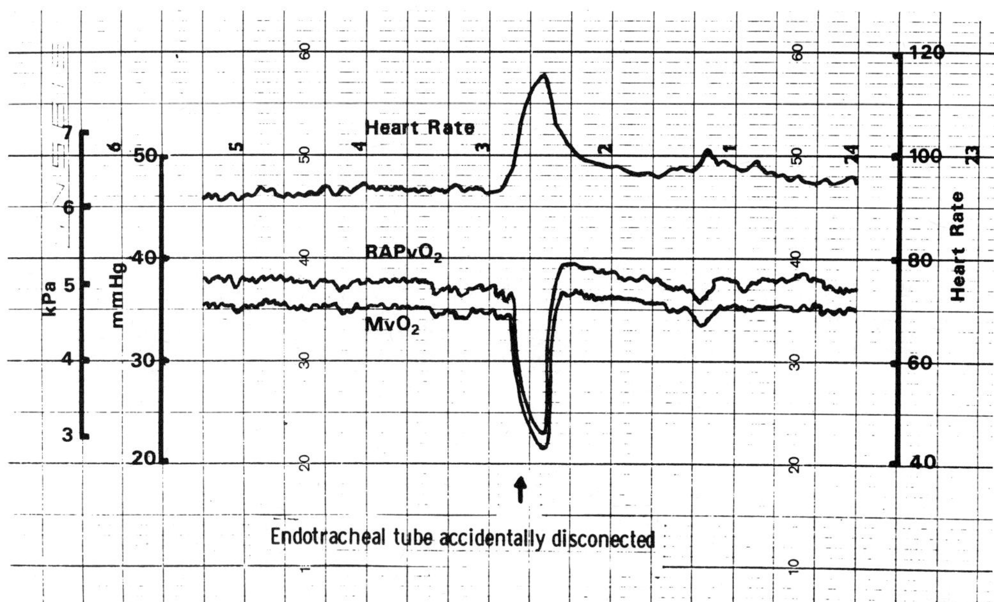

Fig. 10.3. Simultaneous continuous measurement of right atrial and pulmonary artery oxygen tension. (The patient had pneumonia and respiratory failure.)

Continuous Monitoring of Mixed Venous Oxygen Levels as an Index of Cardiopulmonary Performance

The development of a miniaturized Clark electrode (22) has now enabled workers to study *in vivo* oxygen tensions continuously. The electrode consists of a silver cathode surrounded by dried potassium chloride electrolyte and capped by a silver anode. The complete unit is dip-coated in polystyrene and mounted on the tip of a double lumen 5 F PVC catheter. One lumen carries the wire from the tip and the other is used for sampling. The electrical output is relayed to an amplifier and chart recorder via an optically coupled isolator (*Fig.* 10.4).

Insertion

After appropriate skin preparation and using a strict aseptic technique, the catheter is filled with saline and inserted percutaneously via a 12 G cannula (Medicut) into a central or peripheral vein (*Fig.* 10.5). To prevent blood loss between catheter and cannula, we have developed a small collar surrounding the catheter which can be slid into the Medicut hub (*Fig.* 10.6). The catheter is connected via a transducer to an oscilloscope

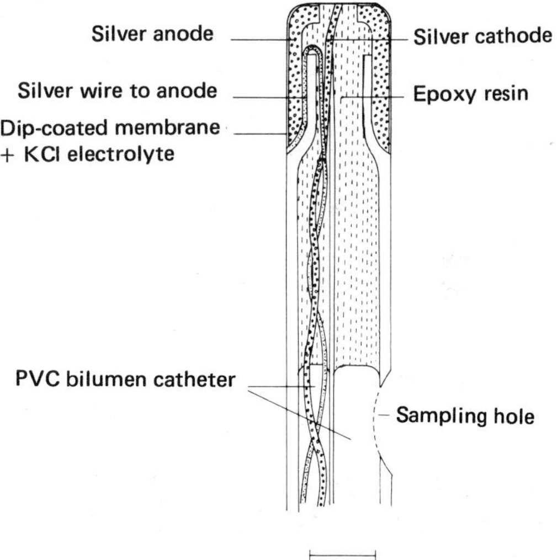

Fig. 10.4. The catheter-tip Po_2 transducer. (*After* Soutter, Conway et al., by courtesy of *Biomedical Engineering*.)

and gently advanced towards the heart until the characteristic pressure traces of atrium, ventricle or pulmonary artery are seen. In patients with low cardiac output states, PA positioning may not be possible. ECG control is important

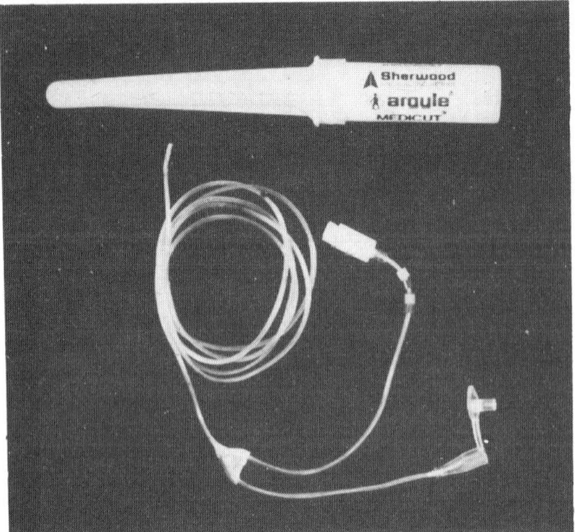

Fig. 10.5 The catheter, showing sampling lumen and electrical output arm. An Argyle Medicut container is included to demonstrate catheter dimensions.

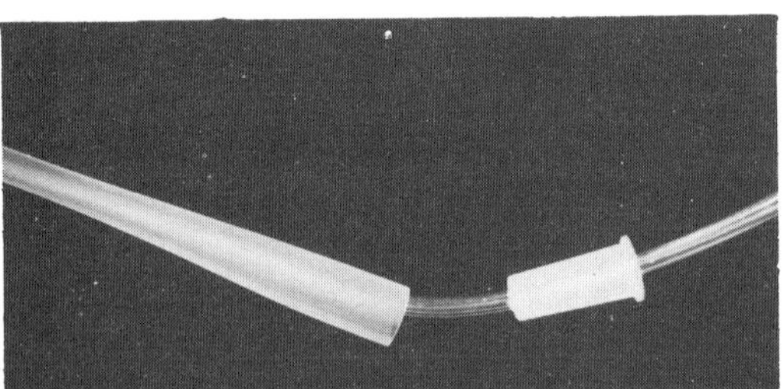

Fig. 10.6. Close-up of catheter collar.

during this procedure as occasional ventricular extrasystoles may occur. The catheter is now secured and a continuous flushing device (Intraflo) connected so that heparinized saline constantly perfuses the system.

Activation

Once in the bloodstream, activation of the electrode occurs by liquification of the dried electrolyte. Completion of the activation process, as indicated by a steady electrical output, is usually within 4 hours, though it is often considerably sooner than this.

Calibration and Catheter Performance

When a steady electrical output is obtained from the catheter, a small volume of blood can be taken from the sampling lumen and oxygen tension measured by blood gas analysis. The visual display and chart recorder can then be calibrated accordingly (*Fig.* 10.7).

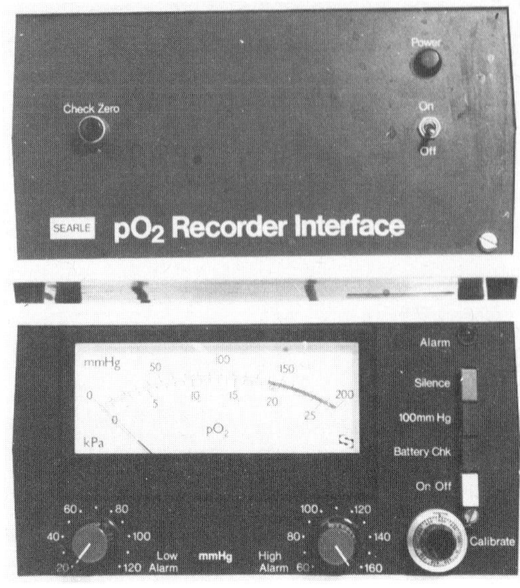

Fig. 10.7. Visual display meter and interface. An optically coupled isolator and battery-driven meter prevent earth leakage current reaching the patient.

Accuracy

From our studies we have found the accuracy of these electrodes to be satisfactory for clinical use. However, where infrequent repeat calibrations are made there is a tendency for drift to occur. In a recent study the data from 70 electrodes were compared with *in vitro* measurements (ABL blood gas analysis) using samples taken from the sampling lumen (23). These electrodes were used for a total of 3687·8 hours and during this time 654 paired observations were made. *Fig.* 10.8 summarizes the paired observations in a correlation table.

Securement

Care in securing the electrode is important to avoid damage to wiring etc. when nursing manoeuvres are carried out. An adequate length of wire between catheter and interface is essential.

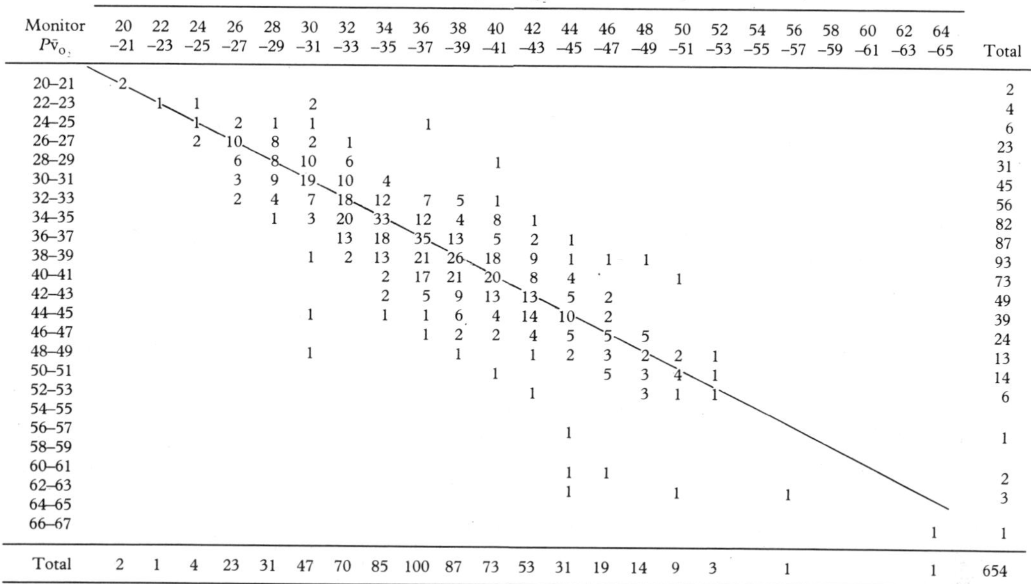

Analyser $P\bar{v}_{O_2}$

Monitor $P\bar{v}_{O_2}$	20–21	22–23	24–25	26–27	28–29	30–31	32–33	34–35	36–37	38–39	40–41	42–43	44–45	46–47	48–49	50–51	52–53	54–55	56–57	58–59	60–61	62–63	64–65	Total
20–21	2																							2
22–23		1	1			2																		4
24–25			1	2	1	1			1															6
26–27			2	10	8	2	1																	23
28–29				6	8	10	6				1													31
30–31				3	9	19	10	4																45
32–33				2	4	7	18	12	7	5	1													56
34–35					1	3	20	33	12	4	8	1												82
36–37							13	18	35	13	5	2	1											87
38–39						1	2	13	21	26	18	9	1	1	1									93
40–41								2	17	21	20	8	4			1								73
42–43								2	5	9	13	13	5	2										49
44–45						1		1	1	6	4	14	10	2										39
46–47									1	2	2	4	5	5	5									24
48–49						1				1		1	2	3	2	2	1							13
50–51											1			5	3	4	1							14
52–53												1			3	1	1							6
54–55																								
56–57													1											1
58–59																								
60–61													1	1										2
62–63													1			1			1					3
64–65																								
66–67																						1		1
Total	2	1	4	23	31	47	70	85	100	87	73	53	31	19	14	9	3		1			1		654

Fig. 10.8. Distribution of $P\bar{v}_{O_2}$ levels and relationship between monitor and analyser results. Figures on the graph represent the number of times the values on the axes corresponded. (Reproduced from Armstrong R. F., Moxham J., Cohen S. L. et al.: Intravenous mixed venous oxygen tension monitoring. *Br. J. Anaesth.* 1981; **53**: 89, by kind permission of the Editor.)

Technical Problems

No serious medical problems have been encountered in using venous oxygen tension electrodes. The insertion and removal procedure have always been uncomplicated and there has been only one significant arrhythmia reported. However, there have been a number of technical problems. In 30 per cent of cases pulmonary artery placement was unsuccessful and right atrial placement was accepted as an alternative. Keeping the sampling lumen patent is an important aspect of electrode management. If the lumen becomes blocked with clot, it is no longer possible to check the accuracy of the electrode and information on intracardiac pressures is lost. In our series 4 per cent of catheters eventually developed blocked sampling lumens, usually as a consequence of inadequate management of the pressurized flushing system. The electrodes frequently remain *in situ* for several days and they are of delicate construction. It is not surprising, therefore, that electrode failures occur due to damage to the wiring from excessive pulling during nursing care manoeuvres. Successful monitoring is only possible if all the staff involved with the patient are aware of the purpose, function and delicacy of the electrode. Ten per cent of our electrodes have failed as a result of accidental trauma.

Transient loss of electrical output is relatively common, occurring in about 10 per cent of electrodes. We presume that this is due to fibrin clots forming on the electrode tip. These output failures are usually self-limiting, but if persistent can frequently be corrected by flushing or by withdrawing the electrode a centimetre or two. Occasionally the output failure persists and the catheter has to be removed. In our studies there have been three occasions when electrodes were faulty prior to insertion and therefore completely failed to activate. Overall, technical failure occurred in 25 of 70 probes, resulting in premature removal after a mean useful life of 48 hours.

Results

One of the advantages of this technique is the continuous nature of the information it provides. This gives a useful account of the progress of the patient's cardiorespiratory performance. The effect of therapy can be objectively assessed and deterioration promptly recognized. Patients who are very ill can be adversely affected by routine nursing manoeuvres, and continuous monitoring detects these cases (*Fig.* 10.9). The response to oxygen therapy or withdrawal (*Fig.* 10.10), changes in ventilation settings, failure of adequate ventilation and deterioration of pulmonary function are all immediately apparent from the continuous $P\bar{v}o_2$ trace at the bedside of the patient. The effectiveness of therapy de-

signed to increase cardiac output can be assessed, and we have used the technique to decide on optimal dopamine infusion rates and even cardiac pacing rates.

When continuous right atrial or pulmonary artery venous oxygen tensions are used to monitor cardiopulmonary performance, it is our practice to keep oxygen tensions as near normal as possible and to avoid any disturbance of the patient that produces a significant fall of $P\bar{v}o_2$.

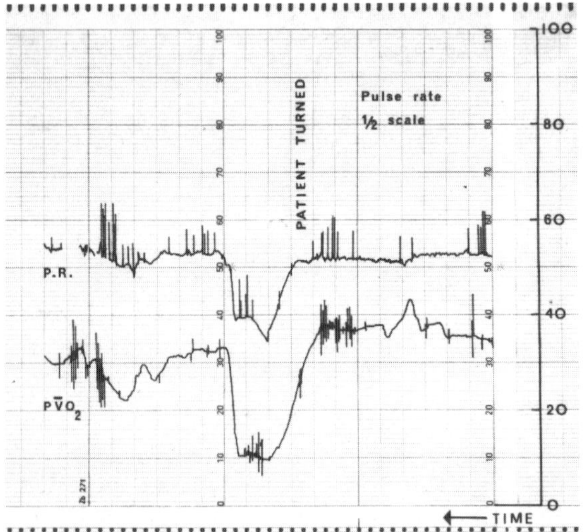

Fig. 10.9. A tracing of the heart rate and $P\bar{v}o_2$ against time to illustrate the effect on these parameters of moving a critically ill patient in bed.

Continuous Monitoring of Mixed Venous Oxygen Saturation

As an alternative to oxygen tension measurement, several monitoring devices now exist utilizing fibreoptic systems for measuring oxygen saturation. The basis of this method is an optical head containing light-emitting diodes. These send alternating pulses of light of different wavelengths along a glass or plastic fibreoptic bundle incorporated in a plastic catheter.

The three transmitted light wavelengths are reflected by haemoglobin in the patient's bloodstream down a second set of fibres in different intensities according to the oxygen saturation. These light pulses are received by a photoelectric device which allows analysis of the relative light intensities and expression as oxygen saturation. Several workers (24, 25) have reported results obtained from this type of system. Problems

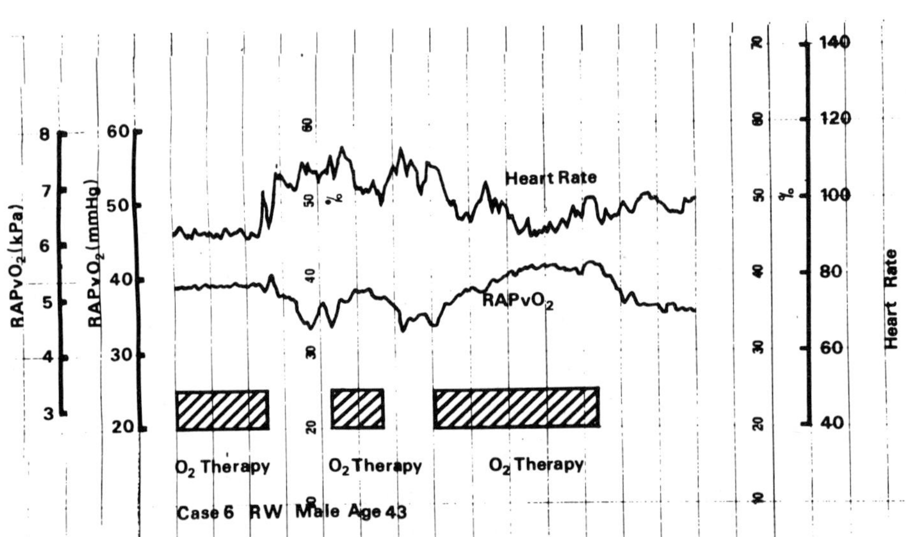

Fig. 10.10. Effect of oxygen therapy and withdrawal on $RaP\bar{v}o_2$ and heart rate. (Reproduced from Moxham J. and Armstrong R. F. (23) by kind permission of the Editor of *Intensive Care Medicine*.)

described include fibre damage, clotting on the tip and positioning of the catheter tip against the vessel wall. Good results have been obtained using catheters incorporating these principles and they are now commercially available (*Fig. 10.11*).

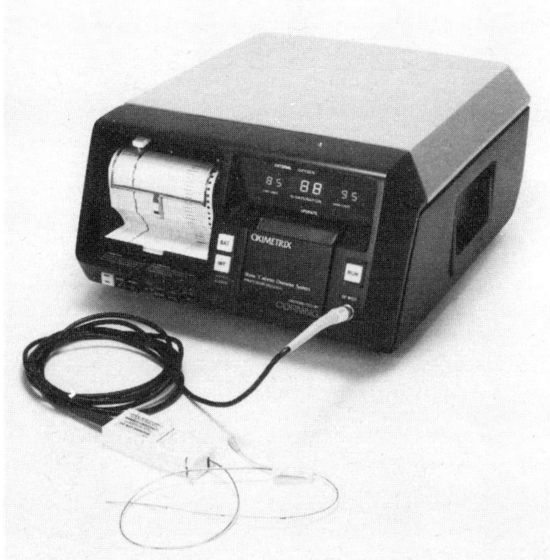

Fig. 10.11. The Oxymetrix system for continuous measurement of oxygen saturation.

References

1. Fick A.: Über die Messung des Blutquantums in den Herzventrikeln. *Phys.-med. Ges. Würzburg* 1870; 9 July.
2. Grehant N., Quinquaud, C. E.: Recherches expérimentales sur la mésure du volume du sang qui traverse le poumon en un temps donné. *C. R. Séanc. Hebd. Soc. Biol.* 1886; **5** (Series 8): 159.
3. Zuntz N., Hagemann O.: Untersuchungen über den Stoffwechsel des Pferdes bei Ruhe und Arbeit. *Landw. J.* 1898; **28**: 1–438.
4. Forssmann, W.: Der sondierung des Rechten Herzens. *Klin. Wochenschr.* 1929; **8**: 2085.
5. Diaz J., Cuenca S.: El sondage del corazón derechio. *Arch. Cardiol. Hematol.* 1930; **2** (March).
6. Cournand A., Ranges H. A.: Catheterisation of the right auricle in man. *Proc. Soc. Exp. Biol. Med.* 1941; **46**: 462–4.
7. Richards D. W., Cournand A., Darling R. C. et al.: Pressure of blood in the right auricle in animals and man: under normal conditions and right heart failure. *Am. J. Physiol.* 1942; **136**: 115.
8. McMicheal J., Sharpey-Schafer E. P.: The action of intravenous digoxin in man. *Q. J. Med.* 1944; **13**: 1123.
9. Boyd A. D., Tremblay R. E., Spencer F. C. et al.: Estimation of cardiac output soon after intra-cardiac surgery with cardio-pulmonary bypass. *Ann. Surg.* 1959; **150**: 613–26.
10. Krauss H., Verdouw P. D., Hugenholtz P. G. et al.: On-line monitoring of mixed venous oxygen saturation after cardio-thoracic surgery. *Thorax* 1975; **30**: 636–43.
11. Kirklin J. W., Theye A. R.: Cardiac performance after open intracardiac surgery. *Circulation* 1963; **28**: 1061–70.
12. Parr G. V. S., Blackstone E. H., Kirklin J. W.: Cardiac performance and mortality early after intracardiac surgery in infants and young children. *Circulation* 1975; **51**: 867–74.
13. Stanley T. H., Isern-Amaral J.: Periodic analysis of mixed venous oxygen tension to monitor the adequacy of perfusion during and after cardio-pulmonary bypass. *Can. Anaesth. Soc.* 1974; **21**: 454–60.
14. Tenney S. M.: A theoretical analysis of the relationship between venous blood and mixed tissue oxygen pressures. *Resp. Physiol.* 1974; **20**: 283–96.
15. Krogh A.: The number and distribution of capillaries in muscles with calculations of the oxygen pressure head necessary to supply the tissue. *J. Physiol.* 1919; **52**: 409–15.
16. Kasnitz P., Druger G. L., Yorra F. et al.: Mixed venous oxygen tension and hyperlactataemia. *JAMA* 1976; **236**: 570–4.
17. Simmons D. H., Alpas A. P., Tashkin D. P. et al.: Hyperlactatemia due to arterial hypoxaemia or reduced cardiac output or both. *J. Appl. Physiol.* 1978; **45**: 195–202.
18. Hiller C., Bone R.: Assessment of correlation between tissue oxygen and mixed venous oxygen. *Am. Rev. Resp. Dis.* 1978; **117**: 126.
19. Cain S. M.: Oxygen delivery and uptake in dogs during anaemic and hypoxic hypoxia. *J. Appl. Physiol. Resp. Environ. Ex. Physiol.* 1977; **42**: 228–34.
20. Suter A. M., Lindauer J. M., Fairley H. B. et al.: The Swan-Ganz catheter. Criteria for wedging. *Crit. Care Med.* 1973; **1**: 119.
21. Lee J., Wright F., Barber R. et al.: Central venous oxygen saturation in shock. *Anaesthesiology* 1972; **36**: 472–8.
22. Parker D., Key A., Davies R. S.: Catheter tip transducer for continuous *in vivo* measurement of oxygen tension. *Lancet* 1971; **1**: 952–3.
23. Moxham J., Armstrong R. F.: Continuous monitoring of right atrial oxygen tension in patients with myocardial infarction. *Intensive Care Med.* 1981; **7**: 157–64.
24. Martin W. E., Cheung P. W., Johnson C. C. et al.: Continuous monitoring of mixed venous oxygen in man. *Anaesth. Analg. (Cleve.)* 1973; **52**: 784–93.
25. Wilkinson A. R., Phibbs R. H., Gregory G. A.: Continuous *in vivo* oxygen saturation in newborn infants with pulmonary disease. *Crit. Care Med.* 1979; **7**: 232–5.

Chapter 11

The Flow-directed Balloon Flotation Catheter

R. B. Hopkinson

In 1970 Swan and his colleagues reported their initial experience with the use of a balloon-tipped flow-directed catheter which could be inserted simply and rapidly into the pulmonary artery without the aid of fluoroscopy (1). This innovation arose from both the work of Bradley, which showed that miniature catheters could be carefully floated in the central venous circulation and pulmonary artery (2) and the realization by Swan that such catheter manipulations would be enhanced by fitting the intravascular tip of the device with an air-filled 'balloon' or 'sail' akin to the fluid-filled balloon catheters introduced to vascular surgery by Thomas Fogarty (3).

This heralded the development of bedside haemodynamic monitoring of the pulmonary–capillary wedge pressure and cardiac output. During the past 10 years the technique has enabled a comprehensive assessment to be made using this sensor linked to suitable transducers without recourse to moving a critically ill patient to a cardiac catheterization room. Any rapid changes in the circulation can be detected and the efficacy of any therapeutic manoeuvre monitored. Swan has estimated that between 1 and 2 million flow-directed catheters have been inserted since 1970 (4). In common with all invasive procedures, this technique has been associated with serious and sometimes fatal complications; the exact incidence is at present unclear. In view of these problems and the cost of the catheter with its disposable supplies, one should not embark on this form of diagnostic intervention without careful consideration.

Indications

Flotation catheters have been inserted in a variety of situations since they came into use.

1. Myocardial infarction complicated by shock, arrhythmias, interventricular septal rupture, papillary muscle necrosis.
2. Hypovolaemia and associated myocardial ischaemia.
3. Perioperatively in major cardiovascular surgery.
4. Major trauma.
5. Adult respiratory distress syndromes.
6. Septic shock.
7. Pancreatitis complicated by shock and pulmonary oedema.
8. Obstetrics—severe pre-eclamptic toxaemia, cardiac disease and inhalation of vomit.

Controversy at present surrounds the precise indications, and Dalen has recently suggested that there has been an inappropriate expansion and subsequent overuse of bedside haemodynamic monitoring with flow-guided balloon catheters (5). He proposes that these catheters should only be used when precise haemodynamic data are needed to determine therapy, and when such data cannot be derived from non-invasive, clinical or radiological evaluation. He also raised another important issue—who should perform this technique? He rightly points out that one would not be allowed to perform right heart catheterization in a catheter laboratory without formal training in the technique. The skills required to insert a Swan–Ganz catheter and interpret the information need to be acquired under supervision. The potential complications must be acknowledged, recognized and treated rapidly when necessary.

Design Characteristics

Flotation balloon catheters are extruded with a double lumen configuration in PVC to a length of approximately 110 cm. The main lumen has an internal diameter of 1 mm, the auxiliary narrow lumen has an internal diameter of 0·4 mm and this communicates with a latex balloon mounted with a special wound thread binding on to the shaft of the catheter. When this is inflated with approximately 0·8–1·5 ml of air, the balloon expands and prolapses slightly beyond the tip of the catheter, thus preventing undue irritation of the subendocardial myocardium on its passage through the heart. The entry ports to the catheter channels are protected by female Luer connections. These catheters vary from about 1·6 to 2·2 mm external diameter (5 F–7 F). Recently, catheters have been extruded with pacing wires and electrodes embedded in the catheter matrix. The catheter, used in conjunction with a standard blood pressure transducer and an appropriate display, enables the monitoring of right atrial (RA), right ventricular (RV), pulmonary artery (PA) and pulmonary artery wedge (PAWP) pressure (*Fig.* 11.1). The terminology used for pulmonary artery wedge pressure varies between centres, e.g.: PAWP, pulmonary artery wedge pressure; PCP, pulmonary capillary pressure; PAOP, pulmonary artery occlusion pressure; PCWP, pulmonary capillary wedge pressure.

Catheterization may be performed via the internal jugular, subclavian, antecubital, external jugular, proximal basilic, femoral or axillary veins. Correct placement is obtained by continuous pressure monitoring using an oscilloscope display. Detection of respiratory fluctuations on the pressure trace indicates entry into the thorax, and the balloon is inflated. The catheter is then advanced, using the blood flow

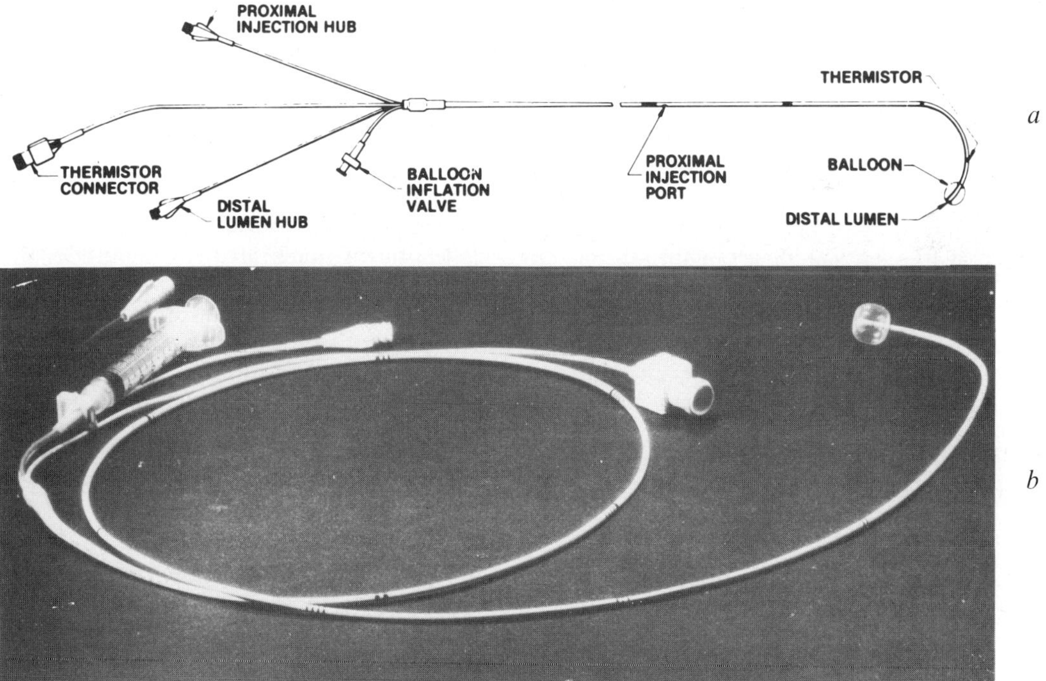

Fig. 11.1. *a*, Diagram of the component features of the Swan–Ganz catheter. *b*, Photograph of the device with the terminal balloon distended with air. (Reproduced by kind permission of American Hospital Supply Corporation and Edwards Laboratories and Dr P. G. Barash, MD, Department of Anesthesiology, Yale School of Medicine, New Haven, Connecticut.)

to carry the catheter tip through the tricuspid valve to the right ventricle and thence through the pulmonary valve into the pulmonary artery.

A family of catheters is available, enabling the measurement of pulmonary artery wedge pressure, pulmonary artery pressure and right atrial pressure. Also available are catheters for thermodilution cardiac output determination which incorporate a thermistor and a right atrial injectate channel; catheters have also been devised for pulmonary angiography, paediatric catheterization, transvenous pacemaking and *in vivo* oximetry.

Theoretical Considerations

Though measurement of central venous pressure is a simple procedure, it has been shown to be misleading as an indicator of myocardial function or of circulating blood volume. If the effective function of the right and left ventricles differs, as in the presence of lung or myocardial disease, the filling pressures of the ventricle will differ, and the central venous or right atrial pressure will no longer reflect left ventricular end diastolic pressure. It is the diastolic pressures in the ventricles that are the most valuable parameter of cardiovascular function on which to base therapeutic decisions. Under most circumstances, pressures recorded within the atrial chambers correlate well with the ventricular diastolic pressures. The 'wedge' pressure thus reflects the pumping pressure of the left ventricle which is the critical determinant of the circulation.

A re-evaluation of the role of central venous pressure (CVP) measurement as a guideline for managing shock and hypovolaemia has shown a poor or absent correlation with pulmonary artery wedge pressure, pulmonary artery end diastolic pressure or left atrial pressure where right and left ventricular function are so disparate in the seriously ill. Not only the absolute CVP, but changes in CVP are often unreliable and provide misleading estimates of left heart filling (6–9). Pulmonary artery monitoring with Swan–Ganz catheters may be considered one of the most important advances in the care of the critically ill patient. Swan has recommended that such catheters should be used whenever measurement of CVP is considered necessary (10).

As systole commences the pressure in the right ventricle (RV) rises, closing the tricuspid valve; then, as the right ventricular pressure exceeds pulmonary artery diastolic pressure, the pulmonary valve opens, allowing ejection of blood from the right ventricle, and the pulmonary artery pressure peaks with that of the right ventricle. With falling right ventricular pressure, the pulmonary valve closes and at the end of systole the right ventricular pressure will fall below that of the pulmonary artery during the initial diastolic phase. Passive flow of blood down the pressure gradient from the right atrium into the right ventricle is augmented by atrial contraction in late diastole. Ventricular contraction recommences and the tricuspid valve closes.

The central venous pulse, like that exhibited by the fluctuations in the internal jugular veins, represents a retrograde transmission of the pressure variations which originate in the right atrium. The positive waves are labelled: 'a', the result of atrial systole; 'c', associated with isovolumic ventricular contraction; 'v', the peak pressure obtained just before opening of the atrioventricular valves.

Recognition of the pressure characteristics of each chamber of the heart and the pulmonary artery is vital to the correct insertion of the Swan–Ganz and other flotation catheters. During each cardiac cycle the low pressure atrium normally produces two positive deflections, whereas the right ventricle produces one positive deflection of much greater magnitude, though the diastolic pressure will normally approximate to that of the right atrial pressure. Pulmonary artery systolic pressure is normally the same as that of the right ventricle, yet the diastolic is greater because of the pulmonary valve (*see* Table 11.1).

The 'Wedge' Pressure

When the balloon-tipped catheter is carried through the pulmonary valve, it will lodge in a branch of the pulmonary artery, thus occluding that branch. The lumen of the catheter will then be in direct communication with the left atrium (LA), via the pulmonary capillary bed. The left atrial pressure, over a pressure range of 6–20 mmHg, will, under most circumstances, adequately reflect left ventricular diastolic press-

Table 11.1. **Normal pressure values for the great veins, right heart and pulmonary artery**

	Pressures (mmHg)
Right atrium	
Mean	−1–+7
Right ventricle	
Systolic	15–25
End diastolic	0–8
Pulmonary artery	
Systolic	15–25
Diastolic	8–15
Mean	10–20
Pulmonary wedge	
Mean	6–12

ure (*see below*). As the balloon is wedged in the pulmonary artery, it no longer reflects the high systolic pressures generated proximally by the right ventricle (*see Fig.* 11.11). When the balloon is deflated (or not in the 'wedge' position), the catheter records pulmonary artery pressures, the pulmonary artery end diastolic pressure (PAEDP) being of particular importance. The pressure trace obtained during insertion of a Swan–Ganz catheter is depicted in *Fig.* 11.2. In the right atrium the pressure is low (CVP); however, as the catheter tip crosses the tricuspid valve, it shows the much higher pressure of the right ventricle, but note the low diastolic pressure.

INSERTION OF BALLOON FLOTATION CATHETERS

The basic equipment which must be assembled prior to the procedure comprises:

1. Catheter
2. Pressure transducer and amplifier
3. Oscilloscope
4. ECG monitor and defibrillator
5. Catheter introducer set
6. Sterile draped trolley

Insertion Technique

The vein to be used for central venous access is identified, the skin prepared and draped. The author's favoured site is the right internal jugular vein. If the patient is conscious, infiltration of a local anaesthetic at and deep to the puncture site should not be forgotten. Using a sterile technique, the catheter is prepared. The catheter sheath is peeled off (as per package instructions) and the proximal end handed to an assistant who inflates the balloon and tests its integrity. During the catheterization procedure the patient should be in a 20° head-down Trendelenburg position.

Inflation of the Balloon

Carbon dioxide drawn through a Millipore filter has been recommended for balloon inflation, because if balloon rupture occurs this gas is rapidly absorbed into the blood. Air is often used, but is contraindicated if there is any possibility of a right-to-left intracardiac shunt or pulmonary arteriovenous fistula. The use of air is more convenient than carbon dioxide which diffuses through the latex balloon at a rate of 0·5 ml/min.

The balloon should *never* be inflated with fluid, because the inflation lumen is very small and it may be impossible to aspirate. The bal-

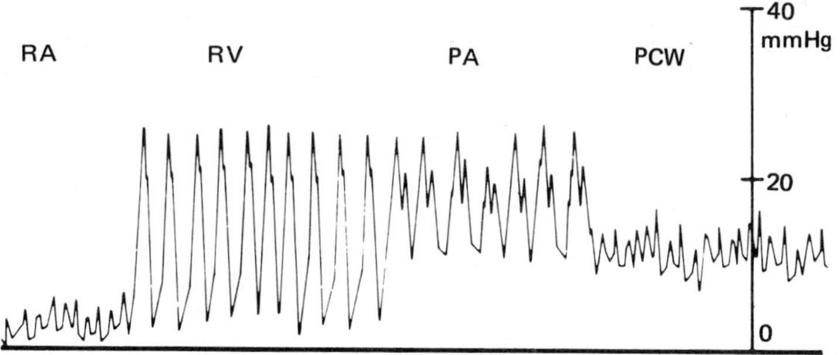

Fig. 11.2. Pressure recordings obtained during advancement of a Swan–Ganz catheter through the chambers of the heart to a wedged position in the pulmonary arterial tree.

loon will also lose most of its flow-direction capacity. Only the smallest syringe that will hold the balloon inflation volume printed on the catheter should be used, and this volume should not be exceeded. This is kept attached to the inflation lumen of the catheter to prevent inadvertent injections of fluid into the balloon. The balloon should always be tested prior to insertion by injection of the required volume of gas (usually 1·5 ml). Over-inflation will cause rupture. If the plunger of the syringe fails to spring back on release, the balloon may have ruptured. Inflation should always be slow as this mitigates against balloon rupture and the remote possibility of a tear in a pulmonary artery.

The pulmonary artery lumen of the catheter is connected to a blood pressure transducer and flushed with dilute heparin solution (500 units per 500 ml of 5 per cent dextrose). A pressure infusor connected to an Intraflow (Sorensen Research) is very convenient because it allows a flow of 3 ml/h to be maintained without significantly affecting the pressures being measured. If a standard intravenous infusion is used, a flow of 25–30 ml/h is necessary to maintain catheter patency. If a triple lumen catheter is used, the third lumen should be flushed and connected to a manometer. (This opens into the right atrium or superior vena cava for central venous pressure measurement.)

It should then be verified that the catheter will pass through the catheter sheath of whichever introducer set is to be used. Introduction of the catheter is effected by a modified Seldinger technique (2,11–13). The vein may be punctured or cannulated and a flexible guide wire passed through the needle or cannula 10 cm into the vein (*Fig.* 11.3). Unless this advances easily, the vein should be punctured again so as to avoid risk of extravascular passage of the introducer. The guide wire should always be secured so that embolism cannot occur (*Figs.* 11.4, 11.5). The needle or cannula is then removed over the guide wire. This is long enough (35–40 cm) to remain in the vein while allowing the vein dilator to be threaded on to it. A small wound with a pointed scalpel blade is made over the guide wire. This facilitates insertion of the vein dilator over which is threaded the catheter sheath. These are railroaded over the wire (which is secured at all times) using a to-and-fro rotating

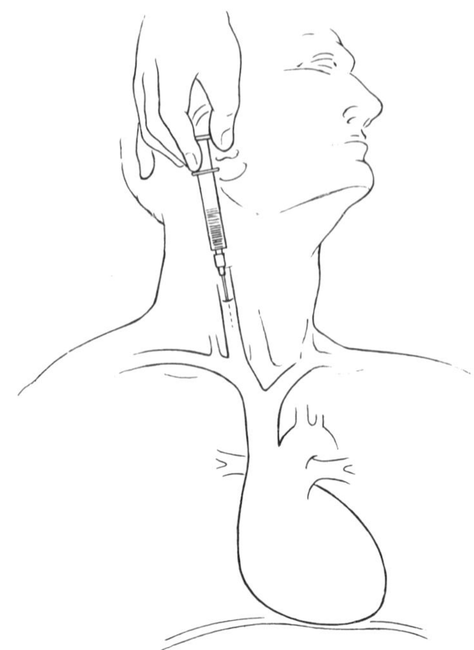

Fig. 11.3. Percutaneous cannulation of the right internal jugular vein performed with a syringe and introducing needle/cannula.

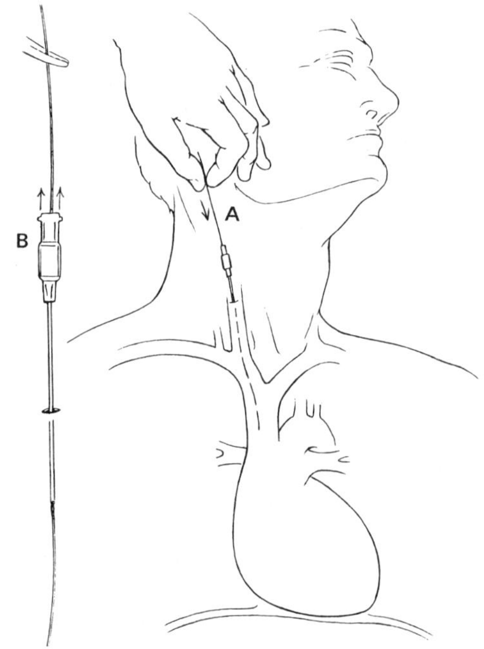

Fig. 11.4. (A) Introduction of the guide wire (gloves and drapes omitted for clarity). *Inset* (B), the guide wire is shown carefully secured with a forceps to prevent embolization occurring as the introducing needle or cannula is withdrawn over the wire.

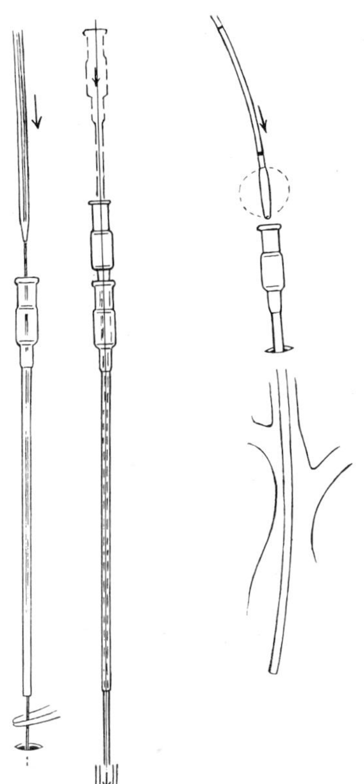

Fig. 11.5. A technique of using the guide wire, introducing sheath and vein dilator prior to passage of the Swan–Ganz catheter into the jugular vein is depicted in the sequence from left to right. Note the importance of carefully securing the guide wire during each manipulation and manoeuvre to prevent its loss into the circulation.

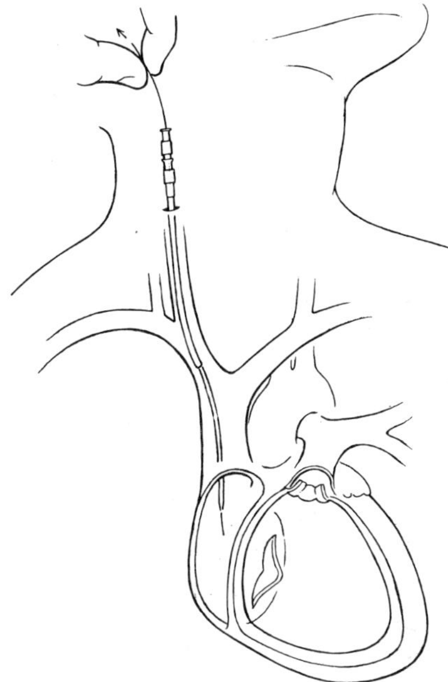

Fig. 11.6. The dilator and sheath have been successfully passed into the jugular vein and superior vena cava; the vein dilator and guide wire are being removed simultaneously. The hub of the device should be protected at this point by a sterile syringe containing heparinized saline.

action as the dilator and sheath are advanced as one unit (*Figs.* 11.5, 11.6). When the catheter sheath is well within the vein, the introducer and wire are withdrawn, leaving the sheath in place. If this is an 8 F sheath, then a 7 F Swan–Ganz catheter may be passed into the vein. Precautions must be taken against air embolism. This procedure, using the internal jugular route, can take as little as 10 minutes to perform (*Fig.* 11.7). Devices exist which preserve a sterile length of catheter and seal the catheter/sheath junction.

The catheter is advanced within the central venous system. Entry into the thoracic cavity may be identified by an increase in respiratory fluctuation of the recorded pressure. The junction of the right atrium and the superior vena cava will be 10–15 cm from the jugular vein, 10 cm from the subclavian vein, 40 cm from the right antecubital fossa, 50 cm from the left

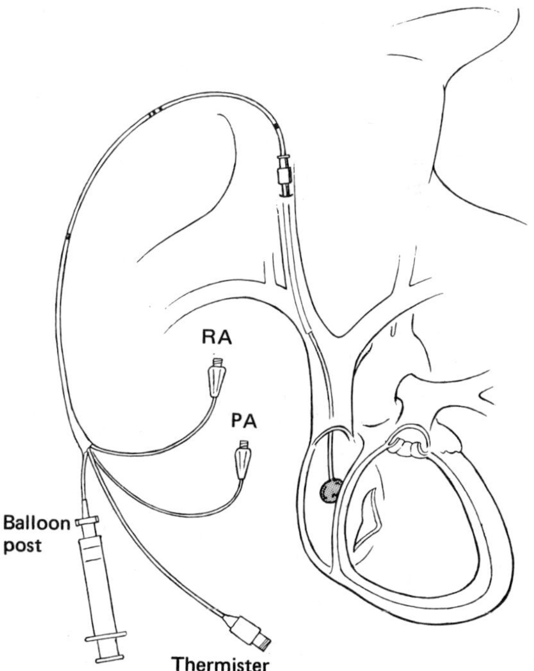

Fig. 11.7. A diagram showing the Swan–Ganz catheter being passed through to the right atrium via the introducing sheath.

antecubital fossa or 30 cm from a femoral puncture site. At this time the pressure excursion observed will normally be about 4 mmHg (*Fig. 11.8*). The balloon is then inflated with the required volume of gas and advanced rapidly, pausing every 10–15 cm while pressures and ECG are monitored on the oscilloscope. Within 10–20 s it will usually pass through the right atrium and right ventricle into the pulmonary artery and thence into the pulmonary artery wedge position. The pressure sequence shown in *Fig.* 11.2 will be displayed on the oscilloscope. As the catheter traverses the right ventricle, the ECG should be observed for ectopic beats (*Figs.* 11.8–11.11).

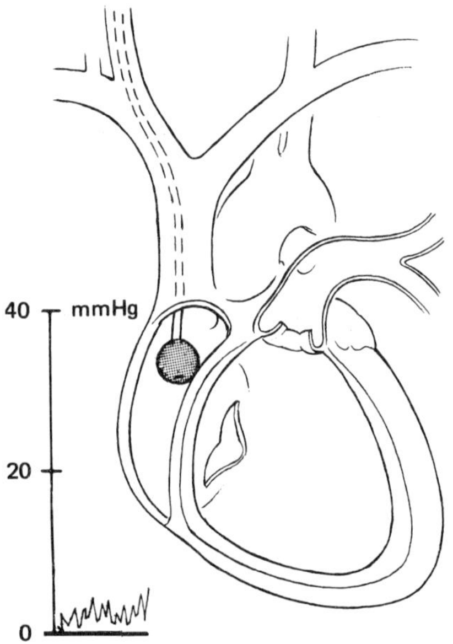

Fig. 11.8. The catheter floats through the superior vena cava and right atrium. The right atrial pressure tracing is shown.

If a pulmonary pressure is not obtained, after advancing the catheter the necessary distance, the balloon should be deflated, the catheter withdrawn to the right atrium and the procedure repeated. Failure is rare, but may occur in patients with a dilated right atrium or ventricle, particularly when the cardiac output is low or there is tricuspid incompetence. The catheter may pass from one cava to the other, if advanced too far before the balloon is inflated, or the catheter may loop and form a knot. A deep inspiration by the patient may facilitate passage. Alternatively, the catheter may be stiffened by

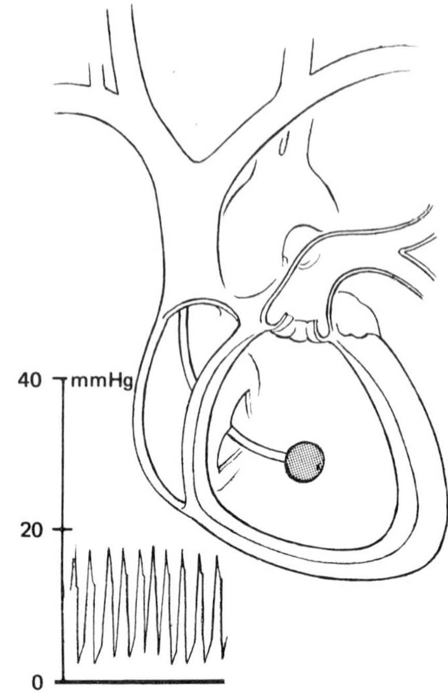

Fig. 11.9. The balloon having passed through the tricuspid valve is carried towards the pulmonary valve. The pressure tracing obtained in the right ventricle is shown.

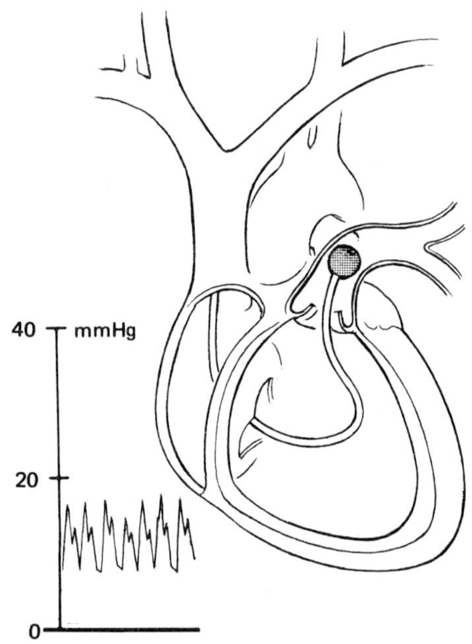

Fig. 11.10. After traversing the pulmonary valve, the characteristic pressure tracing from the pulmonary artery (unwedged) is obtained.

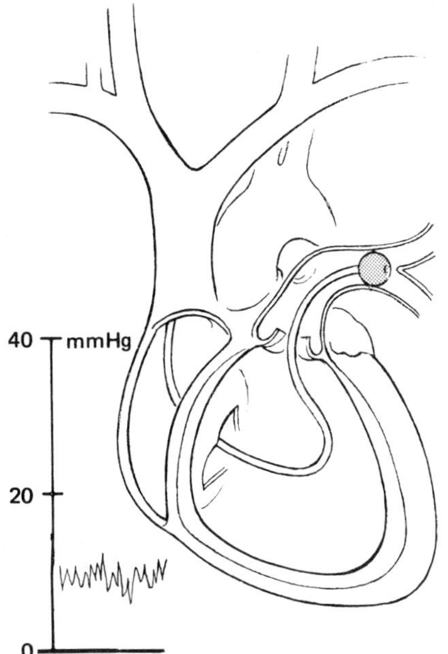

Fig. 11.11. After wedging the balloon in a peripheral radicle of the pulmonary artery, a wedge-pressure recording may be obtained, and other diagnostic manipulations performed with the catheter ports.

perfusion with 5–10 ml of cold intravenous solution.

Once the balloon is lodged in the 'wedge' position it should be deflated. It may then recoil back into the ventricle, in which case the balloon should be re-inflated and the catheter advanced a few more centimetres. With time, the catheter may soften, allowing the transcardiac loop to shorten with migration of the catheter tip into smaller branches of the pulmonary artery and spontaneous wedging. *The pressure contour should be observed continuously so that if a pressure other than that in the pulmonary artery is seen (and this is not eliminated by flushing the catheter) the catheter may be withdrawn 3–4 cm.*

Inflation of the balloon for further determinations should be done slowly and stopped immediately the change to 'wedge' pressure is noted, because the balloon may have migrated into a smaller branch of the pulmonary artery. The pressure generated by a full and rapid inflation of the balloon can rupture the vessel and damage lung parenchyma; this appears to be a particular hazard when the patient has previously suffered from pulmonary hypertension. If a 'wedge' pressure is obtained with a small inflation volume it is safer to withdraw the catheter 3–4 cm. Lengthy periods of balloon inflation are to be avoided as these can cause pulmonary infarction. When the catheter is properly wedged, a pressure excursion of around 2 mmHg will be observed, and in the absence of hypertensive lung disease will approximate to the pulmonary artery end diastolic pressure (PAEDP). Two positive excursions can often be observed during the cardiac cycle with a mean 1–4 mmHg less than that of the pulmonary artery end diastolic pressure.

Damping of the pressure trace may be caused by clotting or air bubbles in the catheter lumen and transducer. Kinking of the lumen may also occur. This will show as a reduction in amplitude of the pulmonary artery pressure which has not been caused by therapy. The mean will be similar to that of the previously recorded pulmonary artery pressure. Having checked the system for bubbles, an attempt should be made to aspirate any clot. If there is any question of the pressure being a 'wedge' pressure, the catheter should be withdrawn. If recurrent damping occurs, the catheter may have to be replaced (14, 15). Also, if a pulmonary artery wedge pressure is recorded at a low balloon volume and inflation continued, a spuriously high pressure will result, possibly related to the over-inflated balloon transmitting its pressure to the catheter tip. Slow inflation of the balloon will avoid this. This is called 'over-wedging'.

Measurement of Pressures

In order to obtain consistent and accurate pressure recordings, the following procedure should be adopted:

The pressure transducer should be placed at a consistent zero reference point, i.e. phlebostatic axis, which can be marked on the patient's chest, and then the transducer system calibrated with a zero point at atmospheric pressure. If possible, a recording of the pressures obtained should be made and kept in the patient's notes for future reference. This also facilitates averaging the measurements over a few heart beats.

The patient would normally be supine for measurement; however, it has been shown that patients can be moved from flat to a 45° Fowler's position without affecting pulmonary 'wedge' pressure or pulmonary artery pressure

(16). In this study the patients were not critically ill.

Pulmonary artery and 'wedge' pressure should be measured at end expiration. The spontaneously breathing patient can be asked to 'count to ten' mentally following a normal expiration so that a measurement may be taken. It has been suggested that patients undergoing mechanical ventilation should have it discontinued for measurements; however, it has been shown that this is unnecessary (17). The same paper concludes that pressures can be accurately determined with a positive end-expiratory pressure (PEEP) of up to $10\,cmH_2O$ pressure. Above these levels the situation remains confused. It has been suggested that the position of the catheter tip within the pulmonary artery (i.e. anterior or posterior) may affect the value, but this has not been substantiated. Always remember to deflate the balloon after measurement of the 'wedge' pressure. It should never be left permanently inflated. The 'wedge' pressure can never be greater than the pulmonary artery end diastolic pressure. If this occurs, pulmonary artery end diastolic pressure has been wrongly assessed, or the catheter is not fully wedged or the balloon is overwedged.

In patients with acute mitral insufficiency the large 'v' wave will obscure the 'a' wave so that transition to 'wedge' pressure may not be obvious. In the shocked patient, pulmonary artery end diastolic pressure approaches the right ventricular diastolic pressure and there may be only a few mmHg difference.

Clinical Applications

Left ventricular function is one of the critical determinants of the systemic circulation of blood. As left ventricular function deteriorates, left ventricular end diastolic pressure will increase and the cardiac output decrease. This will be reflected as an increase in the pulmonary artery wedge pressure. When compensatory mechanisms fail, this will be reflected in the clinical condition of the patient as a falling blood pressure with the signs and symptoms of poor peripheral perfusion. In the past, central venous pressure has been used as an indication of left ventricular function. This will only be the case if the performance of the left and right ventricles is equal, for CVP reflects right ventri-

cular filling pressure. In the critically ill patient this may not be the case. For instance, pulmonary disease may affect the right ventricular pressure without affecting the left, while ischaemic heart disease may raise left ventricular pressures in the presence of a normal central venous pressure. In either condition, the central venous pressure will not reflect the left ventricular end diastolic pressure if there is haemodynamically significant disease. In these circumstances, measurement of the pulmonary artery wedge pressure is necessary to obtain left ventricular end diastolic pressure, i.e. left ventricular filling pressure.

An obstruction between the catheter tip and the left ventricle (such as mitral stenosis or a left atrial myxoma) will invalidate the technique. Also, above a pressure of 25 mmHg, the left atrial pressure tends to be higher. When there is chronic lung disease the left ventricular end diastolic pressure will be higher than the 'wedge' pressure. Normally, the pulmonary artery diastolic pressure is 1–4 mmHg greater than the wedge pressure, a correlation which holds true through the physiological range of pressures so that, once the relationship is established, the former can be used for continuing evaluation. When lung disease is present, the pulmonary artery diastolic pressure will be more than 5 mmHg greater than the wedge pressure, but again the correlation will be constant. The wedge pressure should never exceed the pulmonary artery diastolic pressure; however, erroneously high estimates may be caused by overwedging the catheter. Also, the pulmonary artery diastolic pressure may not be properly identified.

Haemodynamic Parameters

A large series of parameters may be derived from using the flotation balloon catheter, particularly if the thermodilution cardiac output technique is used, and a program has been published for use with a hand-held calculator (18). Calculation of cardiac index, left ventricular stroke work and total peripheral resistance are of value in the therapy of left ventricular failure following myocardial infarction. Vasodilators may be used to increase cardiac output and an optimal wedge pressure determined. The Swan–Ganz catheter may also be used to identify two complications of myocardial infarction, namely ventricular septal rupture and acute mitral incompetence from ruptured chordae tendinae. Abnormally high oxygenation in the pulmonary artery will be found in the former, and a tall 'T' wave in the wedge pressure tracing of the latter.

Cardiac Output Determination by Thermal Dilution

In the past, both the direct Fick procedure and dye dilution techniques have been used for cardiac output determination. However, they are not suitable for rapid and serial measurements at the bedside of the critically ill patient. Fegler introduced the measurement of cardiac output in anaesthetized animals using a thermodilution method in 1954 (19). Branthwaite and Bradley pioneered the introduction of this concept in man in 1968 (20). The routine bedside use of the Swan–Ganz catheter has enabled the introduction of a thermodilution technique for determining cardiac output. Heat (negative heat) is used as an indicator rather than a dye. The addition of a thermistor to the tip of the flow-directed catheter enables the measurement of the fall of temperature that is caused by a chilled solution added to the blood upstream of the thermistor at the central venous pressure or right atrial port. Mixing of the 'tracer' (5 per cent dextrose at 0–5 °C or 22–25 °C) and the blood occurs in the right ventricle and is 'sampled' in the pulmonary artery. Clinical studies have shown an excellent correlation ($r = 0.99$) between dye dilution and thermal dilution techniques (21, 22). The dilution curves obtained by both techniques are similar, except that there is no recirculation to distort the descending limb of the thermodilution curve. Bedside computers are now available to calculate the cardiac output from the curve obtained, and from this the cardiac index (cardiac output/body surface area) may be calculated. The normal values for cardiac index are $2.5–3.5 \, l \, min^{-1} \, m^{-2}$. The thermodilution technique does not require withdrawal of blood from an artery or vein for calibration, and determinations can be performed up to twice per minute. Triplicate cardiac output determinations show a reproducibility of 4 per cent.

In some severely ill patients, fluctuations of pulmonary artery temperature induced by respiratory or cardiac cycles may equal the magnitude of change induced by the 'cold' injection, hence the use of iced dextrose rather than fluid at room temperature to obtain a sufficiently great signal-to-noise ratio. Syringes (10 ml) are filled with 5 per cent dextrose, capped and put in a beaker of sterile fluid immersed in a bath of iced water for at least 45 minutes. After calibrating the cardiac output computer, and if necessary putting a reference probe into one specimen of the iced solution, a cardiac output determination can be performed. A syringe is quickly removed from the ice bath and, with minimal handling of the barrel, the contents injected rapidly (5 s) by either hand or pump into the proximal catheter lumen. Mixing will take place by the time the thermistor is reached, 4 cm from the distal catheter tip in the pulmonary artery. This is connected to the computer, which will calculate the cardiac output. If serial determinations show a variability that exceeds 5 per cent this may be because of:

1. Variations in cardiac rate or rhythm. The ECG should be monitored.

2. Movement of the patient, changing venous return.

3. Variation of body or injectate temperature.

4. A change in haemodynamic state.

If an intracardiac shunt is present, the calculation will be unreliable. This is also true when there is right-sided valvular disease with tricuspid or pulmonary incompetence affecting determination.

Hypovolaemia

Volume replacement can be monitored by the response of the cardiac output and 'wedge' pressure to repeated fluid challenges. An increase of the pressure to normal levels is required. Elevation to 15–18 mmHg will further increase cardiac output but higher values may precipitate pulmonary oedema. When pulmonary oedema exists, from either over-transfusion or left ventricular failure, pressures higher than 30 mmHg may occur. Treatment should be aimed at obtaining a 'wedge' pressure of 15–18 mmHg. A further fall may reduce the cardiac output. If the plasma colloid osmotic pressure is reduced, pulmonary oedema may occur at lower pressures. Puri and colleagues have found radiological evidence of pulmonary oedema present in 80 of 134 patients with reduced plasma protein osmotic pressure compared with 20 of 134 control patients whose plasma oncotic pressure was normal. They also observed that pulmonary oedema was present at a much lower pulmonary artery wedge pressure in the patients with reduced plasma oncotic pressure. Thus, where a reduction in plasma proteins can be demonstrated, correction may be indicated (23).

COMPLICATIONS

During the past 10 years, there has been a low incidence of reported complications associated with the use of balloon flotation catheters. However, it is clear that these potential complications, although rare, are occasionally extremely serious and even fatal. The true incidence of these complications is at present unknown. In the future, it is to be hoped that these will be even further reduced by adopting and following a strict protocol for maintenance of the device, connections and ancillary equipment. Because there are more ports and channels in these devices, scrupulous attention to aseptic technique must be observed at all times. The list of complications reported in the literature is slowly enlarging with the passage of time (*see below*). In reading case reports it is apparent that some of the more severe complications have occurred because catheters may have been left in place for an inappropriate length of time. It is particularly important that these intravascular devices should be removed as soon as possible, with improvement of the patient's condition, and their progress subsequently monitored with non-invasive techniques and clinical examination. It must be remembered that in patients catheterized for longer than 72 hours, the incidence of positive pulmonary blood cultures has been reported to be as high as 50 per cent (24). Swan has recommended that these devices are only left *in situ* for a maximum of 72 hours and replaced unless clinical re-evaluation provides a strong argument for not changing or removing the device (25). Nehme compared variations in insertion techniques and found that the percutaneous internal jugular and subclavian approaches were superior to and associated with fewer complications than the cephalic and basilic vein routes of insertion or cut-down procedures (13).

Complications of Balloon Flotation Catheter Insertion

1. Arterial puncture
2. Pneumothorax
3. Brachial plexus injury
4. Air embolism
5. Cardiac arrhythmias (26, 27)

Major Reported Complications following Catheter Placement

1. Thrombophlebitis (13)
2. Deep venous thrombosis (13)
3. Septicaemia (24)
4. Catheter knotting (28, 29)
5. Balloon rupture
6. Permanent wedging (30)
7. Pulmonary artery rupture (31, 32)
8. Pulmonary haemorrhage (33)
9. Pulmonary embolism (34)
10. Haemoptysis and pneumothorax (35–38)
11. Lung infarction (39, 40)
12. Heart valve trauma (41–43)
13. Pneumoperitoneum (44)

Many of these listed complications are discussed in Chapters 12, 13 and 14. The following events are of particular relevance to balloon flotation catheters.

Cardiac Arrhythmias

Transient arrhythmias during passage of the balloon through the pulmonary valve and the right ventricle are not uncommon. These rhythm disturbances are usually terminated by withdrawal of the catheter but two deaths have been reported (ventricular tachycardia/fibrillation and heart block). Arrhythmias are more commonly associated with displacement of the catheter tip from the main pulmonary artery into the sensitive right ventricular outflow tract. If the balloon is deflated, inflation may stop the arrhythmia.

Balloon Rupture

Thin latex membranes absorb lipoprotein from the blood and lose their elasticity, thus precipitating rupture, particularly if the inflating volumes are exceeded. This is of little consequence, unless air crosses the left side of the heart, when coronary or cerebral embolism could occur. If there is any possibility of a right-to-left shunt, carbon dioxide should be used as the inflating gas.

Knotting

This is especially likely to occur in the finer catheters and with prolonged manipulation, when the shaft will soften. If the catheter is not advanced beyond the distance at which it should have entered the right ventricle, so causing looping and knotting, the complication can be avoided. It has been recommended that advancement of the catheter should be discontinued if the right ventricle has not been entered within 60 cm from the right antecubital fossa, 70 cm from the left antecubital fossa, 35 cm from the internal jugular and subclavian veins, or 50 cm from the femoral vein (22). Furthermore, once the right ventricle has been entered, the catheter tip should reach the pulmonary artery after it has been advanced for no more than a further 15 cm. Should the complication occur, the knot may occasionally be unlooped under fluoroscopic control with the aid of a guide wire (29). Other ingenious techniques have been devised whereby a Teflon sheath is passed over the catheter, the knot tightened until it is of a small dimension and this assembly is then withdrawn back through a small venotomy exposed using a cutdown procedure. Alternatively, via a femoral venotomy, a variety of retrieval forceps, snares and the like have been used to capture the intracardiac catheter; the knot is pulled tight and finally the balloon flotation catheter shaft is cut at the skin level, in the neck, for instance, and the rest of the catheter is withdrawn down through the inferior vena cava and out through the femoral venotomy. All of these procedures need to be carried out under X-ray control (45).

Pulmonary Artery Trauma

Inappropriate inflation of the balloon whilst the catheter tip is located in a peripheral pulmonary artery has caused pulmonary artery rupture and even fatal intrathoracic haemorrhage (*Fig.* 11.12) (46, 47). This, of course, is likely to occur

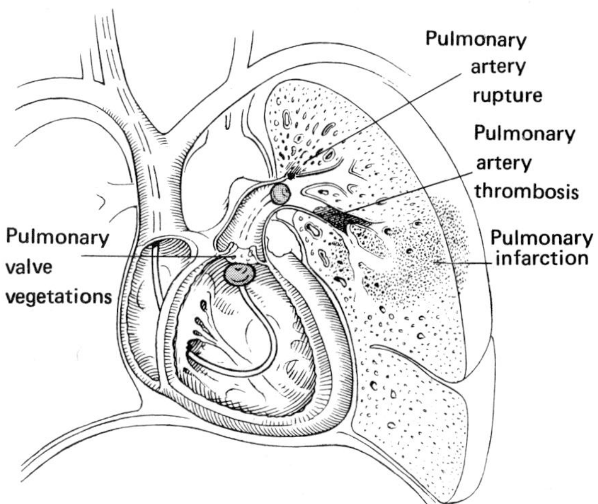

Fig. 11.12. The various pulmonary artery complications of balloon flotation catheters. Vegetations may occur on the valve, pulmonary artery rupture is depicted and haemorrhagic infarction secondary to pulmonary embolism.

if the pulmonary artery is running predominantly in the inter-lobar fissures. The complication may be less severe if a segmental artery tears and the haemorrhage occurs into the lung parenchyma. There have also been reported cases of pulmonary valve damage and insufficiency secondary to mechanical trauma to the pulmonary valve cusps.

Persistent undetected wedging of the catheter may result in small, often unrecognized areas of pulmonary infarction. If solutions are forcibly injected through the catheter to restore a damped trace, the incidence of this complication increases. It can be avoided by continuous monitoring of the catheter tip pressure and taking great care not to leave the balloon inflated for longer than 1 or 2 minutes. The inflation of the balloon should always be slow (0·2 ml increments) and stopped as soon as the 'wedge' pressure is obtained. Slow inflation also reduces the possibility of balloon rupture.

References

1. Swan H. J. C., Ganz W., Forrester J. S. et al.: Catheterisation of the heart in man with the use of a flow-directed balloon-tipped catheter. *N. Engl. J. Med.* 1970; **283**: 447–51.
2. Bradley R. D.: Diagnostic right heart catheterisation with miniature catheters in severely ill patients. *Lancet* 1964; **2**: 941–2.

3. Fogarty T. J., Cranley J. J., Krause J. J. et al.: A method for extraction of arterial emboli and thrombi. *Surg. Gynecol. Obstet.* 1963; **116**: 241–5.

4. Swan H. J. C., Ganz W.: Complications with flow-directed balloon-tipped catheters. *Ann. Intern. Med.* 1979; **91**: 494–7.

5. Dalen J. E.: Bedside haemodynamic monitoring. *N. Engl. J. Med.* 1979; **301**: 1176–8.

6. Forrester J. S., Diamond G., McHugh T. J.: Filling pressures in the right and left sides of the heart in acute myocardial infarction. A reappraisal of central venous pressure monitoring. *N. Engl. J. Med.* 1971; **285**: 190–3.

7. Mond H. B., Hunt D., Sloman G.: Haemodynamic monitoring in the coronary care unit using the Swan–Ganz right heart catheter. *Br. Heart J.* 1973; **35**: 635–42.

8. Civetta J. M., Gabel J. C.: Flow directed pulmonary artery catheterization in surgical patients. Indications and modifications of techniques. *Ann. Surg.* 1972; **176**: 753–6.

9. Pace N. L.: A critique of flow-directed pulmonary arterial catheterisation. *Anaesthesiology* 1977; **47**: 455–65.

10. Swan H. J. C.: Central venous pressure monitoring is an out-moded procedure of limited practical value. In: Ingelfinger F. J., Elbert R. V., Finland M. (ed.): *Controversy in Internal Medicine, II.* Philadelphia: Saunders, 1974: 185–93.

11. Barash P. G., Dizon C. T.: An introducer for intra-operative percutaneous insertion of a Swan–Ganz catheter. *Anaesthesia Analgesia (Cleve.)* 1977; **56**: 444–6.

12. Kaplan J. R., Miller E. D.: Insertion of a Swan–Ganz catheter. *Anaesthesiology Rev.* 1976; Nov., 22–5.

13. Nehme A. D.: Swan–Ganz catheter: comparison of insertion techniques. *Arch. Surg.* 1980; **115**: 1194–6.

14. Shoum S., Kahn R. C., Howland W. S.: A guide-wire technique for replacement of Swan–Ganz catheters. *Anaesthesia Analgesia (Cleve.)* 1980; **59**: 455–6.

15. Brotman S., Wiles C. E., Cowley R. A.: Method for re-introduction of Swan–Ganz catheter. *Arch. Surg.* 1981; **116**: 483.

16. Woods S. L., Mansfield L. W.: Effects of body position upon pulmonary artery and pulmonary wedge pressures in non-critically ill patients. *Heart Lung* 1976; **5**: 89.

17. Davidson R., Parker M., Harrison R. A.: The validity of determination of pulmonary wedge pressure during mechanical ventilation. *Chest* 1978; **73**: 352–5.

18. Shabot M. M., Shoemaker W. C., State D.: Rapid computation of cardiorespiratory variables with a programmable calculator. *Crit. Care Med.* 1977; **5**: 111–17.

19. Fegler G.: Measurement of cardiac output in anaesthetised animals by a thermodilution method. *Q. J. Exp. Physiol.* 1954; **39**: 153–64.

20. Branthwaite M. A., Bradley R. D.: Measurement of cardiac output by thermal dilution in man. *J. Appl. Physiol.* 1968; **24**: 434–8.

21. Weisel R. D., Berger R. L., Hechtman H. B.: Measurement of cardiac output by thermodilution. *N. Engl. J. Med.* 1975; **292**: 682–4.

22. Buchbinder N., Ganz W.: Haemodynamic monitoring: invasive techniques. *Anaesthesiology* 1976; **45**: 146–55.

23. Puri V. K., Weil M. H., Micheals S. et al.: Pulmonary oedema associated with reduction in plasma oncotic pressure. *Surg. Gynecol. Obstet.* 1980; **151**: 344–8.

24. Applefeld J. J., Caruthers T. E., Reno D. J. et al.: Assessment of the sterility of long-term cardiac catheterisation using the thermo-dilution Swan–Ganz catheter. *Chest* 1978; **74**: 377–80.

25. Swan H. J. C., Ganz W.: Use of balloon flotation catheters in critically ill patients. *Surg. Clin. North Am.* 1975; **55**: 506.

26. Geha D.: Persistent arrhythmias associated with placement of a Swan–Ganz catheter. *Anaesthesiology* 1973; **39**: 650–3.

27. Thomson I. R., Dalton B. C., Lappas D. G. et al.: Right bundle-branch block and complete heart block caused by Swan–Ganz catheter. *Anaesthesiology* 1979; **51**: 359–62.

28. Lipp H., O'Donoghue K., Resnekov L.: Intracardiac knotting of a flow-directed balloon catheter. *N. Engl. J. Med.* 1971; **284**: 220.

29. Mond H. G., Clark D. W., Nesbitt S. J.: A technique for unknotting a flow-directed balloon catheter. *Chest* 1975; **67**: 731–2.

30. Meister S. G.: Potential artefact in measurement of left ventricular filling pressure with flow-directed catheters. *Catheterisation Cardiovasc. Diag.* 1976; **2**: 175–9.

31. Chun G. M. H., Ellestead H.: Perforation of the pulmonary artery by a Swan–Ganz catheter. *N. Engl. J. Med.* 1971; **284**: 1041–2.

32. Deren M. M., Barash P. G., Hammond G. L. et al.: Perforation of the pulmonary artery requiring pneumonectomy after the use of a flow-directed (Swan–Ganz) catheter. *Thorax* 1979; **34**: 550–3.

33. Pape L. A., Haffajee C. I., Markis J. E. et al.: Fatal pulmonary haemorrhage after use of the flow-directed balloon-tipped catheter. *Ann. Intern. Med.* 1979; **90**: 344–7.

34. Yorra F. H., Oblath R., Jaffe H.: Massive thrombosis associated with the use of the Swan–Ganz catheter. *Chest* 1974; **65**: 682–4.

35. Lapin E. S., Murray J. A.: Haemoptysis with flow-directed cardiac catheterisation. *JAMA* 1972; **220**: 1246.

36. Krantz E. M., Viljoen J. F.: Haemoptysis following insertion of a Swan–Ganz catheter. *Br. J. Anaesth.* 1979; **51**: 457–9.

37. Kopman E. A.: Haemoptysis associated with the use of a flow-directed catheter. *Anaesthesia Analgesia (Cleve.)* 1979; **58**: 153–6.

38. Farber D. L., Rose D. M., Bassell G. M. et al.: Haemoptysis and pneumothorax after removal of a persistently wedged pulmonary artery catheter. *Crit. Care Med.* 1981; **9**: 494–5.

39. Foote G. A., Schobel S. I., Hodges M.: Pulmonary complications of the flow-directed balloon-tipped catheter. *N. Engl. J. Med.* 1974; **290**: 927.

40. McLoud T. C., Putman C. E.: Radiology of the Swan–Ganz catheter and associated pulmonary complications. *Radiology* 1975; **116**: 19–22.

41. O'Toole J. D., Wurtzbacher J. J., Wearner N. E. et al.: Pulmonary valve injury and insufficiency during pulmonary artery catheterisation. *N. Engl. J. Med.* 1979; **301**: 1167–8.

42. Boscoe M. J., Lange S. de.: Damage to the tricuspid valve with a Swan–Ganz catheter. *Br. Med. J.* 1981; **283**: 346–9.

43. Pace N. L., Horton W.: Indwelling pulmonary artery catheters. Their relationship to aseptic thrombotic endocardial vegetations. *JAMA* 1975; **233**: 893–4.

44. Smith G. B., Willatts S. M.: A hazard of Swan–Ganz catheterisation. *Anaesthesia* 1981; **36**: 398–401.

45. Block P. C.: Snaring of a Swan–Ganz catheter. *J. Thorac. Cardiovasc. Surg.* 1976; **71**: 917–19.

46. McDaniel D. D., Stone J. G., Faltas A. N. et al. Catheter-induced pulmonary artery haemorrhage. Diagnosis and management in cardiac operations. *J. Thorac. Cardiovasc. Surg.* 1981; **82**: 1–4.

47. Barash P. G., Nardi D., Hammond G. et al.: Catheter-induced pulmonary artery perforation. Mechanisms, management and modifications. *J. Thorac. Cardiovasc. Surg.* 1981; **82**: 5–11.

Chapter 12

Complications of Central Venous Catheterization

J. L. Peters and C. P. O. Garrett

The world literature covering this aspect of central venous catheterization in patient care provides a salutary experience and should stimulate all clinicians to improve upon their technique and avoid errors of judgement, whether by omission or commission. Unfortunately, the very nature of hospital staff organization dictates that the maintenance and care of central venous catheter systems always involves numerous individuals. Furthermore, there are multiple components in the infusion system which can fail, fracture, fall apart or become contaminated by micro-organisms. For such a unique clinical arrangement to be successful, it must obey the following verse from 'The Laws of the Navy':

> On the strength of one link in the cable
> Dependeth the might of the chain;
> Who knows when thou mayest be tested?
> So live that thou bearest the strain!
>
> Captain Hopwood

Any weakness involving either the judgement or ability of individuals in the chain of people responsible for the care of the patient, or the chain of plastic components in the infusion system, may lead to disaster.

In view of their importance, the specific problems of sepsis and catheter embolism have been dealt with separately in Chapters 13 and 14. In this chapter we will attempt to highlight the remaining complications and point out means of avoiding these pitfalls where appropriate. Caution, vigilance and gentleness are watchwords which require constant repetition by those engaged in this sphere of patient care, for the old medical aphorism, 'what can happen, will happen', is unfortunately applicable when a retrospective analysis of clinical series and case reports is made.

Some events are unavoidable, as exemplified by the occurrence of ventricular fibrillation occurring after palpation in the region of the carotid sinus, just prior to an attempt at internal jugular vein cannulation (1). Human error is an almost unaccountable factor; nurses can misunderstand the nature of tubes attached to patients, and Goyanes described an incident in which a blood transfusion was attached to a Redivac drain tube and infused into a shoulder wound, whilst the Redivac bottle was connected to an adjacent central venous catheter which promptly filled with venous blood (2). Invariably, such events associated with this sphere of medical practice go unreported in the literature and thus retrospective surveys often fail to provide a satisfactory picture of the magnitude of related complications. It is important to appreciate the severe consequences that can occur following surgical mishaps. Professor F. D. Moore of Boston, a pioneer in the field of surgical metabolism, has recently emphasized the 'high cost of low frequency events' in auditing the anatomy and economics of surgical mishaps (3). Although his colleagues studied the whole range of perioperative complications, the same principles apply to central venous therapy.

The complications associated with central venous catheterization may be conveniently grouped for discussion into three main categories:

1. Immediate—procedure-related events.
2. Malposition—technical failures in placement.

3. Delayed—sequelae arising following a period of catheter placement.

Inevitably, there is some overlap and an attempt has been made to illustrate the way in which the generic problems associated with central venous catheter insertion technique, maintenance and large volume infusions of electrolyte and parenteral nutrition solutions are related (*Fig.* 12.1). The world literature merely indicates the tip of an iceberg, and this is represented by the pyramidal shape in the diagram. Comprehensive reviews have been documented in recent years (4–6). The crucial role of the radiologist in the early recognition of immediate post-insertion abnormalities has also been emphasized by Mitchell and Clark in their excellent and concise review of experience and the literature (7).

Herbst conducted a prospective study of complications at the North Carolina Memorial Hospital, Chapel Hill, and detected an 11 per cent incidence of problems associated with catheter placement. A pattern analysis suggested inexperience on the part of the clinician as the most important cause of complications (8). His work confirmed the findings of Bernard and Stahl, who demonstrated that the non-infective complications using the infraclavicular approach correlated with the clinical experience in the technique (9). There was an 8·1 per cent incidence for those clinicians who had performed less than 50 procedures and a 0 per cent incidence for clinicians who had inserted more than 50 catheters. In 1972, a review of the literature by Borja on the status of infraclavicular subclavian vein catheterization at that time revealed incidences of problems in the range 0·4–9·9 per cent (10). James and Myers reported a 6 per cent complication rate in the following year with the same technique (11). Burri has reviewed the experience of 17 authors and 10 013 subjects who had internal jugular vein catheterization (5). Whilst the overall complication rate is lower than for the subclavian approach, this procedure is also not without risk in inexperienced hands. It is apparent that sporadic case reports will continue to be published when the more difficult procedures are being carried out by unsupervised and untrained junior staff. Thus, in any institution, it is essential that adequate training and peer review are provided, the safest and most resilient equipment used and individual clinicians should not extend themselves in emergency situations by performing operations which are beyond their experience. The concept of risk to the layman has a wholly different meaning, and, for example, Kletz has suggested that a risk of 1 in 10 million per person per year should be considered unacceptable and corrected, regardless of cost (12). It should be noted that the United Kingdom chemical industry deals with any activity that contributes more than 0·4 to the Fatal Accident Frequency Rate (FAFR) per 1000. Lord Rothschild, in the context of risks associated with nuclear power, suggested in 1978

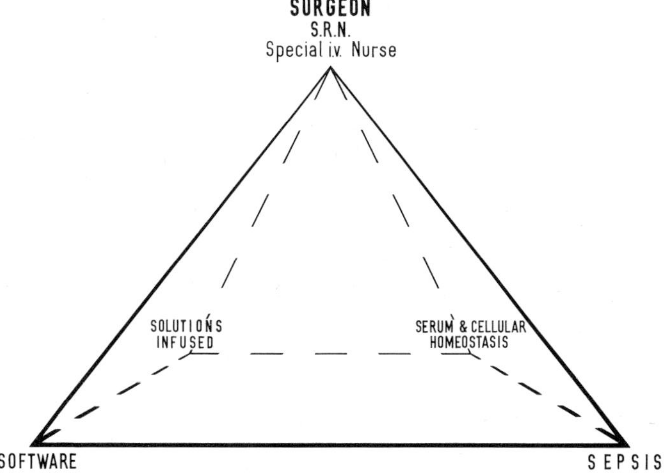

Fig. 12.1. Complications of central venous catheterization and parenteral nutrition.

that a risk in the order of 1 in 10 000 per person per year (roughly that of being killed in a car accident) might be a good starting point for selecting the maximum acceptable level of risk (13). Against this background, the reported figures for serious morbidity and mortality associated with the use of central venous catheters compare very unfavourably indeed.

There can be no room for compromise or complacency in the overall management of these apparently innocuous and simple procedures because, in medicine and surgery, many of the complications to be described may progress to a fatal outcome. Tuition should be mandatory for any tyro, before attempts are made to cannulate veins in the root of the neck. As a radiologist, or cardiologist, one would not be allowed to perform right heart cardiac catheterization without formal training in the technique. Similarly, a cautious awareness of the immediate and delayed problems should temper the enthusiasm for these invasive procedures and ensure that a competent clinician chooses the correct catheter, and decides upon the most appropriate approach for each patient.

IMMEDIATE COMPLICATIONS

The tabulation of complications as shown below (Table 12.1) does not adequately convey the morbidity for individual patients, e.g. the painful expanding haematoma or the rapid development of subcutaneous emphysema causing airways obstruction sufficient to require tracheostomy. Almost all procedure-related complications can be eliminated by careful technique, whilst a few will naturally occur because of variations in human anatomy. Selected references have been provided.

Arterial Puncture

Fortunately, little harm usually arises if this mishap is recognized promptly and treated correctly (25). The blood will escape with force into the syringe, although this may not be so obvious in a hypovolaemic and hypotensive patient (*Figs.* 12.2 and 12.3). The needle should be removed quickly and firm digital pressure applied simultaneously to the vessel for at least 5 minutes by the clock. This invariably controls the haemorrhage and exploration by a surgeon

Table 12.1. **Procedure-related complications of central venous catheterization**

Site of trauma	*Clinical sequelae*
Atrial puncture	Haematoma Carotid artery laceration (14, 15) Subclavian artery perforation (9, 16, 17) Ascending cervical artery laceration (18) Internal mammary artery laceration (19, 20) Pulmonary artery laceration (apical branch) (21) Brachiocephalic false aneurysm (22) Aortic puncture (23) Aortic dissection (24) Arteriovenous fistula (25)
Pleural and mediastinal injury	Pneumothorax (26–30) Haemothorax (21, 31, 32) Haemomediastinum (9)
Venous cannulation	Air embolism (6, 11, 33–40) Catheter embolism (*see* Chapter 14)
Lymphatic vessels	Thoracic duct laceration (41)
Neurological injury	Phrenic nerve (21, 42–44) Brachial plexus injury (27) Recurrent laryngeal nerve injury (45, 46) Horner's syndrome (47) Fatal cerebrovascular episode (48, 49)
Trachea	Endotracheal cuff deflation (31, 50, 51)
Thyroid	Penetration of a thyroid cyst (52)

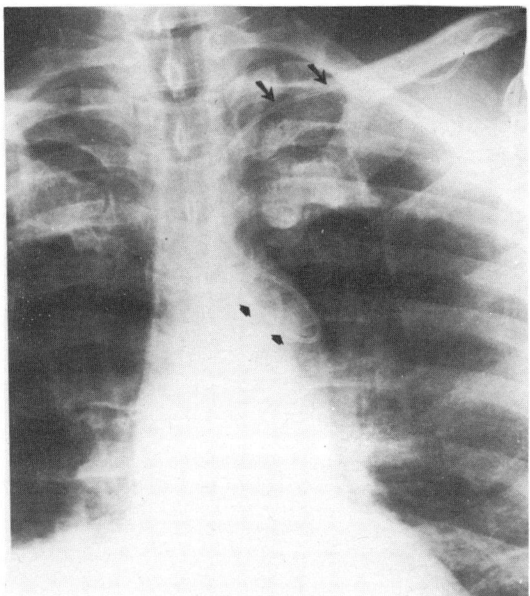

Fig. 12.2. Aortic catheterization from the subclavian artery. A 73-year-old man had surgery for a perforated gastric ulcer. A left subclavian catheter was inserted just before the film. The subclavian catheter has entered the subclavian artery (long arrows) and the tip is situated within the aortic arch (short arrows). (Reproduced by kind permission of Dr S. E. Mitchell and the Editor of the *American Journal of Roentgenology.*)

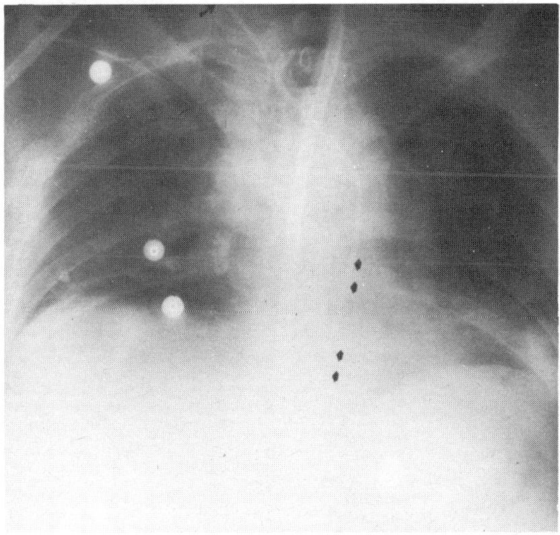

Fig. 12.3. Aortic catheterization from the carotid artery. The right carotid artery has been inadvertently catheterized during right internal jugular vein cannulation. The catheter having been threaded through the right common carotid artery (long arrow) passes into the descending aorta (short arrows). (Reproduced by kind permission of Dr S. E. Mitchell and the Editor of the *American Journal of Roentgenology.*)

is only rarely required. A small apical haematoma may be seen on subsequent chest X-ray films (*Fig.* 12.4). Occasionally, blood will extravasate down to the mediastinum and this region will appear widened on subsequent post-insertion chest X-rays (*Fig.* 12.5). Disastrous haemorrhage may occur if the needle track has communicated with the pleura. The aorta can be injured by the cannula and needle in current use, as exemplified in the case described by McDaniel and Grossman (53). The full spectrum of inadvertent vascular injury is demonstrated in Table 12.1. The possibility of late aneurysm formation or arteriovenous fistula must always be considered. These complications can be eliminated for the infraclavicular approach by using a Doppler ultrasound probe to identify, and hence avoid, the vessel (54).

Pneumothorax

No percutaneous approach to the veins in the root of the neck is free of this complication, and

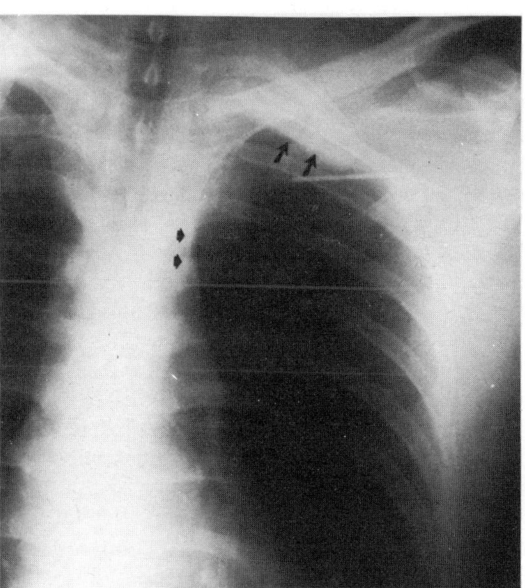

Fig. 12.4. Apical haematoma. A 22-year-old man with burns had a normal chest film 2 weeks earlier. After several unsuccessful attempts at left subclavian catheterization, a catheter was threaded. The catheter tip (short arrows) lies within the mediastinum, too far lateral to be within the innominate vein. A local haematoma overlying the apex of the left lung has formed secondary to vascular injury from multiple catheterization attempts (long arrows). This appearance cleared completely after 1 week.

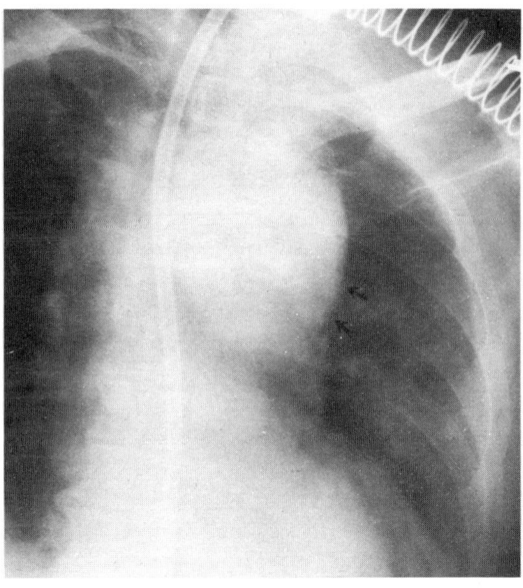

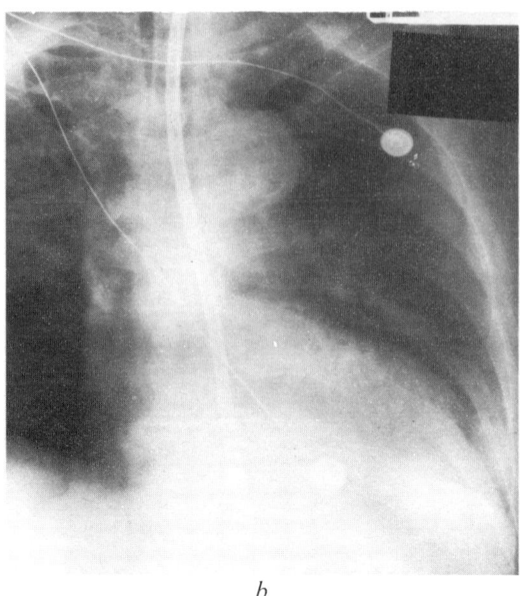

a   *b*

Fig. 12.5. *a*, Mediastinal haematoma. A left subclavian catheterization was attempted in a 79-year-old man. Pulsatile arterial blood was noted to escape from the cannula and the device was removed. There is marked widening of the mediastinum compared with a film taken 2 days earlier (*b*). The possibility of an aortic dissection was considered, but the speed of resolution was more in favour of a mediastinal haematoma. (Reproduced by kind permission of Dr S. E. Mitchell and the Editor of the *American Journal of Roentgenology.*)

indeed Oosterlee and Dudley recently advocated a simple method of exposing and puncturing the subclavian vein under direct vision (55). The operation may be performed under local anaesthesia, with a 2-cm long incision being made under the mid-point of the clavicle. The fibres of the pectoralis muscles and clavipectoral fascia are separated, the vein identified, cannulated and the catheter tunnelled to a distant site on the anterior chest wall. Pneumothorax accounts for approximately 30 per cent of reported complications in the literature (*Fig.* 12.6). The extent of pulmonary collapse varies and reported pneumothoraces have been partial, total, under tension and even bilateral. This latter catastrophe occurs when one pneumothorax is created and an immediate attempt is made to cannulate the contralateral vein. Pneumothoraces are particularly dangerous if induced when the patient is receiving mechanical ventilation, a pneumomediastinum and massive subcutaneous emphysema may develop, which can require tracheostomy (27). The development of a pneumothorax may be delayed, and this should be borne in mind in the presence of insidious deterioration in the patient's cardiorespiratory

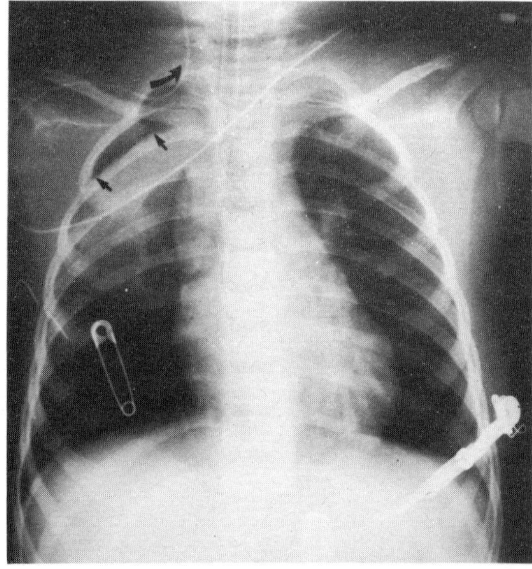

Fig. 12.6. This shows a small apical pneumothorax on the right (short arrows) created following an attempted subclavian vein catheterization. The catheter has, in addition, been misplaced into the right internal jugular vein. The pneumothorax resolved following the insertion of a chest drain. The subclavian route should not be a primary choice in children.

function (56). The development of a tension pneumothorax with the rapid onset of death has been reported sporadically in the literature, usually when catheterization attempts have been made at the beginning of surgical procedures. The vast majority of such events are treated successfully and without late sequelae by the careful insertion of a chest drain followed by a period of underwater-seal drainage. A high index of suspicion must always be maintained and the diagnosis must be made early in order to avoid the serious effects of a tension pneumothorax. Many now recommend serial chest X-rays in inspiration to be performed if a central venous nutrition catheter has been inserted prior to major surgery.

Air Embolism

This serious and potentially fatal hazard should never be allowed to occur nowadays during the insertion procedure. Aubaniac (57) and Yoffa (17) both recognized the possibility of air embolism occurring when they described their original techniques for inserting central venous catheters. The complication was first noted by Baden in 1964, who reported three cases (33). Air was heard to rush into the circulation, although no untoward reaction was noted. The first fatal air embolism occurring during the insertion of a central venous catheter was described in 1969 by Levinsky (34), and examples of subsequent case reports are listed in the references of Table 12.1. Since then, the nursing and medical profession has virtually eliminated this problem by always placing the patient in a 20–30° head-down tilt during the procedure. Borja et al. (38) emphasized that it is not sufficient simply to elevate the legs alone, since one of their patients suffered a fatal air embolism when the standard precaution was omitted. A co-operative patient can provide a further safeguard by performing a Valsalva manoeuvre during the cannulation procedure. The potential for air to enter rapidly into the circulation should never be underestimated, especially when the patient is hypovolaemic, tachypnoeic or in a recumbent position. Any vacillation on the part of the clinician during the cannulation procedure can result in a significant bolus of air entering the great veins. The introducing catheter hub should never be left unguarded for more than a fraction of a

second. Some newer catheters, e.g. Flexi-cath (H. G. Wallace Ltd), have been fitted with an integral compressible hub in order to facilitate this manoeuvre. The problem of air embolism is highlighted later in the section of this chapter on delayed complications.

Neurological Injury

Signs of neurological deficit have appeared immediately after insertion procedures in the peripheral nerves, cranial nerves and the central nervous system. Fortunately, these events are extremely rare, but they do serve to highlight the care that must be exercised by the clinician in selecting the correct line of approach when performing percutaneous cannulations. This is particularly the case for the internal jugular vein, and it is vital that the introducing cannula and needle assembly are not inserted to an inappropriate depth beyond or medial to the vein. The episodes of cerebral infarction reported presumably arose following embolization from arteriosclerotic plaques in the carotid or vertebral arteries which were dislodged, either by manipulation or needle puncture.

Tracheal, Thyroid and Lymphatic Trauma

Injury to these structures in the neck can easily arise, especially in children, unless particular care is taken during the advancement of the needle. It is wise to avoid cannulation attempts close to the confluence of the internal jugular vein and subclavian vein on the left side of the neck because of the variable course of the thoracic duct in this situation. Penetration of the trachea has usually been reported by anaesthetists after the cuffs on the recently inserted endotracheal tubes deflate.

Summary

This necessarily brief synopsis will hopefully emphasize to the beginner the need for caution when engaged in these techniques. The factors that appear to influence the incidence and severity of these procedure-related complications include the experience of the operator, the unknown anatomical variations in the patient and the presence of hypovolaemia. It is extremely important that the patient is placed in the

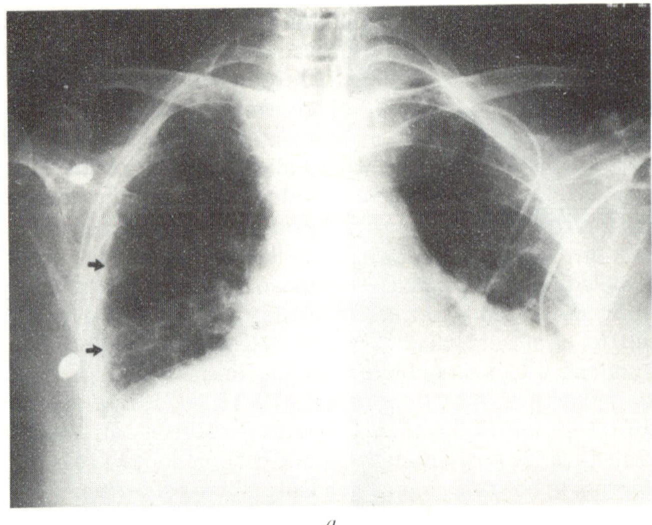

a

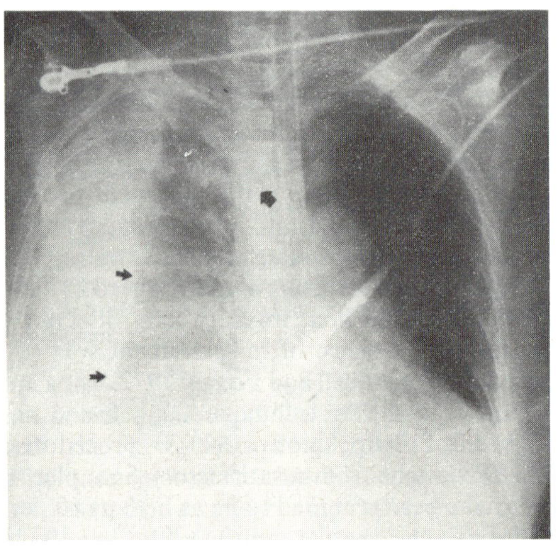

b

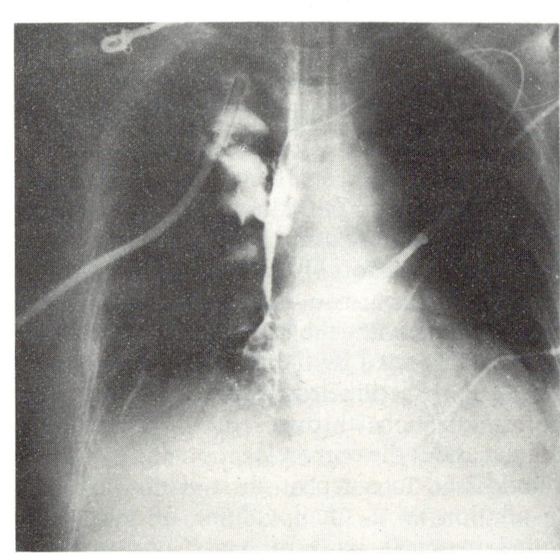

c

Fig. 12.9. *a*, Following the insertion of a left infraclavicular subclavian catheter into a 67-year-old lady for the purposes of parenteral nutrition, slight dyspnoea developed (short arrows indicate a developing right hydrothorax). *b*, The difficulty in breathing progressed and a further film revealed a large right-sided pleural effusion (short arrows) and an acute angulation of the central catheter inserted into the left subclavian vein and superior vena cava (broad arrow). This suggested that the central catheter had perforated the junction of the innominate vein and superior vena cava. *c*, This, in fact, had occurred; the effusion was cleared rapidly via an intercostal chest drain and the intrapleural situation of the catheter shown by contrast radiography. On retrospective analysis of the insertion procedure, a free reflux of blood was not obtained when the administration set controls were open and the bag of infusion fluid lowered below the level of the patient's heart. This is a cardinal test of correct intravascular placement.

Malatinsky et al., in the Postgraduate Medical School of Bratislava in Czechoslovakia, have also presented a comprehensive review of their own work and analysed X-rays performed routinely for aberrant placement and loop formation (73):

Route of insertion	Incidence of malposition
External jugular vein	30%
Internal jugular vein	5·7%
Infraclavicular subclavian vein	5·5%
Supraclavicular subclavian vein	1·4%
Total incidence	5·3%
Loop formation	2·9%

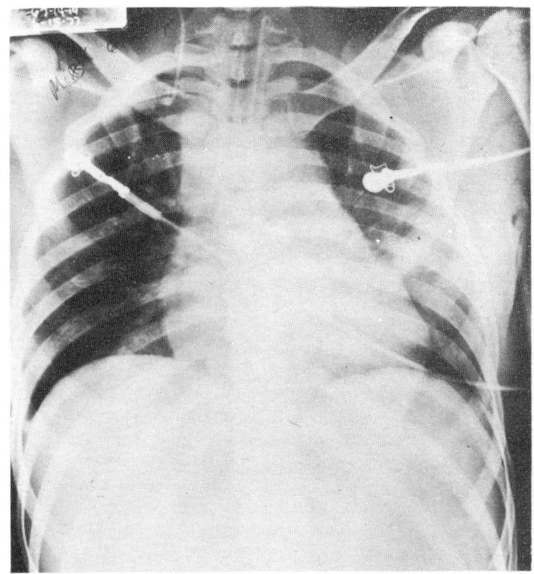

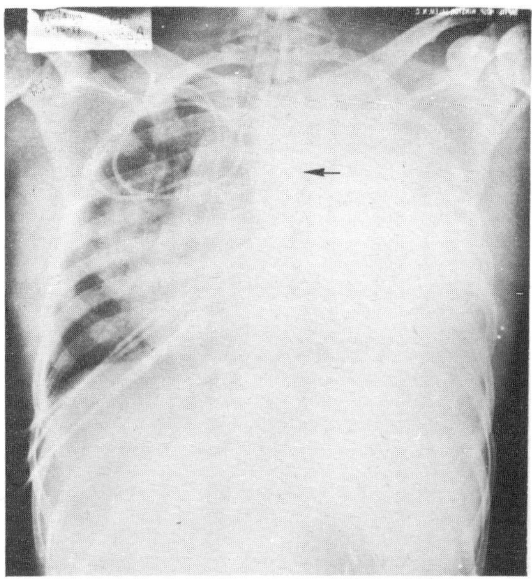

Fig. 12.10. A chest X-ray taken shortly after attempted cannulation of the right internal jugular vein. The patient had been injured in a road traffic accident, requiring splenectomy and drainage of a retroperitoneal haematoma. Easy aspiration of blood had occurred, but the catheter could not be advanced satisfactorily. (Reproduced by kind permission of Dr R. B. Hopkinson, Dr C. E. Parkin and the Editor of *Anaesthesia and Analgesia: Current Researches.*) (*Figs.* 12.10, 12.11 and 12.12 highlight the diagnostic difficulties encountered when patients have been involved in trauma likely to have produced concomitant intrathoracic pathology.)

Fig. 12.11. A left internal jugular vein cannulation was performed in the same patient as shown in *Fig.* 12.10. A tension hydrothorax developed and the tip of the catheter was proved to be situated in the pleural cavity by the use of a contrast study and was seen lying adjacent to the left side of the T4 vertebral body. (Reproduced by kind permission of Dr R. B. Hopkinson, Dr C. E. Parkin and the Editor of *Anaesthesia and Analgesia: Current Researches.*)

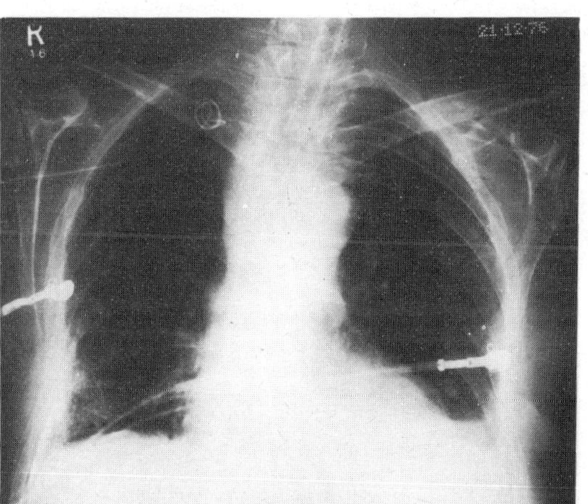

Fig. 12.13. A post-insertion chest X-ray taken with the arm in 90° of abduction following passage of a long central venous catheter from the antecubital fossa reveals a complex loop formation in the subclavian vein.

Fig. 12.12. Resolution of the problem occurred after insertion of bilateral intercostal chest drains and continuing resuscitation involving the use of a Swan–Ganz catheter inserted via the right subclavian vein. (Reproduced by kind permission of Dr R. B. Hopkinson, Dr C. E. Parkin and the Editor of *Anaesthesia and Analgesia: Current Researches.*)

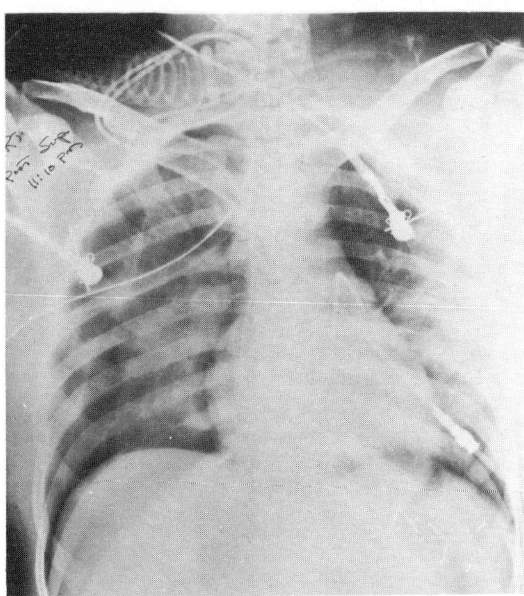

Fig. 12.12.

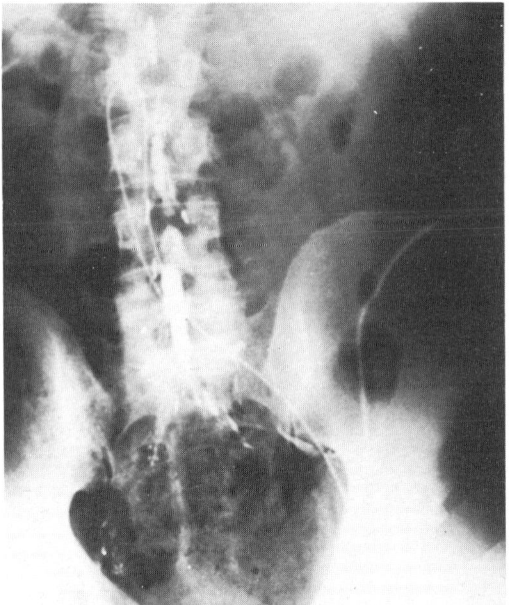

Fig. 12.14. A catheter tunnelled down the left side of the anterior abdominal wall and passed into the vena cava through a branch of the long saphenous vein has unfortunately looped back on itself and this required readjustment under the image intensifier. (The patient had undergone a previous myelogram.)

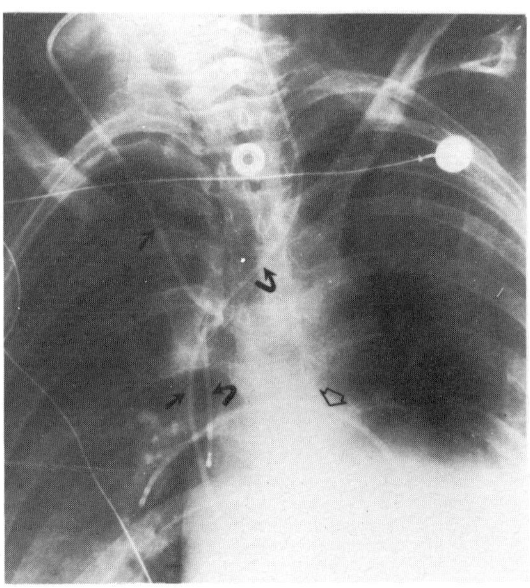

Fig. 12.15. Knotted central venous catheters. A Swan–Ganz catheter inserted via the right internal jugular vein is seen coursing into the right pulmonary artery (hollow arrow). A second catheter, a transvenous pacemaker, has been inserted via the left internal jugular vein and the catheters became knotted in the superior vena cava (solid arrows).

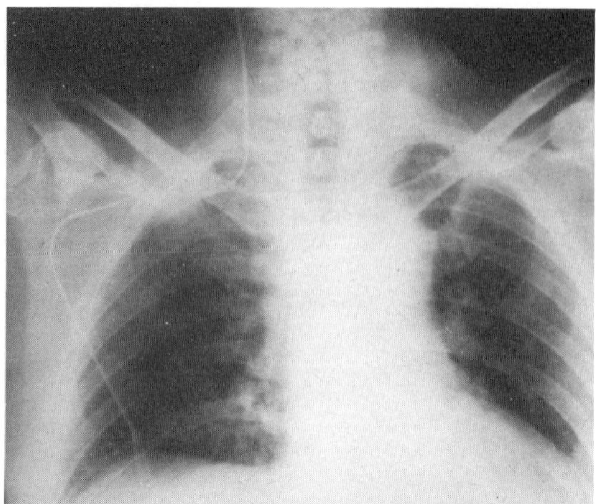

Fig. 12.16. Malposition into the internal jugular vein.

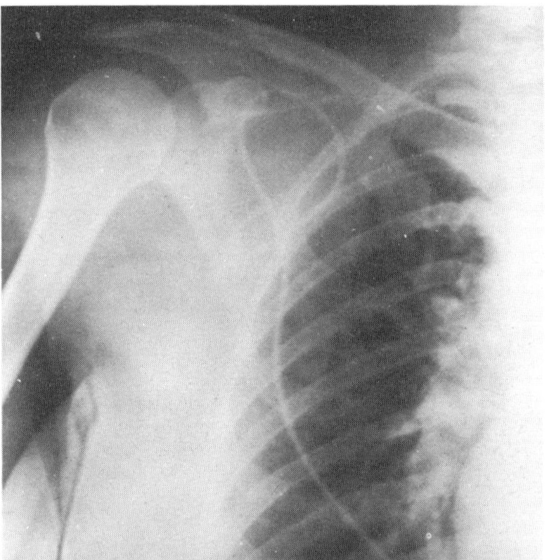

Fig. 12.17. Malposition of a Hickman catheter inserted via the right cephalic vein. The silicone tubing has found its way into another tributary of the subclavian vein in the subscapular region.

The vast majority of such incidents are of no consequence provided that the malposition is recognized by X-ray and corrected (*Fig.* 12.22). The authors prefer to use an image intensifier and screen the catheter into position whenever possible. This must be done before a tunnelling procedure is contemplated. Very little extra time is required and the patient is saved from further unnecessary manipulations of the catheter system. Central catheters which pass up into the

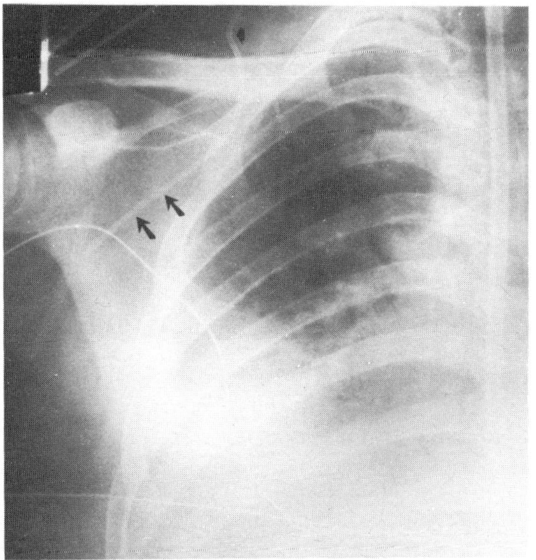

Fig. 12.18. Axillary vein placement from the external jugular vein. A right internal jugular vein catheterization was attempted by the central approach. At the insertion point (short arrow) the catheter lies too far lateral to be within the internal jugular vein and was probably into the right external jugular vein. The catheter tip passed into the axillary vein (long arrows), a common malposition of the external jugular vein approach. (Reproduced by kind permission of Dr S. E. Mitchell and the Editor of the *American Journal of Roentgenology.*)

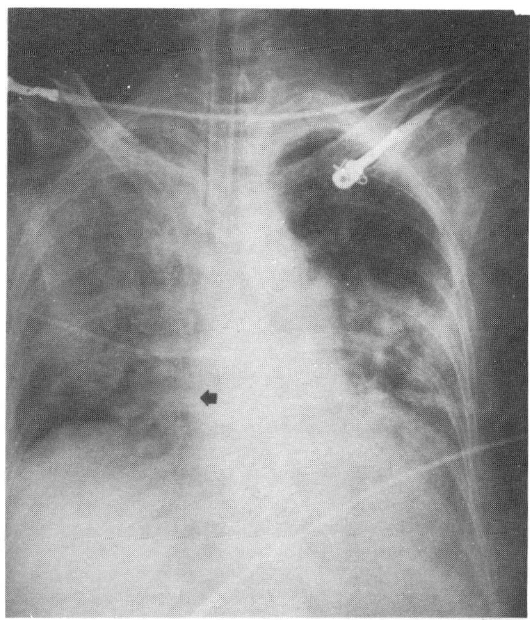

Fig. 12.20. A catheter inserted via the right infraclavicular subclavian route is too far advanced and the tip is situated within the right atrium.

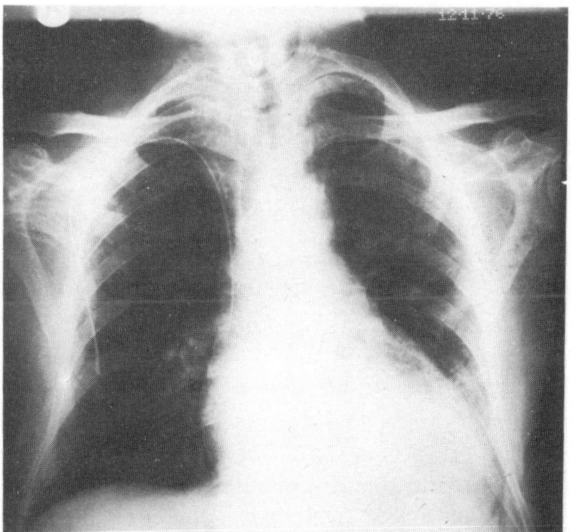

Fig. 12.21. A right infraclavicular subclavian catheter with the tip in the inferior reaches of the superior vena cava. A more suitable position is approximately level with the aortic knuckle.

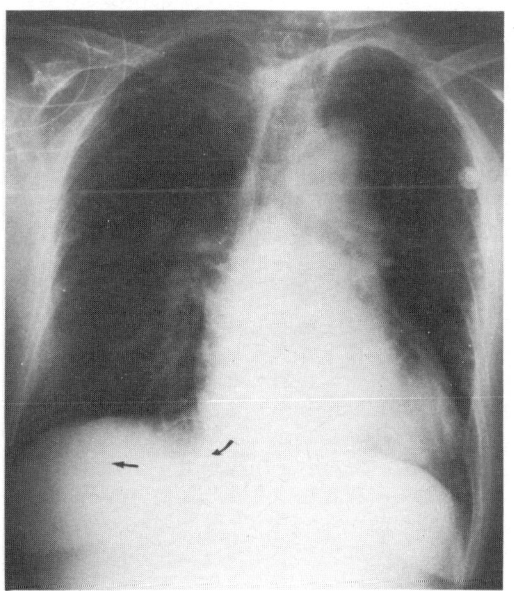

Fig. 12.19. This miniature oxygen electrode has been inserted too far and has passed through into a branch of the right hepatic vein.

internal jugular vein may cause the conscious patient to complain of the 'ear-gurgling' sign as the infusion is commenced (74). Whilst this may seem an interesting and amusing clinical finding,

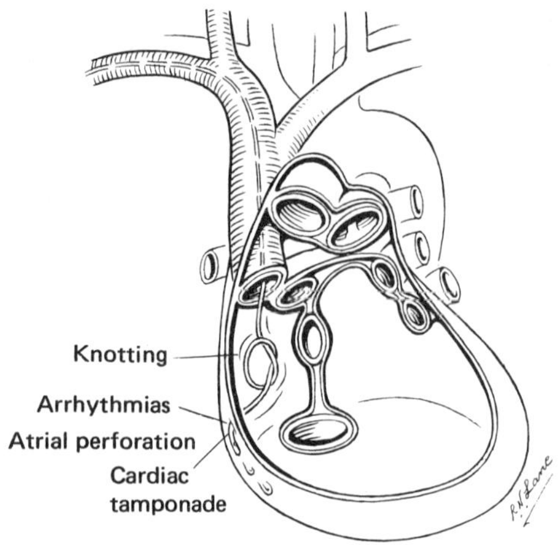

Fig. 12.22. Over-advancement of a long central venous catheter can easily lead to knotting, atrial irritation and perforation with resultant cardiac tamponade from either leakage of blood or the infusion of intravenous fluids.

there are very real dangers of infusing pharmacologically active drugs in a retrograde fashion via the internal jugular vein. Hyperosmolar solutions may cause thrombosis and this can cause serious intracranial sequelae. Klein et al. reported the onset of headaches and coma following the initiation of lignocaine therapy for premature ventricular beats following a myocardial infarction, which resolved spontaneously within an hour when the drug was given by a peripheral vein (75).

Summary

The incidence and importance of aberrant central venous catheters has recently been comprehensively reviewed by Dunbar et al. (76). This problem may result in inaccurate venous pressure measurement, thrombosis at the catheter tip, pneumothorax, chylothorax, hydrothorax, pericardial tamponade, arrhythmias and the extravasation of infusion fluids into the heart, lungs or mediastinum. Furthermore, retrograde infusion of potentially toxic or unphysiological solutions into the cerebral or hepatic veins can have serious sequelae. Almost all of such events can be prevented by precise radiological location of the initial catheter tip position and careful subsequent clinical surveillance.

DELAYED COMPLICATIONS

Past experience has shown that catheter-related

sepsis is the most frequent delayed complication and accordingly this has been dealt with separately in Chapter 13. There are, however, a variety of important non-infectious mechanical problems that may arise during periods of prolonged catheter placement, namely: air embolism; venous thrombosis; vascular perforation; nerve injury; sepsis, osteomyelitis, abscess and fistula formation.

Air Embolism

A review of the literature reveals that during the past 10 years there has been an increasing awareness of the importance of this problem occurring during the period of intravenous infusion or monitoring (48). Grant, in his monograph, has emphasized this problem by discussing it first in the section devoted to complications (6). It is interesting to note that in the series described by him, from Duke University Medical Center, North Carolina, a fatal case of air embolism had occurred. It is also the present authors' experience that once such a clinical mishap occurs, it is never forgotten. Although the hazard is a relatively infrequent event, the clinical consequences for the individual patient are devastating. Furthermore, there are still inadequacies in equipment currently available which contribute directly to the initiation of this complication, and therefore the problem can be considered to be 'technogenic'. Earlier in this chapter the ease with which air can enter the central circulation during the insertion procedure was described. Indeed, it has been known for centuries that air can rapidly enter the circulation and result in death. The first observation of the fatal potential of intravenous air was described in 1667 by Redi, the Italian naturalist (77). Beauchesne reported the first fatal case of air embolism following surgery on the neck in 1818 (78). Magendie reported his experience with air embolism in 1821 (79), whilst in 1844, Erichsen correlated changes in the heart sounds with the onset of venous air entry (80).

The serious nature of air accidents occurring during transfusion was first highlighted by Simpson in 1942 (81). The exact dose of intravenous air which can cause death in man is not known. The rate at which air enters the circulation appears to be more important, and a bolus of 100 ml of air has been known to cause death in an adult (82). In 1902, Mariani treated a patient with an injection of 160 ml of air per hour without any detrimental effect (83). In 1916, Tunnicliffe and Stebbing, physicians at King's College Hospital, London, administered intravenous oxygen to 3 patients as a treatment for cyanosis (84). The rationale behind the introduction of these experiments was the urgent need to find a means of providing respiratory support for men being gassed in France during World War I. Their 'therapeutic' dose was 10 ml/min and 'toxic' effects were observed at 20 ml/min. Gurgling heart sounds were noted and transient quadriplegia was produced in one case.

The undesirable pathophysiological consequences of air gaining entry to the circulation have been observed in a wide variety of clinical circumstances (85–88). The cyclical negative pressures generated within the thoracic cavity during respiration facilitate the rapid entry of air via any laceration in the vein wall. This is particularly likely to occur if the patient is sitting, hypovolaemic, tachypnoeic or being ventilated mechanically. Because central venous catheters traverse the most proximal valves guarding the great veins, and their tips lie within the thoracic cavity, air can easily be conducted to the heart if the catheter hub is left unguarded during the insertion procedure, and the patient has not been placed in a 20–30° head-down tilt, or if accidental disconnection of the administration tube from the catheter hub occurs. Ordway has shown experimentally that supralethal doses of air can enter the circulation through cannulas presently in clinical use (89). He noted that with a negative intrathoracic pressure of $-5\,cmH_2O$, 80 ml of air per second can flow through a 14 G cannula. He also suggested that doses that are not lethal may accumulate in the central veins and then 'burp' into the circulation as a bolus. The mechanisms by which air enters the circulation has been carefully investigated from both a theoretical and practical standpoint (90). Central venous catheters in effect create a wound in a neck vein if they are left unprotected against the entry of air from the atmosphere (*Figs.* 12.23, 12.24).

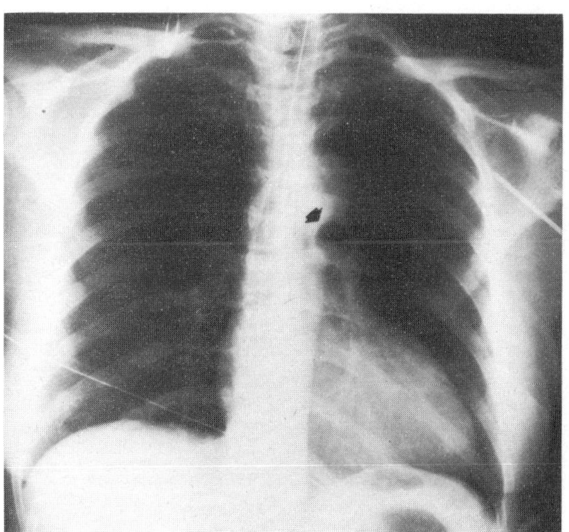

Fig. 12.23. Air embolism. A 57-year-old woman had a left subclavian line inserted for hyperalimentation. A few days later she developed sudden hypotension and syncope. A portable chest X-ray showed air in the pulmonary artery. A hole was found in the tubing to the central line through which air was sucked into the circulatory system. Fortunately, the patient survived this complication. (Reproduced by kind permission of Dr S. E. Mitchell and the Editor of the *American Journal of Roentgenology.)*

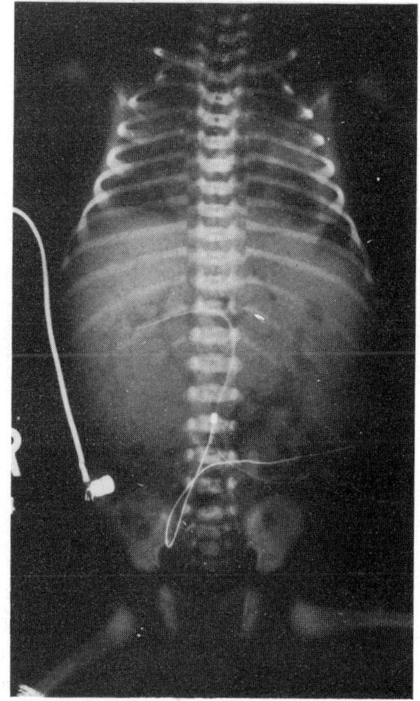

Fig. 12.24. A fatal case of air embolism following entrainment through a disconnected umbilical vein catheter. Air can be seen in the portal venous system, the right atrium and right ventricle. Paradoxical systemic embolization had also occurred and air is present in the left ventricle. (Reproduced by kind permission of the Editor of the *British Journal of Intravenous Therapy.)*

The incident that has most frequently caused air embolism associated with central venous catheters has been disconnection of the junction between the catheter hub and the administration set. Such events have occurred both with the infusion sets fitted with simple Luer taper fittings and Luer 'lock' mechanisms. Air does not always enter the venous circulation; if the central venous pressure is in the high range, then either haemorrhage from the catheter may occur or the lumen will simply become occluded by thrombus following disconnection of the infusion system. Alternatively, the attention of the nursing staff may be drawn to the patient because the infusion fluid may be found leaking into or around the dressings. The incidence of disconnection of central venous systems is high and has been noted in the most sophisticated medical centres (91). A confidential survey carried out in 1979 revealed an awareness of this problem in 90 per cent of the intensive care nursing staff who were questioned in the United Kingdom. An attempt has been made to put this

event into clinical perspective. Human error or accidents leading to misconnection, disconnection, hub fracture, stress fractures or defects in the infusion system can all lead to fatal air embolism. The presence of three-way stopcocks in which a port is left unguarded provides an additional risk to the patient who may turn this to the open position if in a confused state; or conversely the nursing staff may omit to return the tap to the closed position following an injection. Such mistakes easily happen in a busy clinical environment. There have been 22 cases of air embolism occurring following disconnection of the catheter hub from the attached infusion system (7, 89, 92–102). There were 5 deaths in this group and 4 patients suffered serious neurological sequelae in the form of coma, convulsions or hemiplegia. Seven of the remainder were resuscitated successfully after varying degrees of cardiorespiratory collapse. No details of the eventual outcome were provided for the other patients. Air embolism with a fatal outcome has also occurred after attempted

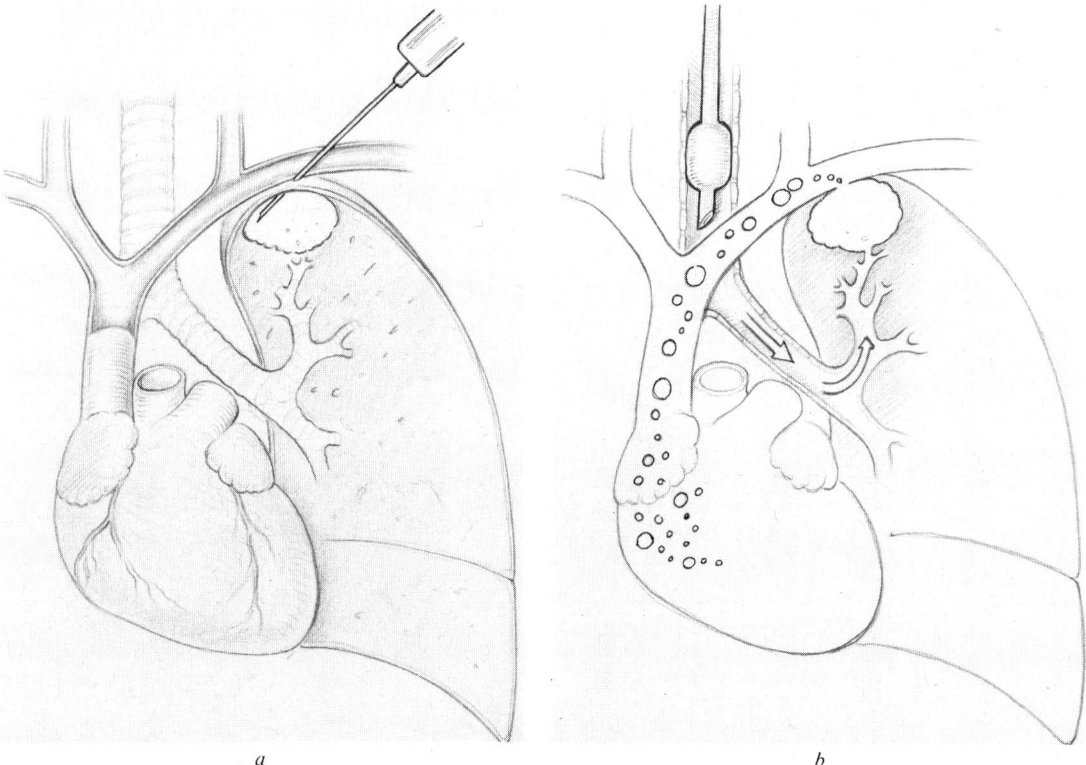

a   b

Fig. 12.25. *a*, Air embolism can follow the creation of a fistulous track between a vein and an apical bulla if this occurs at the beginning of surgery. Following intubation and ventilation of the patient, air entrainment into the circulation can occur (*b*).

subclavian catheterization injured an apical emphysematous bulla on the lung surface resulting in a communication between the lung and subclavian vein along the needle track. The procedure was carried out at the commencement of a surgical operation in which positive pressure ventilation was used via an endotracheal tube and air fluxed into the circulation (*Fig.* 12.25) (103). Air can be easily vented into the circulation by infusion pumps, and a fatal episode followed air being aspirated through an air inlet on bottles containing antibiotics which were being dripped in a piggy-back fashion through a central line (38).

The ways in which air can gain entry to an infusion system can easily be predicted. Any defect which affects the hydraulic integrity of the catheter from its tip right back to the container of the infusate is a potentially lethal route for air to gain access to the heart (*Figs.* 12.26–12.28). In addition to separation of the hub, air has gained entry through holes in the intravenous tubing (7), three-way stopcock ports inadvertently left in the 'open' position (102) and also through an introducing catheter which has been left in the subclavian vein (104). In the latter instance, the definitive central catheter slipped out of the introducing cannula lumen, leaving a patent tube through which air gained entry (104). Finally, air has even gained entry via the track of

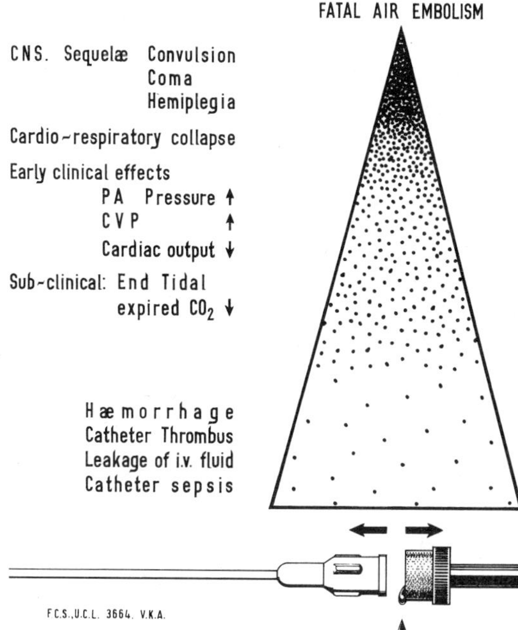

Fig. 12.26. The potential complications of central venous catheter misconnection or disconnection from infusion apparatus and the clinical sequelae.

a central venous catheter after its removal; thus, the wound should be covered by an occlusive dressing for several days (105).

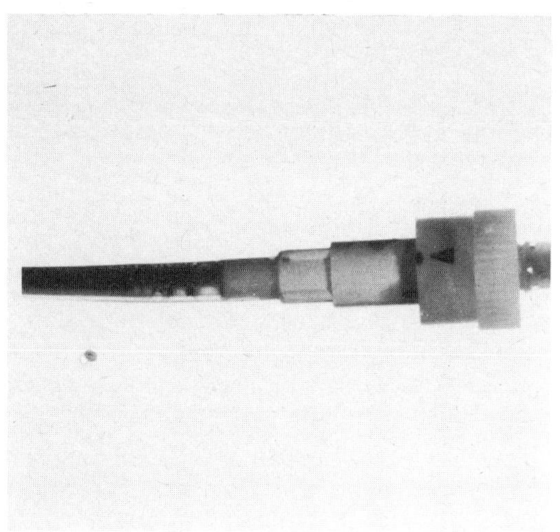

a

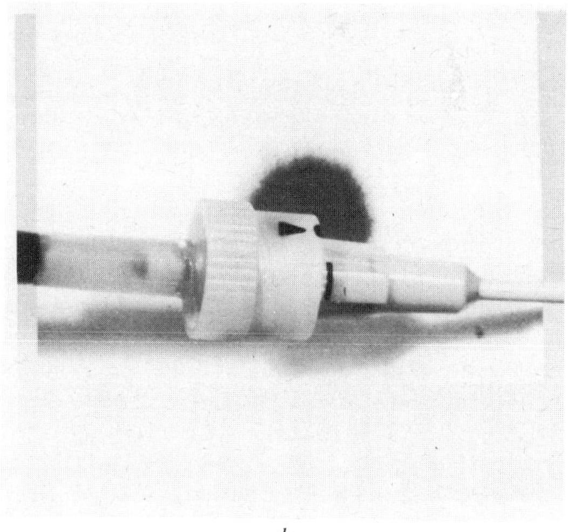

b

Fig. 12.27. This central catheter hub and administration set junction look to be intact until tested by aspiration when air bubbles can be seen entering the assembly and passing down the lumen of the central catheter (*a*). Similarly, a Luer-lock central catheter hub and administration set junction which appears to be intact easily leaks fluid, as shown in this dye test (*b*). (Reproduced by kind permission of the Editor of *The Lancet*.)

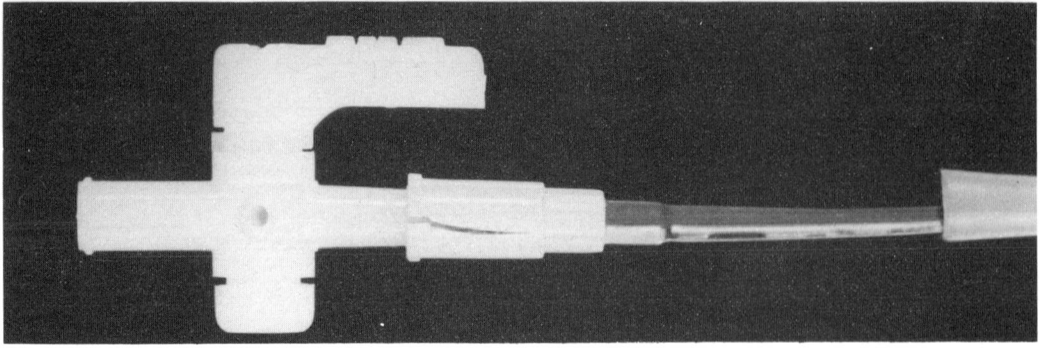

Fig. 12.28. A three-way stopcock has been inserted into the hub of a central venous catheter which carries a stress fracture. This defect was sufficient to result in the entrainment of air into the circulation of a patient receiving mechanical ventilation. He developed a left hemiplegia from which a slow recovery was made. The three-way stopcock is another potential source of air entry if used in central venous infusion systems. (Reproduced by kind permission of the Editor of *The Lancet.*)

The manufacturers have a responsibility to provide safeguards against such 'technogenic' complications. The aim in the design of extra-corporeal administration systems should be to simulate the human circulation as far as possible; superfluous injection ports should be eliminated from infusion lines or cannulas whenever possible by the medical and nursing staff taking a careful interest in the choice of catheter and administration sets, and choosing apparatus most appropriate for each individual patient. Furthermore, rapid progress needs to be made in order to achieve safer locking mechanisms between components in the intravenous systems (100, 106). The ease with which components can be disconnected or misconnected is alarming. Wear and tear arises in clinical practice when infusion sets are changed and reconnected at regular intervals to the catheter hubs. Erosion and distortion of plastic occurs quickly and the screw-thread mechanisms can override or fail completely, leaving the junction looking safe to the casual observer, when in fact, the slightest traction will separate the components and allow air to enter the patient (*Figs.* 12.29, 12.30) (106, 107). The plastic components used in these junctions, extension tubes and stopcocks, have the inherent property to creep apart with the passage of time. Irving has also recently reported that the Luer-lock mechanism is not infallible (108). Such design failures are difficult for plastic engineers to foresee since their bench is not an adequate test bed for clinical equipment. Patients may be confused at times and interfere with their 'life-line'; they must be able to move about the bed, and this creates unusual stresses upon infusion lines and associated junctions. Finally, of necessity, nursing staff constantly change and manipulate infusion lines so that the potential for misconnection because of human error is an ever-present reality. It would be difficult for an engineer to predict and provide a design which would be effective against the 'pacemaker twiddler's' syndrome (109, 110). Adhesive tape is widely used to provide a safeguard against separation of connections, yet this material is often contaminated and has been associated with catheter infection. It must therefore be considered to be unsatisfactory (111). Disconnection of intravenous equipment was noted to be a significant problem in an audit performed in the USA (112).

Even if the intravenous infusion route were rendered foolproof against the risk of air entry, embolism into the circulation can occur in bizarre circumstances through catheters placed in the central veins. Jacobsen and his colleagues recently described a fatal event in a patient with a LeVeen peritoneo-jugular shunt for ascites and portal hypertension. Colonoscopy for the removal of a polyp in the caecum was performed and the patient collapsed and subsequently died. A post-mortem examination revealed a caecal perforation and air had gained entry to the right ventricle via the LeVeen shunt (113).

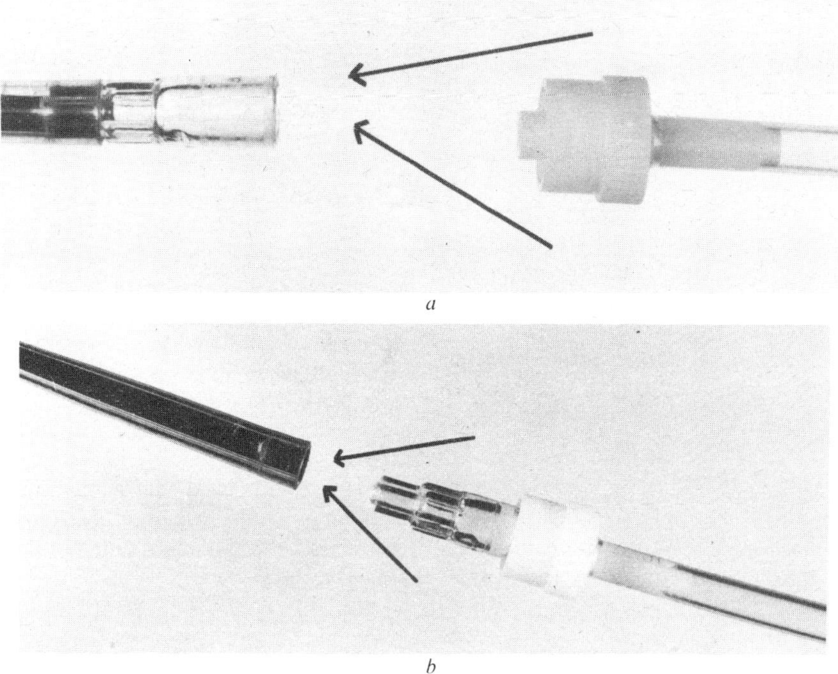

Fig. 12.29. *a*, Air may enter the central venous catheter lumen and human circulation from a simple disconnection of Luer-lock mechanisms, or (*b*) the hub may disconnect from the shaft of the central catheter, allowing air to enter via this defect. The use of fixed-collar Luer-lock mechanisms results in daily twisting forces being applied to the catheter shaft and hub junction.

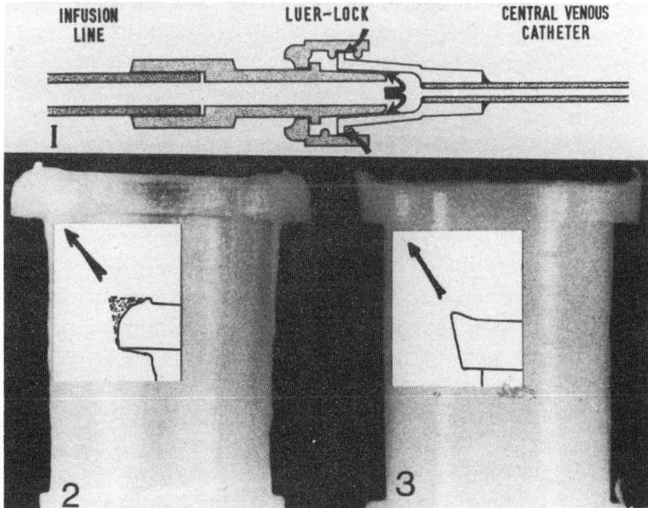

Fig. 12.30. The inadequacies of the Luer-lock mechanism are highlighted. Wear and tear of the threads can occur and unless the Luer male taper fitting sits firmly in the female hub, then a potential space exists in the lock mechanism around which fluid and hence air or bacteria may gain entry to the system. The fixed-collar Luer-lock mechanism can actually prevent correct alignment of the Luer taper fitting from being achieved (**1**). **2** and **3** show a central catheter hub subjected to 4 days' use and the inset pictures reveal the way in which the hub has been worn away by the administration set threads. A new central catheter hub is shown in **3**. The change in shape of the hub edges was sufficient to cause slipping of the thread and failure of the Luer-lock mechanism, resulting in a non-fatal air embolism.

Infusion Pumps and Air Embolism

Fatal incidents have been reported because of air being pumped into patients without the alarms sounding (114). Indeed, in one case the patient's physiological monitoring system sounded before that of the pump providing the fluid. The use of conventional pumps will always carry the risk of air being dragged into the circulation either from the vented container or burette compartment. The potential exists for air to be sucked in through any defect of the tubing distal to the pump. Warnings have also been issued in the United Kingdom concerning air gaining entry after the use of non-vented semi-rigid containers when using a positive displacement pump to administer intravenous fluids (115).

Management of Air Embolism

Air embolism probably occurs more frequently than medical and nursing personnel imagine. Durant et al. (116) and Nicholson (117) made the point that the true incidence of death from air embolism is impossible to determine since often the diagnosis is not made and the cases go unreported. The clinical manifestations of venous air embolism depend upon the rate and amount of air which has entered the circulation. Mechanical obstruction of the pulmonary outflow tract occurs (*see Fig.* 12.23), with the creation of a 'mill wheel' murmur. The central venous pressure rises, the respiratory rate increases and the patient may develop a central chest pain with cyanosis. Ultimately, the cardiac output falls, the systemic blood pressure falls and the peripheral pulses quicken and become thready before syncope occurs as a result of cerebral ischaemia. It must also be remembered that in neonates a patent foramen ovale exists and may be present in as many as 20 per cent of adult patients, leading to paradoxical arterial air embolism, which in many respects can be more serious (*see Fig.* 12.24) (118). In 1947, Durant et al. carried out important experiments on this hazard; they differentiated between the clinical electrocardiographic features of venous and arterial air embolism. In dogs, as little as 0·025 ml of air in a coronary artery can produce an ischaemic disturbance in the myocardium. Following arterial air embolism, the patient may complain of sudden dizziness or faint, quickly

lose consciousness and may have a convulsion. Various neurological deficits may be observed, e.g. nystagmus, hemiplegia or loss of vision. Pathognomonic signs of arterial air embolism are the presence of air in the retinal vessels, a well-defined pallor of the tongue following the entry of air into the lingual artery, 'marbling' of the skin and air bleeding from tissues. If open cardiac massage is being performed, air can be detected in the left ventricle and coronary artery. Air can be detected also in X-rays of the chest and skull. It is easy to see how collapse from this cause can be attributed erroneously to heart disease or some other condition (116). To clarify the relationship between air embolism and sudden death, a post-mortem chest X-ray is a valuable aid and Simpson has emphasized the need for a careful autopsy examination if the problem has been suspected. Needless to say, the pathologist should be informed of any preceding clinical events.

Once the diagnosis is established, any defect noted in the infusion system should be immediately corrected. If the problem is emanating from an administration set or pump defect, these should be disconnected from the central venous catheter and a sterile syringe inserted into the hub. If the defect is in the catheter itself, then this will have to be clamped proximal to the hole. The Durant manoeuvre should be carried out and the patient quickly placed in the head-down position, lying on the left side. This will prevent air travelling to the brain and, if an embolism is small and detected early, rapid recovery can be expected. The adoption of this position should release the air block in the pulmonary outflow tract. Should these measures fail, then an attempt can be made to aspirate the air using the central catheter, but this is not usually successful. A patent airway should be maintained and endotracheal intubation and manual ventilation established with oxygen. Finally, an emergency thoracotomy may have to be considered and the air vented by aspiration and manual manipulations. If the patient's circulation has stopped, this procedure must be carried out within minutes for a successful outcome to be achieved. The usual cardiac resuscitation measures will also have to be employed as appropriate.

Thus, there is still a great need for a safer, more sophisticated infusion system in order to eliminate the hazard of air embolism from peripheral or central intravenous therapy. In the study by Bos (101), an incidence of 2 per cent for air embolism was noted and this figure is similar to the experience of University College Hospital, London. Every effort has to be made to eliminate unnecessary risks of this magnitude.

Thrombosis

This problem can arise either in the lumen of the catheter or the venous system of the patient. Thrombosis generated within the catheter lumen may be initiated by kinks which may cause intermittent cessation in the flow of the infusate. Blood will then reflux back into the catheter over a short distance and clot is formed. This is an undesirable state of affairs which can be serious if the catheter is meant to carry inotropic drugs necessary for cardiac support and the problem goes unrecognized. Many people now advocate daily intermittent injections of low-dose heparin (e.g. Hepsal, 10 i.u./ml). No catheter material is exempt from this problem, and it has been noted with Hickman–Broviac silicone catheters (119) and other varieties of narrow-gauge silicon catheters (40). Once a significant thrombus occludes such an important line, it can be dangerous to attempt its removal by forcibly injecting saline down the catheter because the catheter may 'balloon' and rupture or fragment into the circulation. Recently, the introduction of Streptokinase (Kabikinase; Kabi-Vitrum) or Urokinase (Abbokinase; Abbott Laboratories) has proved effective for the dissolution of thrombus occluding catheters.

The genesis of thrombosis within the major veins in association with central venous catheters has long been recognized. Such devices must alter the flow patterns of blood in the locality of the venous puncture site, and the intravascular configuration of the catheter tubing is of critical importance. The formation of loops, kinks or knots will predispose to thrombus formation (34, 120). Late displacement of catheters into loop shapes after originally being correctly positioned has also been known to lead to thrombosis of the subclavian vein (121). The materials used for peripheral venous cannulas have been shown to be of significance in the aetiology of thrombophlebitis (122). It would seem prudent to use either a

silicone, FEP (fluoroethylene propylene) or polyurethane catheter, rather than a device made from PVC (polyvinyl chloride). Particular care should be taken if tubing meant for some other function (e.g. nasogastric aspiration) is used in an emergency for the purpose of central venous access (123). Most of these devices are composed of PVC and have an inappropriately large diameter for prolonged venous placement. Catheters which do become kinked or looped in a major vein tend to reduce the lumen to a slit shape and further impede venous return. The mechanical and chemical irritation of the vessel wall by the catheter may be compounded by the local effect of hyperosmolar solutions entering the vessel from the catheter tip and the presence of hypercoagulable state in some groups of patients. Thus, the trinity of requirements first introduced by Virchow in 1856 is ever present after central catheters are inserted (124).

Bansmer reported an incidence of 48 per cent for major venous thrombosis associated with catheters inserted into the inferior vena cava (125). The importance, incidence and aetiology of central venous thrombosis in burned patients was highlighted in a post-mortem study from Brooke Army Medical Center, Fort Sam Houston, and the lethal nature of suppurative thrombophlebitis emphasized (126). The incidence of thrombosis associated with internal jugular vein catheters is low and this has been attributed to the relatively straight course of the vein and the high blood flow (5). Cases have been reported by Schuster (127), Steffelaar (128) and Nottage (129). Recently, a case of bilateral thrombosis of the internal jugular vein was recorded after multiple percutaneous cannulation attempts (130).

Subclavian-axillary vein thrombosis occurs infrequently, and the incidence has been reported at 0·24 per cent and 0·29 per cent respectively (5, 6). Unilateral swelling of the face, neck and supraclavicular fossa is usually noted (*Fig.* 12.31). In the arm, the characteristic triad of swelling, pain and venous prominence may develop rapidly. The extent of oedema is variable and is usually most notable in the upper arm and shoulder region. In women, swelling of the breast may be a feature. Primary subclavian vein thrombosis is a rare entity (131, 132) and was first described as a 'gouty phlebitis' by Sir James Paget in 1875 (133). Subsequently, Von

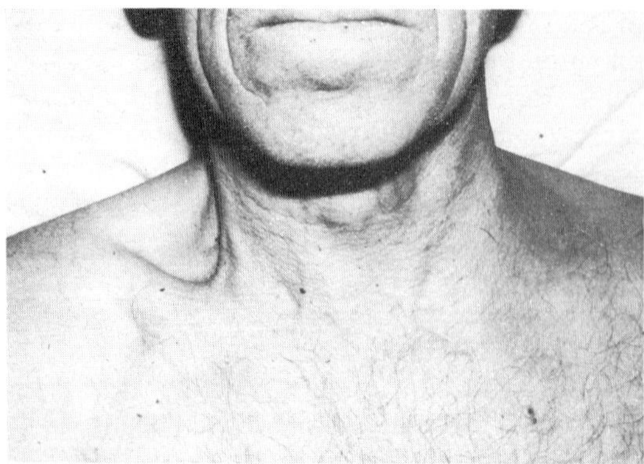

Fig. 12.31. A subclavian and axillary vein thrombosis has developed on the left side following prolonged placement of a brachial central venous catheter. Note the swelling in the supraclavicular region of the posterior triangle of the neck compared to the scaphoid fossa on the right side.

Schroetter also described the condition in 1884 (134), and hence it gained from Hughes (131) the eponym of 'Paget–Schroetter's syndrome'. The condition has been attributed to stress, trauma, effort and strain. A most important diagnostic feature is whether or not there is an anatomical structure that may be causing compression. The subclavian vein thrombosis associated with central catheters falls into the classification of 'secondary' subclavian–axillary vein thrombosis and it is worth remembering that there may be additional and alternative causative factors contributing to the development of the venous

occlusion; these include (132):

Direct injury—penetrating or blunt.
Extrinsic compression—neoplasm, lymphadenopathy, retrosternal goitre, ascending aortic aneurysm.
Thrombophlebitis in the distal arm: chemical; infectious; thromboangiitis obliterans; Trousseau's syndrome.
Intrathoracic infections.
Extension of thrombosis from superior vena cava.
Congestive cardiac failure.
Shock.
Dehydration.
Hypercoagulable states.

It is most important to consider whether or not the subclavian vein is patent before catheterization is attempted. This is of particular relevance if there have been previous catheters in place for a prolonged period of time. The necessity of performing venography where any doubt exists about this point has recently been emphasized following a study in Copenhagen (135). Doppler ultrasound may also be used to determine patency of the vein prior to any insertion attempts (136). Radionuclide intravenous angioscanning may be performed using technetium-99^m (*Fig.* 12.32). Grant has demonstrated the formation of fibrin sheaths on subclavian catheters after relatively short periods of placement (6).

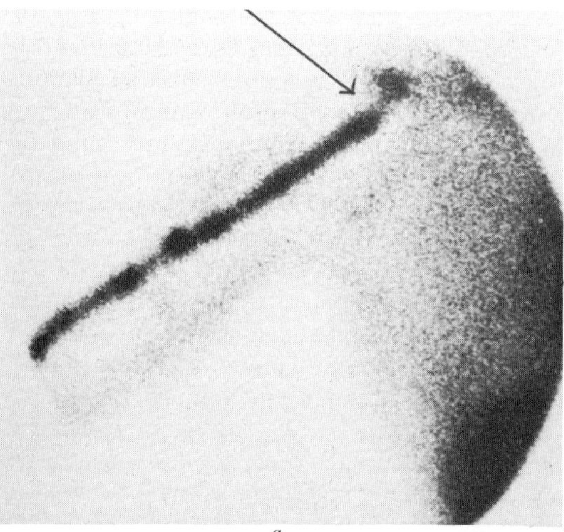

a

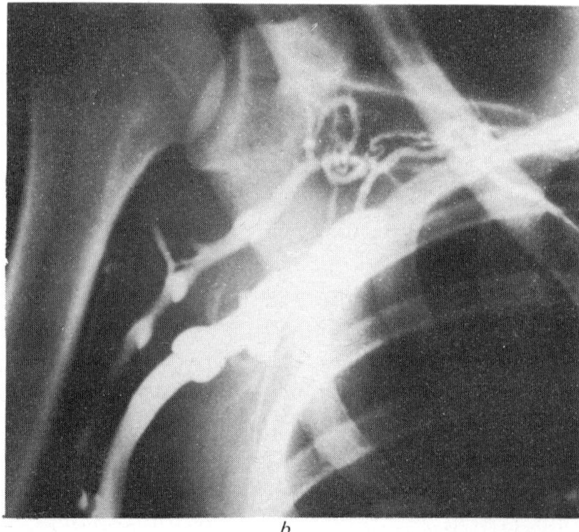

b

Fig. 12.32. *a*, A technetium-99^m venoscan revealing an obstructed right axillary and subclavian vein. The corresponding venogram is shown in (*b*). This figure also highlights the valves of this region and the very variable anatomy of the entrance of the cephalic vein into the subclavian vein.

The treatment of subclavian–axillary vein thrombosis depends very much upon the other co-existing clinical problems which the patient faces. The catheter should be removed, the tip cultured for micro-organisms and, if possible, intravenous heparin therapy should be started. It may be appropriate to institute intravenous Urokinase (Abbokinase; Abbott Laboratories) or Streptokinase (Kabikinase; Kabi-Vitrum) therapy. Although this is expensive, the morbidity from this condition over a long period of time is quite considerable (6, 132). The limb should be rested and elevation is of benefit to some patients. An appropriate analgesic should be prescribed. The most serious developments are the relentless extension of the thrombus into the superior vena cava (*Fig.* 12.33) and the

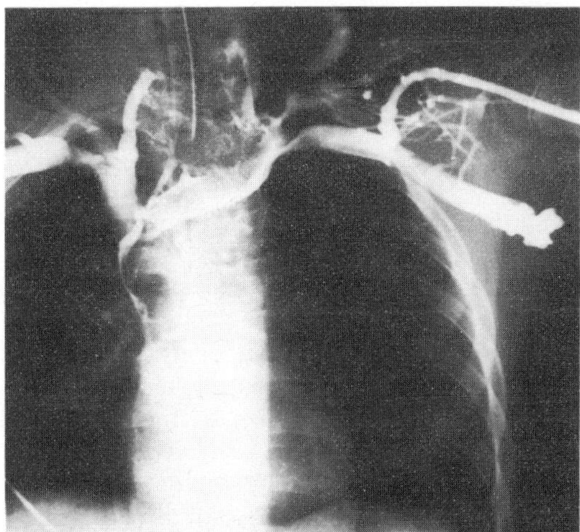

Fig. 12.33. A superior vena cavogram was obtained by injecting contrast medium into the antecubital vein. It reveals obstruction of the superior vena cava by an extensive thrombus that also can be seen filling the left innominate vein. There is minimal opacification of collateral venous pathways, and the azygos vein is not visible. (Reproduced by kind permission of Dr L. I. Bonchek MD and the Editor of the *Journal of Thoracic and Cardiovascular Surgery*.)

development of a suppurative thrombophlebitis or pulmonary embolism. In one such case, which developed after infusion of antibiotics through a subclavian catheter, Bonchek and his colleagues were able to perform a successful emergency thrombectomy (137). Singh has also performed similar surgery in a case in which the thrombus extended into the right atrium and had caused recurrent pulmonary embolism (138). All the major studies have emphasized the

definite risk of major pulmonary embolism occurring with central catheter-related thrombosis. The development of this problem must be taken seriously and the most appropriate therapeutic measures instituted; evidence of lung infarction should be sought if indicated, using ventilation–perfusion scans or chest radiography. Occasionally, satisfactory pulmonary angiograms can be achieved using the central catheter as the injection route of the contrast medium.

Vascular Perforation

The problem of central venous catheters eroding through the walls of important vascular structures in the mediastinum has been known for some time. Indeed, Claude Bernard can be credited with having described the first recorded complication associated with central venous catheterization when he performed an autopsy upon a dog and noted that the right ventricle had been perforated by the glass tube he had used to cannulate the jugular vein (139). Intrapericardial haemorrhage had occurred and caused the death of the animal. Goodwin reported a fatality following cardiac catheterization and, although no definite perforation could be found, the pericardial sac contained 150 ml of bloody fluid. An area of discoloured epicardium was seen, but no perforation tract could be demonstrated (140). Brown and Kent recorded the perforation of the right ventricle by a segment of a polyethylene catheter (141). In 1964, Dalgaard reported the case of a patient with a right ventricular perforation in whom death apparently resulted from cardiac tamponade during cardiac catheterization (142). Further perforations of the right atrium by pieces of catheter tubing were detected by both Johnson (143) and Doering et al. (144). A death resulting from hydropericardium secondary to delayed atrial perforation on the eighth postoperative day from an intact indwelling polyethylene catheter inserted from a vein in the right arm was first reported by Friedman and Jurgeleit in 1968 (145).

Since that time, Defalque has been able to document from the literature at least 45 cases of cardiac tamponade resulting from the use of central venous catheters in a comprehensive review of the problem (146).

No particular route or catheter type is exempt from this potentially fatal complication. In the series reported, one patient died under anaesthesia, others died quietly whilst in bed and the majority developed tamponade insidiously over periods of time varying from hours to days following the insertion of the catheter. The mortality rate was noted to be 78 per cent and both Defalque and other workers (147–149) suspect that many more cases go unreported. Whilst sudden cardiac arrest can occur, most patients suffer the onset of cyanosis with the development of venous engorgement in the head, neck and face. They started to complain of nausea, shortness of breath, retrosternal or epigastric pain and eventually become restless, confused or comatose. As the condition progresses, tachycardia, arterial hypotension, paradoxical pulse, muffled heart sounds and oliguria develop. As the pulmonary venous drainage is impaired, the appearance of signs suggesting pulmonary oedema can lead to errors of diagnosis.

The autopsies revealed perforations at a variety of sites—the subclavian vein, superior vena cava, right atrium, right ventricle, coronary sinus and pulmonary artery. Catheters can enter the coronary sinus when there is a left-sided superior vena cava (*see Fig.* 2.12, p. 18). Approximately 300–500 ml of blood were sufficient to produce death when present in the mediastinum or pericardium. Delayed perforation is likely to occur when the catheter tip lies in the atrium, so damaging the endocardium with each contraction; the catheter then becomes fixed to the thrombus which it produces and slowly necroses the heart wall. Another mechanism by which perforation of the heart or great veins can occur is catheter migration, associated with head, arm and trunk movement. There is good experimental evidence that catheters can move to and fro for distances of up to 10 cm (150). If extravasation of hyperosmolar solutions occurs, up to five times their volume of free water may be drawn into the tissues of the pericardium or mediastinum.

The diagnosis of vascular perforation must be considered whenever any of the previously mentioned symptoms manifest themselves, or when the central venous pressure measurements are abnormally high. Normal pressure measurements and respiratory oscillations can, however, persist in patients who are developing hydro-mediastinum (65, 151). Confirmation of this serious development can be obtained by echocardiography, chest X-ray, both plain and after the gentle injection of 2–5 ml of contrast medium (e.g. meglumine iothalamate 60 per cent w/v, Conray 280 or Hexabrix 320).

Prevention

The problem should be almost eliminated by the application of a few simple precautions. A soft, pliable and inert catheter material should be chosen. Relatively short catheters are often used for the jugular route, but if these are passed percutaneously into the subclavian vein, then the distortion of these devices can cause pressure necrosis of the superior vena cava (152). Central venous catheters should not be placed in the right atrium and only routine X-ray control of the placement can ensure that the catheter tip has not entered the heart. Catheters advanced into the coronary sinus have been known to cause major thrombosis of this vessel with the subsequent development of cardiac tamponade (4). The present authors prefer to screen catheters electively using an image intensifier and contrast medium whenever possible. Defalque has pointed out that introducing a length of catheter equal to the measured external distance from the point of insertion to the manubriosternal junction is grossly misleading with regard to the position of the catheter tip. Post-insertion check chest X-rays of brachial catheters should be taken with the arm in 90° of abduction, so that a precise location of the furthest point of the intravenous advancement is illustrated. Central venous catheter tips should remain in the upper segment of the superior vena cava or even in the innominate vein, above a sagittal X-ray plane drawn through the third rib, the T5–T6 interspace or 2 cm below the inferior clavicular border. Regular checks of the central venous catheter for the presence of backflow or of respiratory oscillation must be made. The presence of grossly abnormal pressure readings suggesting atrial or ventricular placement, and the appearance of arrhythmias, should give an early warning of the dislocation of the catheter from the vein. The catheter should be firmly secured to the skin surface, either with a suture or a sheet of Op-Site.

Another useful trick is to make a mark upon the shaft of the catheter with an indelible ink pen and a similar mark on the adjacent skin so that the nursing staff can detect any creep or piston movement into or out of the vein.

Once this problem has been suspected, there must be no delay in confirming the diagnosis. The central infusion should be stopped and an attempt may be made to aspirate the pericardial sac with a sterile syringe and three-way stopcock. This may successfully restore the cardiac output. The catheter should then be withdrawn for a few centimetres into the right heart and a further 2–5 ml of contrast medium injected in order to detect a myocardial leak and the catheter then removed. If no improvement is obtained after catheter aspiration, needle pericardiocentesis should be performed via the xiphisternal approach. In rare cases, operative intervention will be required and pericardiectomy performed (146).

Thoracic Duct Injury

Immediate laceration of the thoracic duct following insertion has already been described earlier (41), and there has also been a fatal case which followed accidental migration of a long brachial venous catheter into the thoracic duct (153). Thrombosis of the lymphatic channel occurred, resulting in the development of a fatal chylothorax.

Ascites

This unusual event was observed as a delayed complication following malposition of a subclavian central catheter into the pleural space in a patient who had undergone a oesophagogastrectomy for carcinoma through a transverse abdominal laparotomy and a separate right thoracotomy. After the commencement of the intravenous nutrition infusion, the patient gradually developed ascites and subsequently a hydrothorax because of the abnormal communication existing between the chest and abdomen (154). Hepatic vein thrombosis has also been reported (155); this could lead to a form of Budd–Chiari syndrome with jaundice and ascites.

Nerve Injury

Dislocation of a catheter out of the subclavian or jugular vein can result in the infusate being delivered into the soft tissues of the root of the neck. If neurotoxic drugs are also injected inadvertently via such a catheter, severe neurological injury may result. Briscoe and his colleagues described such a case in which the anterior branches of the cervical nerves and cranial nerves IX–XII were involved (156).

Sepsis, Osteomyelitis, Abscess and Fistula Formation

As one might expect, percutaneous attempts at cannulation of the veins around the root of the neck may result in the bones and joints being touched or entered. Even with the most meticulous of skin preparation, a risk of initiating infection exists. Lee and Kerstein reported such a case of osteomyelitis and septic arthritis occurring after subclavian catheterization (157). Abscess formation has occurred in the chest wall following malposition of a parenteral nutrition catheter into the internal mammary vein (158). A central venous catheter, being a foreign body, has the potential to cause a pressure and chemical necrosis of adjacent tissue. Hyperosmolar nutrient solutions enhance this effect, and Brennan described a rare case of veno-bronchial fistula formation (159). The patient suddenly coughed up 'sweet tasting' sputum, which was positive for sugar on biochemical testing.

SUMMARY

An international review of the early, intermediate and late complications associated with central venous catheterization reveals that these procedures should no longer be considered to be innocuous minor operations. Clinicians and nursing staff need to have an acute awareness of the morbid and mortal complications in order to be able to recognize and prevent their development at the earliest possible stage (160). It is imperative that those clinicians proficient in the art supervise junior staff closely during attempts at catheterization and, furthermore, housemen should preferentially choose the simplest and safest route of insertion. Individuals and wards should try to maintain a record or audit of such procedures and any related complications so that they may serve to educate future staff in the department and so be avoided. Endless repetition of the safe basic operative technique and placement checks should eliminate the vast majority of problems discussed. It is an ironic fact that the procedure, first introduced by Forssmann because of his dissatisfaction with the complications of pneumothorax, myocardial laceration and cardiac tamponade caused by direct percutaneous puncture of the heart in the resuscitation of moribund patients (161), should be associated with the very same problems unless the 'most stringent safeguards are employed.

References

1. Sprigge J. S., Oakley G. D. G.: Carotid artery palpation during internal jugular vein cannulation and subsequent ventricular fibrillation. *Br. J. Anaesth.* 1979; **5**: 807.
2. Goyanes A. D., Lomanto C. L., Boyan C. P.: Complications of catheterisation for central venous pressure. *Anaesth. Analg.* 1969; **48**: 563.
3. Couch N. P., Tilney N. L., Rayner A. A. et al.: The high cost of low frequency events. The anatomy and economics of surgical mishaps. *N. Engl. J. Med.* 1981; **304**: 634–7.
4. Ryan J. A.: In: Fischer J. E. (ed.): *Total Parenteral Nutrition*. Boston, Mass.: Little, Brown, 1976: 55–100.
5. Burri C., Ahnefeld E. W.: *The Caval Catheter*. Berlin: Springer-Verlag, 1978: 39–65.
6. Grant J. P.: *Handbook of Total Parenteral Nutrition*. Philadelphia: Saunders, 1980: 57–69.
7. Mitchell S. E., Clark R. A.: Complications of central venous catheterisation. *AJR* 1979; **133**: 467–76.
8. Herbst C. A.: Indications, management and complications of percutaneous subclavian catheters. *Arch. Surg.* 1978; **113**: 1421–5.
9. Bernard R. W., Stahl W. M.: Subclavian vein catheterisations: a prospective study. (i) Non-infectious complications. *Ann. Surg.* 1971; **173**: 184–90.
10. Borja A. R.: Current status of infraclavicular subclavian vein catheterisation. *Ann. Thorac. Surg.* 1972; **13**: 615–24.
11. James P. M., Myers R. T.: Central venous pressure monitoring: complications and a new technique. *Am. Surg.* 1973; **39**: 75–81.
12. Kletz T. A.: What risks should we run? *New Scientist* 1977; May: 320.
13. Lord Rothschild: *Risk*. (Richard Dimbleby Lecture.) *Atom* 1979; **268**: 30.
14. Mostert J. W., Kenney G. M., Murphy G. P.: Safe placement of central venous catheter into internal jugular vein. *Arch. Surg.* 1970; **101**: 431–2.
15. Brinkman A. K., Costley D. O.: Internal jugular venepuncture. *JAMA* 1973; **223**: 182–3.
16. Buchman R. J.: Subclavian venepunction. *Military Med.* 1969; **134**: 451–3.
17. Yoffa D.: Supraclavicular subclavian venepunction and catheterisation. *Lancet* 1965; **2**: 614–17.
18. Wisheart J. D., Hassan M. A., Jackson J. W.: A complication of percutaneous cannulation of the internal jugular vein. *Thorax* 1972; **27**: 496–9.
19. Larsen H. W., Lindahl F.: Lesion of the internal mammary artery caused by infraclavicular percutaneous catheterisation of the subclavian vein. *Acta Chir. Scand.* 1973; **139**: 571–2.
20. Oakes D. D., Wilson R. E.: Malposition of a subclavian line. *JAMA* 1975; **233**: 532–3.
21. Holt S., Kirkham N., Myerscough E.: Haemothorax after subclavian vein cannulation. *Thorax* 1977; **32**: 101–3.
22. Shield C. F.: Pseudoaneurysm of the brachiocephalic arteries: a complication of percutaneous internal jugular vein catheterisation. *Surgery* 1975; **78**: 190–4.
23. Schwartz A. J.: Percutaneous aortic catheterisation—a hazard of supraclavicular internal jugular vein catheterisation. *Anaesthesiology* 1977; **46**: 77.
24. Allsop J. R., Askew A. R.: Subclavian vein cannulation: a new complication. *Br. Med. J.* 1975; **1**: 262–3.
25. Lefrak F. A., Noon G. P.: Management of arterial injury secondary to attempted subclavian vein catheterisation. *Ann. Thorac. Surg.* 1972; **14**: 294–8.
26. Mogil R. A., Delaurentis D. A., Rosemond G. P.: The infraclavicular venepuncture: value in various clinical situations including central venous pressure monitoring. *Arch. Surg.* 1967; **95**: 320–4.
27. Smith B. E., Modell J. A., Gaub M. L. et al.: Complications of subclavian vein catheterisation. *Arch. Surg.* 1965; **90**: 228–9.
28. Walker M. M., Saunders R. C.: Pneumothorax following supraclavicular venepuncture. *Anaesthesiology* 1969; **24**: 453–60.
29. Matz R.: Complications of determining the central venous pressure. *N. Engl. J. Med.* 1965; **273**: 703.
30. Maggs P. R., Schwaber J. R.: Fatal bilateral pneumothoraces complicating subclavian vein catheterisation. *Chest* 1977; **71**: 552–3.
31. Yarom J.: Subclavian venepuncture. *Lancet* 1964; **1**: 45.
32. Schapira M., Stern W. Z.: Hazards of subclavian vein cannulation for central venous pressure monitoring. *JAMA* 1967; **201**: 327–9.
33. Baden H.: Perkutan Kateterisation of V. subclavia. *Nord. Med.* 1964; **75**: 590–3.
34. Levinsky W. J.: Fatal air embolism during insertion of CVP monitoring apparatus. *JAMA* 1969; **209**: 966.
35. Flanagan J. P., Gradisar I. A., Gross R. J. et al.: (Letter.) *N. Engl. J. Med.* 1969; **281**: 1426.
36. Johnson C. L., Lazarchick J., Lynn H. B.: Subclavian venepuncture: preventable complications; report of two cases. *Mayo Clin. Proc.* 1970; **45**: 712.
37. Jernigan W. R., Gardner W. C., Mahr M. M.: Use of internal jugular vein for placement of central venous catheter. *Surg. Gynecol. Obstet.* 1970; **137**: 520–4.
38. Borja A. R., Shruck L., Pejo S.: Unusual and fatal complications of infraclavicular subclavian vein catheterisation. *Int. Surg.* 1972; **57**: 42–5.

39. Conahan T. J.: Air embolism during percutaneous Swan–Ganz catheter placement. *Anaesthesiology* 1979; **50**: 360–1.

40. Ross A. H. M., Anderson J. R., Walls A. D. F.: Central venous catheterisation. *Ann. R. Coll. Surg. Engl.* 1980; **62**: 454–8.

41. Khalil K. G.: Thoracic duct injury: a complication of jugular vein catheterisation. *JAMA* 1972; **221**: 908–9.

42. Epstein E. J., Quereshi M. S. A., Wright J. S.: Diaphragmatic paralysis after supraclavicular puncture of subclavian vein. *Br. Med. J.* 1976; **1**: 693–4.

43. Obel I. W. P.: Transient phrenic nerve paralysis following subclavian venepuncture. *Anaesthesiology* 1970; **33**: 369–70.

44. Drachler D. H., Koepke G. H., Weg J. G.: Phrenic nerve injury from subclavian vein catheterization; diagnosis by electromyography. *JAMA* 1976; **236**: 2880–1.

45. Moosman D. A.: The anatomy of infraclavicular subclavian vein catheterisation and its complications. *Surg. Gynecol. Obstet.* 1973; **136**: 71–4.

46. Butsch J. L., Butsch W. L., Da Rosa J. F. T.: Bilateral vocal cord paralysis: a complication of percutaneous cannulation of the internal jugular vein. *Arch. Surg.* 1976; **111**: 828.

47. Tarikh R. K.: Horner's syndrome: a complication of percutaneous catheterisation of the internal jugular vein. *Anaesthesia* 1972; **27**: 327–9.

48. McGoon M. D., Benedetto P. W., Greene B. M.: Complications of percutaneous central venous catheterisation: a report of two cases and review of the literature. *Johns Hopkins Med. J.* 1979; **145**: 1–5.

49. Hurwitz B. J., Posner J. B.: Cerebral infarction complicating subclavian vein catheterisation. *Ann. Neurol.* 1977; **1**: 253–64.

50. Blitt C. D., Wright W. A.: An unusual complication of percutaneous internal jugular vein cannulation, puncture of an endotracheal tube cuff. *Anaesthesia* 1974; **40**: 306.

51. Klipper W. S., Waite H. D., Tomlinson C. O.: Endotracheal cuff perforation complicating subclavian venepuncture. *JAMA* 1974; **228**: 693.

52. Kosters B., Bertels D.: Erfahrungen mit der Subclaviakatheterisierung auf der Wachstation. *Med. Ernähr.* 1970; **11**: 63.

53. McDaniel M. M., Grossman M.: Aortic dissection complicating percutaneous jugular vein catheterisation. *Anaesthesiology* 1978; **49**: 213–14.

54. Peters J. L., Belsham P. A., Kurzer M. et al.: The use of the Doppler ultrasound as an aid to subclavian vein catheterisation. *Am. J. Surg.* 1982; **143** (3): 391–3.

55. Oosterlee J., Dudley H. A. F.: Central catheter placement by puncture of exposed subclavian vein. *Lancet* 1980; **1**: 19–20.

56. Mitchell A., Steer H. W.: Late appearance of pneumothorax after infraclavicular subclavian vein catheterisation. *Br. Med. J.* 1980; **2**: 1339.

57. Aubaniac R.: L'injection intraveneuse sous claviculaire; advantages and technique. *Presse Méd.* 1952; **60**: 1456.

58. Smith G. B., Willatts S. M.: A hazard of Swan–Ganz catheterisation. *Anaesthesia* 1981; **36**: 398–401.

59. Fassolt A., Braun U., Schaub S.: Klinische Erfahrungen mit der Infraclavicularen Venenkatheterismus. *Schweiz. Med. Wochenschr.* 1968; **98**: 461.

60. Walker M. M., Sanders R. C.: Pneumothorax following supraclavicular subclavian venepuncture. *Anaesthesia* 1969; **24**: 453–60.

61. Refetoff S.: Iatrogenic hydrothorax. *Ann. Intern. Med.* 1965; **63**: 869–72.

62. Koch M. J.: Bilateral intravenous hydrothorax. *N. Engl. J. Med.* 1972; **286**: 218.

63. Rudge C. J., Bewick M., McColl I.: Hydrothorax after central venous catheterisation. *Br. Med. J.* 1973; **3**: 23–5.

64. Carvell J. E., Pearce D. J.: Bilateral hydrothorax following internal jugular vein catheterisation. *Br. J. Surg.* 1976; **63**: 381–3.

65. Hopkinson R. B., Parkin C. E.: Hydrohaemothorax following percutaneous internal jugular vein cannulation recognized by intravenous pyelography. *Anaesth. Analg.* 1978; **57**: 507–11.

66. Brandt R. L., Feley W. J., Fink G. H. et al.: Mechanism of perforation of the heart with production of hydropericardium by a venous catheter and its prevention. *Am. J. Surg.* 1970; **119**: 311–16.

67. Fenn J. E., Stensel H. C.: Certain hazards of the central venous catheter. *Angiology* 1969; **20**: 38–43.

68. Belani K. G., Buckley J. J., Gordon J. R. et al.: Percutaneous cervical central venous placement: a comparison of the internal and external jugular vein routes. *Anaesth. Analg.* 1980; **59**: 40–4.

69. McConnell R. Y., Fox R. T.: Experience with percutaneous internal jugular-innominate vein catheterisation. *California Med.* 1972; **117**: 1.

70. Shang W., Rosen M.: Positioning central venous catheters through the basilic vein. *Br. J. Anaesth.* 1973; **45**: 1211.

71. Langston C. S.: The aberrant central venous catheter and its complications. *Diagnostic Radiol.* 1971; **100**: 55–9.

72. Burri C., Gasser D.: *Der Vena Cava-Catheter.* Berlin: Springer-Verlag, 1971: 126.

73. Malatinsky J., Kadlic T., Májek M. et al.: Misplacement and loop formation of central venous catheters. *Acta Anaesth. Scand.* 1976; **20**: 237–47.

74. Gilner L. I.: The 'Ear-gurgling' sign. *N. Engl. J. Med.* 1981; **296**: 1301.

75. Klein H. O., Segni E. D., Kaplinsky E.: Unsuspected cerebral perfusion: a complication of the use of a central venous pressure catheter. *Chest* 1978; **74**: 109–10.

76. Dunbar R. D., Mitchell R., Lavine M.: Aberrant locations of central venous catheters. *Lancet* 1981; **1**: 711–15.

77. Cited in: Larsen C. P.: Venous air embolism. Report of four cases. Suggested method of treatment. *Am. J. Clin. Pathol.* 1951; **21**: 247.

78. Bichat M. F. X.: *Physiological Researchs into Life and Death.* Translated by F. Gold with notes by F. Magendie. Boston: Richardson & Lord, 1827: 188.

79. Magendie F.: Sur l'entrée accidentelle de l'air dans les veines. *J. Physiol. Pathol.* 1821; **1**: 192.

80. Erichsen J. E.: On the proximate cause of death after the spontaneous introduction of air into the veins,

with some remarks on the treatment of that accident. *Edinb. Med. Surg. J.* 1844; **61**: 1.

81. Simpson K.: Air accidents during transfusion. *Lancet* 1942; **1**: 697–8.

82. Yeakel A. E.: Lethal air embolism from plastic blood storage container. *JAMA* 1969; **204**: 267.

83. Mariani: Cited by Cole F. C.: Intravenous oxygen. *Anaesthesiology* 1951; **12**: 181.

84. Tunnicliffe F. W., Stebbing G. F.: Intravenous injection of oxygen gas as a therapeutic measure. *Lancet* 1916; **2**: 321.

85. Gottlieb J. D., Ericsson J. A., Sweet R. B.: Venous air embolism: a review. *Anaesth. Analg. Curr. Res.* 1965; **44**: 773.

86. Alexander J. I., Lewis A. A. M.: Air embolism during mastectomy. *Anaesthesia* 1969; **24**: 618–19.

87. Buckland R. W., Manner J. M.: Venous air embolism during neurosurgery. *Anaesthesia* 1976; **31**: 633–43.

88. Stoney W. S., Alford W. C., Burrus G. R. et al.: Air embolism and other accidents using pump oxygenators. *Ann. Thorac. Surg.* 1980; **29**: 336–40.

89. Ordway C. B.: Air embolism via CVP catheter without positive pressure: presentation of a case and review. *Ann. Surg.* 1974; **179**: 479–81.

90. Barth L., Richter J.: Untersuchen zum mechanismus der luftembolie im Bereich der Halsvenen des Menschen. *Anaesthetist* 1971; **20**: 430–6.

91. Colley R.: Education of the hospital staff. In: Fischer J. E. (ed.): *Total Parenteral Nutrition.* Boston, Mass.: Little, Brown, 1976: 123.

92. Lucas C. E., Irani L.: Air embolus via subclavian catheter. *N. Engl. J. Med.* 1969; **281**: 966.

93. Hoshal V. L., Fink G. G.: The subclavian catheter. *N. Engl. J. Med.* 1969; **281**: 1425.

94. Green H. L.: Air embolism as a complication during parenteral nutrition therapy. *Am. J. Surg.* 1971; **121**: 614.

95. Parsa M. H., Ferrer J. H. (ed.): *Safe Central Venous Nutrition.* Springfield, Ill.: Thomas, 1974: 68.

96. Ferrer J. M., Parsa, M. H.: Fatal air embolism via subclavian vein. *N. Engl. J. Med.* 1970; **282**: 688.

97. Walls A. D. F.: In: Baxter D. H. and Jackson G. M. (ed.): *Clinical Parenteral Nutrition.* Proceedings of a clinical nutrition workshop. University of Liverpool: Liverpool Medical Institute, 1977: 182.

98. Grace D. M.: Air embolism with neurological complications. A potential hazard of central venous catheters. *Can. J. Surg.* 1977; **20**: 51.

99. Colqhoun B. P. D.: Simple device to prevent disruption of centrally placed intravenous catheters. *Can. J. Surg.* 1977; **20**: 565.

100. Peters J. L., Armstrong R.: Air embolism occurring as a complication of central venous catheterisation. *Ann. Surg.* 1978; **187**: 375–8.

101. Le Bos L. P., Weterman I. T.: Total parenteral nutrition in Crohn's disease. *World J. Surg.* 1980; **4**: 163–5.

102. Peters J. L.: Intravenous systems, a need for change? *Br. J. Intravenous Ther.* 1980; **1**: 43–5.

103. Mattox K. L., Bricker D. L.: Air embolism following subclavian vein catheterisation. *Texas Med.* 1970; **66**: 74.

104. Ross S. M., Freedman P. S., Farman J. V.: Air embolism after accidental removal of intravenous catheter. *Br. Med. J.* 1979; **1**: 987.

105. Paskin D. L., Hoffren W. S., Tuddenham W. T.: A new complication of subclavian vein catheterisation. *Ann. Surg.* 1974; **179**: 266.

106. Peters J. L.: Central venous catheter Luer-locks. *Lancet* 1978; **2**: 430–1.

107. Metcalfe E., Griffiths D., Peters J. L. et al.: Air embolism and intravenous catheters. *Br. Med. J.* 1979; **1**: 1630.

108. Irving M., Tresadern J.: The benefits of central vein feeding and long term access to the circulation. *Acta Chir. Scand.* 1980; Suppl. 507: 399.

109. Bayliss C. E., Beanlands D. S., Baird R. J.: The pacemaker twiddler's syndrome. *Can. Med. Assoc. J.* 1968; **99**: 371–3.

110. Tegtmeyer C., Deignan J. M.: Cardiac pacemakers: a different twist. *AJR* 1976; **126**: 1017–18.

111. Bauer E., Densen P.: Infection from contaminated Elastoplast. *N. Engl. J. Med.* 1979; **300**: 370.

112. Cooper J. B., Newbower R. S., Long C. D. et al.: Preventable anaesthetic mishaps; a study of human factors. *Anaesthesiology* 1978; **49**: 399–406.

113. Jacobsen W. J., Briggs B. A., Thorp R. et al.: Air embolism in association with LeVeen shunt. *Crit. Care Med.* 1980; **8**: 659–60.

114. Schofield A.: Hazard Notice (HN) (79) 34. London: DHSS, 1979.

115. Schofield A.: Hazard Notice (HN) (76) 74. London: DHSS, 1976.

116. Durant T. M., Long J., Oppenheimer M. J.: Pulmonary (venous) air embolism. *Am. Heart J.* 1957; **33**: 269–81.

117. Nicholson M. J.: Emergency treatment of air embolism. *Lahey Clin. Bull.* 1954; **56**: 239–47.

118. Gronert G. A., Messick J. M., Cucchiara R. F. et al.: Paradoxical air embolism from a patent foramen ovale. *Anaesthesiology* 1979; **50**: 548–9.

119. Thomas J. H., MacArthur R. I., Pierce G. E. et al.: Hickman–Broviac catheters; indications and results. *Am. J. Surg.* 1980; **140**: 791–6.

120. Bozetti F.: Subclavian venous thrombosis secondary to indwelling catheters for parenteral nutrition. *Surg. Ital.* 1977; **7**: 210–15.

121. Novitsky N., Jacobs, P.: Late displacement of central venous catheter resulting in vascular obstruction. *Br. Med. J.* 1980; **1**: 156.

122. Dinley R. J.: Venous reaction related to in-dwelling plastic cannulae: a prospective clinical trial. *Curr. Med. Res. Opin.* 1976; **3**: 607–17.

123. Westaby S., Gillies I. D. S.: Ryle's tube for rapid intravenous transfusion. *Lancet* 1979; **1**: 360–1.

124. Virchow R.: *Gesammelte Abhandlungen zur Wissenschaftlichen Medicin.* Frankfurt: Verlag Von Meindinger Sohn and Comp., 1856.

125. Bansmer G., Keith D., Tesluk H.: Complications following use of indwelling catheters of inferior vena cava. *JAMA* 1958; **167**: 1606–11.

126. Warden G. D., Wilmore D. W., Pruitt B. A.: Central venous thrombosis: a hazard of medical progress. *J. Trauma* 1973; **13**: 620–6.

127. Schuster W., Vennebusch D.: Vena cava superior thrombose nach anlegen einers jugularis interna katheters. *Anaesthetist* 1978; **27**: 546–7.

128. Steffelaar J. W.: Obductie bevindingen met betrekking tot centrale vene catheters (CVC). *Ned. Tijdschr. Geneeskd.* 1975; **119**: 339.

129. Nottage W. M.: Iatrogenic superior vena cava syndrome, a complication of internal jugular vein catheterisation. *Chest* 1976; **70**: 566.

130. de Bruijin N. P., Stadt H. H.: Bilateral thrombosis of internal jugular veins after multiple percutaneous cannulations. *Anaesth. Analg.* 1981; **60**: 448–9.

131. Hughes E. S. R.: Venous obstruction in the upper extremity (Paget–Schroetter's syndrome). *Int. Abstr. Surg.* 1949; **88**: 89.

132. Swinton N. W., Edgett J. W., Hall R. J.: Primary subclavian-axillary vein thrombosis. *Circulation* 1968; **38**: 737–45.

133. Paget J.: *Clinical Lectures and Essays.* London: Longmans Green & Co., 1875.

134. Von Schroetter L.: Erkrankungen der Gefasse. In: *Nathnagel Handbuch der Pathologic und Therapie.* Vienna: Holder, 1884.

135. Axelsson C. K., Efsen F.: Phlebography in long-term catheterisation of the subclavian vein. A retrospective study in patients with severe gastrointestinal disorders. *Scand. J. Gastroenterol.* 1978; **13**: 933–8.

136. Peters J. L., Kenning B. R., Garrett C. P. O. et al.: Doppler ultrasound, an aid to percutaneous subclavian vein catheterisation. *Br. Med. J.* 1980; **281**: 618.

137. Bonchek L. I., Geiss D. M., Farley G. M.: Emergency thrombectomy for acute thrombosis of superior vena cava. *J. Thorac. Cardiovasc. Surg.* 1979; **77**: 922–4.

138. Singh A. K., Dykhuizan D. L., Varges L. L.: Acute superior vena cava obstruction with intracavitatory thrombosis: A complication of central venous catheterisation. *Cardiovasc. Dis. Bull. Texas Heart Inst.* 1979; **6**: 308–12.

139. Bernard C.: *Lecons sur le Chaleur Animale.* Paris: Baillière et Fils, 1876: 42–81.

140. Goodwin J. F. Fatality following cardiac catheterisation injury. *Br. Heart. J.* 1953; **15**: 330–5.

141. Brown C. A., Kent A.: Perforation of right ventricle by polyethylene catheter. *South. Med. J.* 1956; **1**: 466–7.

142. Dalgaard J. B.: Fatal right ventricular perforation during cardiac catheterisation. *Acta Med. Scand.* 1964; **175**: 697–702.

143. Johnson C. F.: Perforation of right atrium by a polyethylene catheter. *JAMA* 1966; **135**: 584–5.

144. Doering R. B., Stemmer E. A., Connelly J. E.: Complications of indwelling venous catheter with particular reference to catheter embolus. *Am. J. Surg.* 1967; **114**: 259–66.

145. Friedman B. A., Jurgeleit H. C.: Perforation of atrium by polyethylene CV catheter. *JAMA* 1968; **203**: 1141–2.

146. Defalque R., Campbell C.: Cardiac tamponade from central venous catheters. *Anaesthesiology* 1979; **50**: 249–52.

147. Hoffman W. I.: Wounds of the heart from central venous catheters. *J. Trauma* 1971; **11**: 193.

148. Homesly H. D., Zelenik J. S.: Hazards of central venous pressure monitoring: pericardial tamponade. *Am. Heart J.* 1972; **84**: 135–6.

149. Thomas C. S., Carter J. W., Lowder S. C.: Pericardial tamponade from central venous catheters. *Arch. Surg.* 1969; **98**: 217–18.

150. Wickbom G., Brodin M., Krog M.: Cardiac tamponade—a serious complication to central intravenous infusions. In: Abstracts of the 1st European Congress on Parenteral and Enteral Nutrition. Stockholm, 2–5 September 1979: 69.

151. Dobios T. J., Magovern G. J., Gay T. C.: Cardiac tamponade complicating percutaneous catheterisation of subclavian vein. *Surgery* 1975; **78**: 261–3.

152. Guest J., Leiberman D. P.: Late complications of catheterisation for intravenous nutrition. *Lancet* 1976; **2**: 805.

153. Hinkley M. E.: Thoracic duct thrombosis with fatal chylothorax caused by a long venous catheter. *N. Engl. J. Med.* 1969; **280**: 25.

154. Allsop J. R., Askew A. R.: Subclavian vein cannulation: a new complication. *Br. Med. J.* 1975; **1**: 262–3.

155. Raffensperger J. G., Ramenovsky M. L.: A fatal complication of hyperalimentation. A case report. *Surgery* 1970; **68**: 393.

156. Briscoe C. E., Bushman J. A., McDonald W. I.: Extensive neurological damage after cannulation of internal jugular vein. *Br. Med. J.* 1974; **1**: 314.

157. Lee Y. H., Kerstein M. D.: Osteomyelitis and septic arthritis: a complication of subclavian vein catheterisation. *N. Engl. J. Med.* 1971; **285**: 1179–81.

158. Oakes D. D., Wilson R. E.: Malposition of a subclavian line. *JAMA* 1975; **233**: 532–3.

159. Brennan M. F., Sugarbaker P. H., Moore F. P.: Venobronchial fistula: a rare complication of central venous catheterisation for parenteral nutrition. *Arch. Surg.* 1973; **106**: 871.

160. Henzel J. H., De Weese M. S.: Morbid and mortal complications associated with prolonged central venous cannulation. *Am. J. Surg.* 1971; **121**: 600–5.

161. Forssmann W.: Die Sondierung des Rechten Herzens. *Klin. Wochenschr.* 1929; **8**: 2085.

Chapter 13

Sepsis and Central Venous Catheter Systems

R. N. Grüneberg

Serious infection has long been known to follow the creation of a wound in a vein. During the Middle Ages, venesection was widely practised for the treatment of disease. In the sixteenth century Ambroise Paré treated Charles IX of France for a phlebitis which lasted for 3 months after bleeding (1) whilst in 1696 Mareschal, surgeon to the King of France and founder of the Royal Academy of Surgery in France, observed the death of a 'foreign gentleman' from this cause (2). The prevalence of serious inflammation involving veins made Cruveilhier consider that 'phlebitis dominates all pathology' (3). By this he meant that it was the most common source of sepsis that he saw at autopsy. Intravenous infusion has now become an indispensable feature of modern medical therapy; however, infection, especially infusion and catheter-related septicaemia, remains a life-threatening hazard. Contamination of an intravenous infusion or monitoring system can occur at virtually any point, from the time of manufacture of the equipment until the infusion is terminated in hospital.

The relationship between the longevity of venous cannulation, bacterial colonization and the incidence of thrombophlebitis emerged some time ago. The beneficial effects of using plastic administration tubing instead of rubber were also noted in the same study (4). There has been a continuing development of interest in this aspect of patient care during the past 20 years as the use both of peripheral and central venous infusions has proliferated. It is interesting to note that during the 1950s and 1960s the hazard of infusion-related infection was largely unappreciated, and, indeed, the 1962 edition of the American Hospital Association's Monograph *Control of Infection in Hospitals*, did not mention intravenous therapy as a potential source of infection (5). Attention was focused on the problem in the early 1970s when several outbreaks of septicaemia occurred in which bacterial contamination of the fluid containers was traced to the manufacturing process. A full review of this subject has been completed by Maki et al. working at the Center for Disease Control, Atlanta, in the United States (6). More recently, a similar appraisal of the problem has been made in the United Kingdom by Phillips et al. (7). Thus, decisions on whether to set up central venous lines are always a question of balancing possible benefits and possible risks. Perhaps the most important of the risks is infection resulting from contamination by micro-organisms at any point in the system. Once contaminated, the intravenous catheter and its adherent fibrin sleeve will act as an intravascular nidus for the growth of bacteria or fungi which can be rapidly transmitted direct to the heart, great blood vessels and intracardiac valves and so be disseminated to any part of the body by secondary bloodstream spread (8). Furthermore, it must be appreciated that some pathogens grow luxuriantly in infusion fluids at room temperature, attaining concentrations exceeding 10^5 organisms per ml in less than 24 hours. Central venous catheters are consequently an ever-present portal of infection and must be recognized as a potential source of septicaemia.

Quite apart from the obvious hazards of establishing a direct pathway from the patient's environment to his very heart, there are other reasons why this procedure may carry more than the usual infective risks. First, the patient is likely to be in poor condition, or the desirability of central venous catheterization would not have arisen. It is probable that the underlying clinical circumstances will prejudice the patient's chances of recovery from microbial invasion, should this occur. Many surgical patients requiring central venous catheterization may have significant protein–calorie malnutrition and evidence of impaired cellular and humoral immunological defence mechanisms. Secondly, the patient will probably be situated in a hospital ward or specialized unit with its own established flora of highly pathogenic micro-organisms, nowadays often resistant to many antibiotics. Thirdly, because of the other medical conditions present, it is very probable that the patient will be treated with antibiotics which may themselves predispose to colonization with unusual organisms in place of the patient's own accustomed bacteria. These new organisms, commonly resistant to antibiotics and derived from the unit's resident bacterial flora, may have a greater propensity for tissue invasion than do the patient's own microbes. Fourthly, it is probable that both the patient and the infusion system will receive a great deal of handling from nursing and medical staff, physiotherapists, radiographers and numerous others involved in intensive medical care. The effect of all this human contact is to multiply the opportunities for patient-to-patient transfer of locally prevalent (usually antibiotic-resistant) organisms on the hands of the staff. When such patients are gathered together in one unit, as in intensive care units or in premature baby units, it is probable that the nursing and other staff will be over-committed and will in consequence pay less than adequate attention to basic routines aimed at prevention of cross-infection, such as hand washing, with inevitably increased chances of outbreaks of hospital infection (*Fig.* 13.1).

From what has been said so far it might seem that the hazards are so enormous that central venous cannulation should rarely be undertaken. Clearly, such a view would be quite inappropriate, but a decision to insert a central line should always be taken with a lively awareness of the infective risks. Established infection in central venous catheters and systems carries a high morbidity and mortality, but with reason-

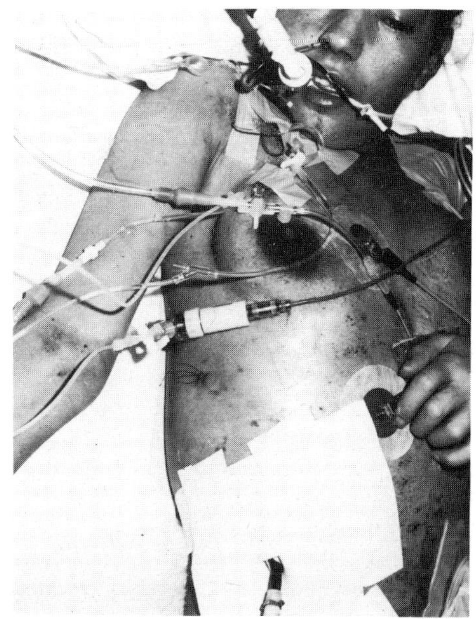

Fig. 13.1. An extreme clinical situation: this patient has developed severe septicaemia and shock secondary to intra-uterine and pelvic infection. Note the multiple portals for entry of nosocomial infection via three-way stopcocks, side-ports and poorly fitting connections. The central catheters are in close proximity to a nasogastric, endotracheal and abdominal drainage tube, as well as an intestinal stoma.

able care the chance of such infection can be kept to an acceptably low level.

Endogenous and Exogenous Infection

The organisms causing infection in central lines may be derived from the patient's own flora (endogenous infection) or from extraneous sites (exogenous infection). Nowadays it is realized that this classification omits a very important intermediate mechanism by which the patient's bowel flora is progressively changed from the moment that he is admitted to hospital, the new flora being characteristic of the ward to which he is admitted and reflecting the time for which he has been subject to the new environment (9). The new faecal flora may then be the source of apparently endogenous infection. What is really happening is a faecal–faecal–lesion type of cross-infection with a great likelihood of transferring organisms with greater pathogenicity, invasiveness and antibiotic resistance than the patient's normal flora with which he was happily co-existing before his admission to hospital.

Endogenous infection will mostly be with organisms present on the skin, notably with coagulase-positive staphylococci (*S. aureus*), coagulase-negative staphylococci (*S. albus* or *S. epidermis*), haemolytic streptococci, such as *S. pyogenes* or *S. faecalis*, and Gram-negative rods derived from the gut flora such as *E. coli* and *Proteus mirabilis*. If the site chosen for insertion is a warm moist one such as the groin, there will be much greater likelihood of the skin being colonized by coliform organisms such as *E. coli*, Proteus spp., klebsiellas or pseudomonads. Prior use of broad spectrum antibiotics such as members of the ampicillin (amoxycillin) group will greatly increase the chance of colonization with the more inherently antibiotic resistant organisms such as Klebsiella spp. and pseudomonads. This has already indicated two ways in which the chance of infection of central lines can be reduced: by choosing a dry flat area of skin for insertion rather than a moist skin fold, and by avoiding the use of broad spectrum antibiotics such as ampicillin and amoxycillin in areas where there are patients concentrated in whom infection with klebsiellas and pseudomonads would be likely and particularly damaging. For this reason, in my own hospital the clinicians and microbiologists have agreed to avoid the use of these antibiotics in high dependency areas such as the intensive care unit and the premature baby unit. By this action alone, the chances of patients becoming infected with these highly antibiotic-resistant but otherwise usually non-pathogenic organisms can be much reduced. It is safer from the infection prevention standpoint to insert a line through the skin of the forearm or the neck than through a skinfold such as the axilla or groin. In addition, it should be remembered that sites below the waist are much more heavily loaded with faecal organisms than are sites elsewhere. This fact was learned shortly after the introduction of plastic intravenous devices, and several groups reported episodes of suppurative thrombophlebitis and septicaemia (10–14).

Exogenous infection may be caused by the same types of organism as those listed as causing endogenous infection but is more likely to be caused by the locally established hospital pathogens. Thus, the staphylococci will be strains of *S. aureus* of particular bacteriophage types with a propensity to cause outbreaks of hospital sepsis. Very commonly such staphylococci will be resistant to tetracycline as well as to other antibiotics such as the penicillinase-sensitive penicillins. Exogenous infections nowadays are much more commonly caused by Gram-negative rods than by Gram-positive cocci. Possible pathogens include all the common faecal aerobic rods such as *E. coli*, Proteus spp., klebsiellas and pseudomonads. Occasionally, outbreaks of sepsis occur with less common organisms such as *Serratia marcescens*, Providencia spp., Acinetobacter spp. and the more unusual species of pseudomonas. These reflect local prevalences and antibiotic usage. Thus, outbreaks of nosocomial (hospital) infection with serratia are not infrequent in the USA and in some countries in continental Europe, but scarcely ever occur in the United Kingdom. The importance of recognition that the most important cross-infecting pathogens are Gram-negative lies in appreciating that they: (*a*) are easily spread on hands which are inadequately washed and dried; (*b*) thrive in many disinfectants; (*c*) prosper in moist sites; and (*d*) are often multiply antibiotic-resistant. Herein lie many of the clues to successful avoidance of infection of central venous lines.

Sometimes infections of central venous lines are caused not by bacteria but by fungi, most commonly yeasts such as the candida species (*C. albicans* and occasionally other variants, e.g. *C. parapsilosis*) or *Torulopsis glabrata*. This nearly always occurs in very debilitated, often immunosuppressed patients who have received prolonged antibiotic treatment, particularly broad spectrum antibiotics, cytotoxic drugs, steroids or radiotherapy. The outlook is poor in such cases, partly because of the surrounding circumstances and partly because of the relative ineffectiveness (and sometimes danger) of antifungal chemotherapy. Occasionally, it is possible to see the fungal colonies growing on the luminal wall of the removed catheter when this is opened (using aseptic technique, *Fig.* 13.2). Such a finding should lead to immediate microscopy of the colonies since this will permit a speedier diagnosis to be reached and so enable the clinician to start appropriate antifungal chemotherapy 1 or 2 days earlier than would otherwise be possible.

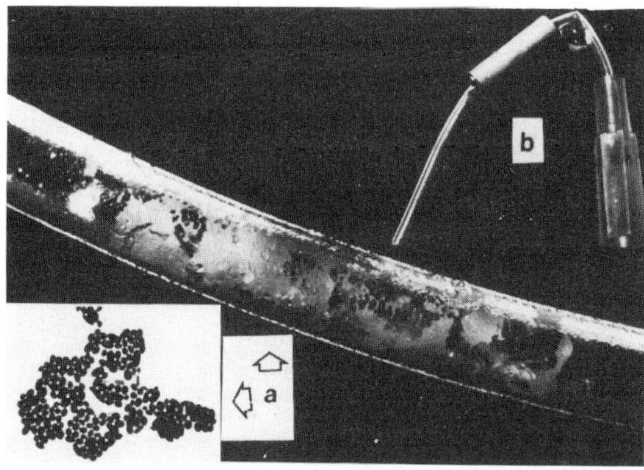

Fig. 13.2. *a,* Colonies of candida can be seen within the lumen of this catheter and were found on microscopy. *b,* The catheter had become colonized via a microstress fracture which the nursing staff had temporarily sealed with adhesive tape. (Reproduced by kind permission of the Editor of the *British Journal of Anaesthesia.*)

Candida Septicaemia

This problem has become more apparent since the advent of total parenteral nutrition (15–18). Although this organism is a normal saprophytic commensal of the respiratory tract, alimentary tract and vagina, it can become a potent nosocomial pathogen if colonization of urinary catheters and central venous catheters or associated connections should occur. Venous blood samples may be unhelpful in establishing the diagnosis, even in the presence of septicaemia; in such circumstances, arterial blood cultures may be of more value (12). The disease often has an insidious onset and, once established, tissue invasion of the heart, retina, kidneys and spleen usually occurs. Candida endophthalmitis can be recognized on fundoscopy and the patient usually complains of eye pain and loss of vision to a varying degree. After the detection of the organism in the urine or sputum, the clinician must have a high index of suspicion that systemic infection has occurred in patients receiving prolonged parenteral nutrition.

Aseptic Technique

When central venous manometer or parenteral feeding lines are set up, the procedure should be performed with the utmost care and there can be no room for compromise. Ideally, a line should be inserted in a relatively safe environment, such as an operating theatre. If that is not possible, a separate treatment room is preferable to the open ward. The proposed site should be carefully palpated and marked before the skin is prepared. It should be recognized that no antiseptic will sterilize the skin completely, the aim being to reduce the bacterial population as much as possible. The skin should be washed with soap and water and thoroughly dried. Hairy areas should be shaved using a sterile disposable razor taking care not to inflict any microabrasions. Thereafter an antiseptic should be used which will leave the skin dry. Alcoholic povidone-iodine or alcoholic chlorhexidine are suitable. The area should then be surrounded with sterile towels applied with full operating theatre technique. The entire procedure from then on should be performed by the gowned, masked and gloved operator using the most careful aseptic technique. Insertion of a line should never be attempted by the operator acting alone; at least one assistant is essential. As in any surgical procedure, there should be as little movement as possible in the operating room, as few non-essential attendants as possible and the handling of the insertion site should be kept to an absolute minimum. The external end of the line should be left in such a way as to permit the necessary procedures being carried out without moving the line longitudinally through the skin. It is preferable then to spray the area of skin immediately adjacent to the catheter exit site with dry povidone-iodine powder (e.g. Disadine, Stuart Pharmaceuticals). A small square of sterile gauze dry dressing should be then placed around the catheter and over the exit site before, finally, the dressing is completed by the application of a transparent sheet of polyurethane adhesive film (e.g. Op-Site, Smith & Nephew). This dressing allows the nursing staff, and indeed the patient, to inspect the catheter exit wound regularly.

The technique used may be a simple through-cannula percutaneous puncture or a surgical cut-down procedure. The use of a skin tunnel technique (reviewed in Chapter 9) should be considered since this offers the opportunity of lengthening the life of the catheter and because the greater distance created between the skin entry site and the point of catheter entry into the superior vena cava appears to reduce the chance of infection being introduced to the bloodstream from the skin. The creation of a skin tunnel has particular relevance if the patient has a co-existing tracheostomy.

Once the line has been established, it should be left undisturbed as much as is practicable. The skin wound should be inspected through the transparent Op-Site and dry gauze dressing. This allows early erythema or exudate to be easily detected. The danger signs of impending catheter-related sepsis are: pain at the site of insertion, lymphangitis or phlebitis proximal to the insertion site and fever. If any of these are noted, the wound should be examined, again using aseptic technique. Apparent blockage of a line should also give rise to suspicion of infection, and recently it has been noted that patients sometimes develop a degree of glucose intolerance. Obstruction to flow may occur because of kinking or thrombosis, but can also be due to the deposition of fibrin at the site of microbial infection. Thus, there may also be a role for intermittent low-dose heparin therapy injected via the infusion line in reducing catheter-related infection (19).

While a line is in position, it should not be used for any purpose other than that originally intended. If the line was set up for haemo-dynamic monitoring purposes, it should not be used for intravenous feeding or for the administration of antibiotics or blood transfusions. Traditionally, central venous catheters have not been used for diagnostic blood samples which can readily be collected from other sites, although Werner Forssmann envisaged such a role following the experiments upon himself (20). More recently, the Hickman–Broviac silicone catheters have been used for the administration of a wide variety of bolus intravenous drug injections, the infusion of blood products and central venous blood sampling without mishap in patients suffering from leukaemia and allied disorders. The rationale for this is sound in such patients since each and every needle puncture is invariably followed by a painful haematoma which in turn may act as a nidus for subcutaneous infection. It must be emphasized, however, that in order to use central catheters in this way, an exceptionally strict aseptic ritual must be carried out by the relevant clinical and nursing personnel. It is wise to restrict such activities to specific members of staff and units in order to avoid all gratuitous interference with the infusion system and reduce to a minimum the opportunities for introducing infection. At the earliest possible moment that the line can be removed without detriment to the patient's well-being, it should be dismantled. During this procedure, as on every other occasion, a strict aseptic technique should be used and the tip of the line should be cut off aseptically and sent for bacteriological culture. In addition, the rest of the catheter and hub should be sent to the microbiology laboratory in a dry sterile pot so that the lumen of the hub and shaft may be cultured. It is possible for the line to be infected without this being suspected clinically.

Clinical Investigation of Suspected Catheter-related Sepsis

When infection is suspected, blood cultures should be collected and a swab taken from the skin wound for bacteriological examination. Blood culture should be taken by the usual technique, making a fresh venepuncture in a vein distant from that in which the line lies. If there is more than a suspicion that the line is infected, the entire line should be removed from the patient. The tip of the line should be cut off aseptically and sent to the microbiology laboratory for culture as previously described. It is unwise to remove the old catheter and replace it with a new sterile device over a Seldinger guide wire if the catheter has been blocked and this is considered to be due to an infected fibrinous plug; the lumen of the new catheter will almost certainly be contaminated in the process. This manoeuvre should be reserved for the rare instances when a catheter starts to develop a stress fracture and replacement into another central venous access site is not feasible.

Patients with central venous catheters situated in their circulatory system who develop pyrexia merit a further full clinical examination in addition to inspection of the central venous infusion system. Often, the fever may be due to some unrelated cause. The oropharynx and parotid glands should be inspected, the chest auscultated and an X-ray performed if indicated. Surgical wounds must be re-examined and urine cultures taken, especially if a urethral catheter has been in place. Other peripheral infusion sites should be examined for evidence of inflammation. In the postoperative surgical patient, the usual sites for occult abscess formation must be considered and, naturally, a rectal examination performed to exclude a pelvic abscess. The central venous catheter may be 'innocent' and indeed may be vital for the patient's continued pharmacological and nutritional support at that time. Therefore, a full spectrum of the relevant bacteriology specimens must be sent off, including: sputum, a wound swab, an MSU, in addition to the blood cultures. Furthermore, any three-way stopcocks must be sent for culture at the same time. Since an infected central venous catheter will intermittently liberate bacteria into the circulation, the symptoms and signs are very much those of a bacterial endocarditis. Accordingly, the fingers, nailbeds and fundi must be inspected carefully and it is a wise precaution to listen carefully to the heart at regular intervals during the patient's period of catheterization so that the clinician can detect the development of any new murmurs. The need for a continuing central venous line should be reviewed at regular intervals. If it is decided that a line needs to be re-inserted in a patient who has suffered an episode of catheter-related sepsis, this should preferably be performed after an interval of the appropriate systemic antibiotic therapy administered by a peripheral infusion.

Patients who have several potential sources of infection and pyrexia after major surgery, e.g. wound sepsis, urinary or respiratory tract infection, and require a central venous catheter for parenteral nutrition, present a difficult problem. The technical difficulties of catheter replacement may make it undesirable to remove the device; it is essential, however, to exclude the central venous catheter as a primary source of intravascular sepsis. Wing et al. described the value of performing quantitative bacteriological culture and analysis of blood withdrawn simultaneously from a distant peripheral vein and from the lumen of the central catheter (21). Detection of increased colony counts from the central catheter blood culture samples compared to those from the peripheral blood confirmed that the catheter was indeed responsible for the septicaemia. This technique may well prove to be of value in the future management of such situations (*Fig.* 13.3).

An episode of proven microbial infection of a central venous line should be investigated jointly by clinician, nurse, infection control nurse and

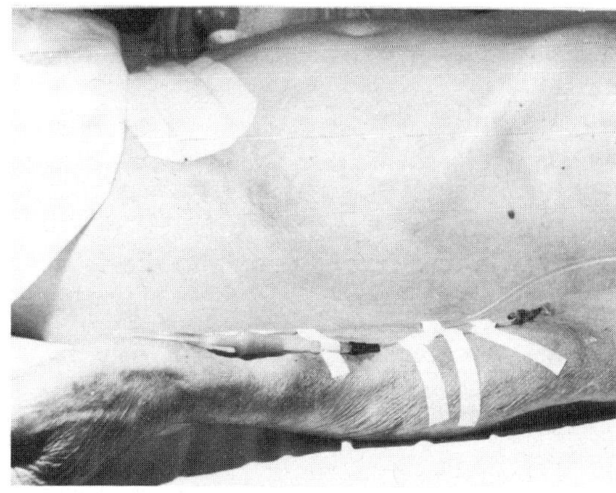

Fig. 13.3. A catheter shown to be the source of systemic infection. Note the inadequate dressing and the position of the introducing cannula with its tip still present within the vein. The introducing cannula lumen is filled with old blood which acts as a perfect nidus for bacterial colonization.

microbiologist in an attempt to establish possible causes. If it is the local usage to have all intravenous infusions inspected daily by an intravenous drip nurse or team, then all patients with central venous lines should be similarly reviewed daily. The team investigating episodes should consider the circumstances in which the line was inserted, the nature of any accessory connections and procedures related to the devices; other relevant circumstances, such as any antibiotic treatment; how well locally defined procedures have been complied with; and the likely source of the organisms isolated. The episode should be treated with at least as much seriousness as would infection in a clean neurological or orthopaedic wound. If there is the slightest suspicion that the infusion fluids could be the source of infection, then the relevant administration sets, bottles and fluid sachets should be saved for microbiological analysis. If more than one case of infection occurs in a unit or if infections occur in the lines of more than one patient attended by the staff member, the most rigorous inquiry should be made by the control of infection officer. The purpose of this inquiry is not to apportion blame but to try to tighten up on any laxity of discipline or procedure in the interest of the safety of patients.

Careful records of all episodes should be kept by the infection control nurse and by the microbiologist for epidemiological and for medicolegal reasons. The clinician in charge of a patient whose central venous line becomes infected should be informed of all the material findings. No opportunity should be missed of publicizing the lessons learned locally. If the details are unusual, the case should be published so that the hazard is notified to a wider relevant audience. Three-way stopcocks and devices that possess injection ports should not be used adjacent to the skin surface and central catheter unless absolutely necessary. The functional integrity of central venous infusion systems is of vital importance and the ease with which small air bubbles can enter the central catheter lumen and hence carry bacteria is clearly shown in *Figs.* 13.4 and 13.5. Furthermore, the meniscus of fluid which is left in the side-port provides a suitable culture medium for the growth of micro-organisms. The importance of such devices used for haemodynamic monitoring of patients in the genesis of septicaemia is well recognized (22). Oberhammer has recently shown in a small patient study that 55 per cent of side-ports on cannulas harboured bacteria (23). Studies in the United States have also revealed high levels of bacterial contamination in three-way stopcocks (24, 25). Clinical bio-engineers are now becoming involved in the appraisal of devices for use in intravenous systems (26).

Laboratory culture of central line tips should

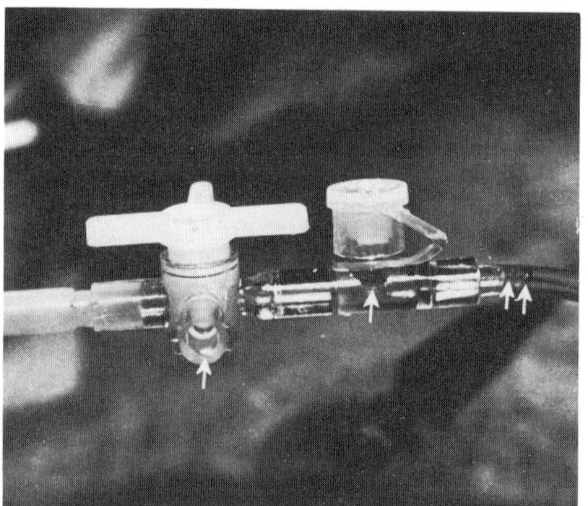

Fig. 13.4. Portals of bacterial entry into the circulation through unguarded three-way stopcocks, side-ports and fragile Luer slip fittings. Bacteria may be carried into the circulation within air bubbles.

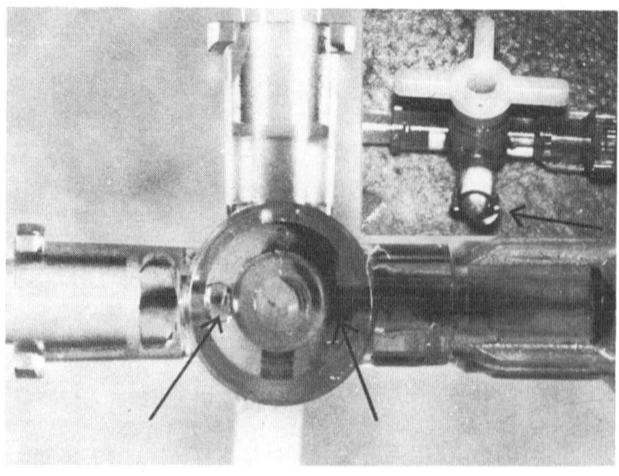

Fig. 13.5. The meniscus of fluid on the outside of a three-way stopcock provides a perfect culture medium for bacterial proliferation when in close proximity to the skin surface and handled frequently. The interstices of the mechanism harbour old blood and air bubbles.

always be performed whenever a line is removed from a patient, regardless of the reason. Some microbiologists may also wish to perform cultures upon samples taken from the lumen of the catheter hub and shaft. Full investigation of episodes should only be undertaken when cultures are positive since phlebitis, obstruction to flow, local pain and fever can all occur for non-infective reasons. The identification of the organism causing the infection will be helpful in tracking down its source. It may be that the same organism has caused several infections, in which case a search will be mounted for possible common sources. Alternatively, several infections may be caused by different organisms, in which case the search will be for breakdowns in procedure. Whatever the nature of the organism, information on its susceptibility to antibiotics will be very important as a guide to treatment. The cultural methods used by the laboratory will have to be such as to grow even small numbers of organisms, so the catheter tip should be flushed through and the washings cultured in nutrient broth, shaken hard and incubated at 37 °C for up to a week.

Treatment Guidelines

Treatment of suspected infection of a central venous line should be swift and determined. As already indicated, blood cultures and catheter tip cultures should be set up before antibiotics are given, and if appropriate, a new central venous line may be set up in another vein. It is preferable to allow a short period of time to elapse before this is performed in order to minimize the opportunity for further secondary infection of the new device. The results of culture and sensitivities will not be available for some time, so initial treatment will have to be undertaken without laboratory guidance. The principles of antibiotic choice are to choose bactericidal antibiotics (as in infective carditis); to choose a combination of drugs that will be effective against the likely pathogens listed previously (with respect to chemotherapy, fungal infection should be ignored initially); to administer the drugs parenterally; to give sufficient to be effective; and to start at once. Usually, a combination of penicillin G (or flucloxacillin) and gentamicin is appropriate. Dosage is not easily defined in patients who are likely to have central venous lines in position; allowances should be made for body weight, urinary output and renal function. The usual mistake with gentamicin is to give too little because of the fear of ototoxicity or nephrotoxicity. Under circumstances such as these, such anxieties are misplaced. An initial dose of 160 mg of gentamicin (for an adult) can safely be given even to a patient in renal failure. Thereafter, further dosage will be modified by serum gentamicin assays. An adult with normal renal function (not always present in those with central venous lines in position) usually needs around 120 mg of gentamicin 8-hourly by intramuscular injection to maintain his trough serum gentamicin level (just before the next dose is given) in the range 1–2 µg/ml. Penicillin G should usually be given in a dose of 1 g intramuscularly every 6 hours. Penicillin tends to accumulate in the blood of patients with defective renal function and may reach neurotoxic levels with epileptiform fits. In such patients the dose may have to be reduced, and serum penicillin assays may be a useful guide. The effect of the sodium administered with the penicillin should be considered in patients with cardiac or renal failure. Flucloxacillin should be given in a dosage of 500 mg 6-hourly.

When the sensitivities to antibiotics of the infecting organism are known, the treatment will be modified accordingly. It will usually be possible at that stage to use one antibiotic rather than two. Treatment should be continued for at least 3 days after the patient has become persistently afebrile. There is often a reluctance to remove an obviously infected central venous line and to try to overcome the problem by relying on antibiotics. This temptation should be resisted, for attempts to sterilize an infected lesion of any sort with antibiotics in the presence of a foreign body such as a catheter are almost doomed to failure. Very rarely an exit site skin tunnel infection may be successfully treated in this way.

Should infection with bacteria occur in a central venous line, the consequence may be very severe. At the least there may be local inflammation and purulence at the puncture site. This is usually easily managed by removal of the line, local application of disinfectants, such as povidone-iodine, and appropriate chemotherapy. A more serious event is the establishment of infective suppurative phlebitis in the cannulated vein, with or without regional lymph gland enlargement. This requires the same therapeutic steps as well as the possibility that analgesics, phenylbutazone and even anticoagulants may be needed. Surgical excision of the offending vein may need to be performed. The worst eventuality is the establishment of an infected thrombus in the lumen of the catheter. This may then result in the continuing release of numbers of bacteria into the bloodstream or even the occasional detachment of infected emboli into the blood. The consequences of this will include fever and toxaemia, often with rigors, usually with a neutrophil leucocytosis. Metastatic abscesses may occur in many different organs with consequent variation in the clinical picture. The development of such a severe clinical picture should raise the question in the clinician's mind that a suppurative phlebitis has become established in the great veins of the mediastinum and thoracic inlet. Careful contrast radiography studies must be performed and a vascular surgical opinion sought since, if this proves to be the diagnosis, the outlook is grave. Thrombectomy, using balloon catheters, may be successful if combined with an aggressive antibiotic therapy. On rare occasions, infected major veins have been successfully excised as a life-saving measure. Disseminated intravascular coagulation may occur and will need appropriate attention. This may then aggravate the clinical situation by compounding the underlying cardiac or renal problems. The consequent steps needed in the treatment of hypotension, renal, hepatic and cardiac failure, haemolysis, marrow depression and central nervous system effects are outside the scope of this chapter. Inability to prevent these severe if rare complications of central venous line infection may result in toxaemia, multiple system failure and death.

Filters

A recent report from the National Co-ordinating Committee on Large Volume Parenterals revealed that, in the USA, approximately 10 million in-line final filters were used annually (27). It was estimated that 100 million devices would be required annually if every intravenous infusion were filtered in an effort to minimize further the entry of particulate matter, micro-organisms and air into the human circulation. This committee recommended that filters should be used in patients who are receiving hyperalimentation therapy and considered for use in patients who have an impaired immune defence mechanism and to whom many additives are to be given in the intravenous fluid. Filters were not recommended for use when drugs in concentrations of less than $5\,\mu g/ml$ and/or where the total amount is less than $5\,mg$ over a 24-hour period unless studies confirmed that the specific drug was not absorbed or adsorbed to the intravenous solution container, administration set and filter.

The widespread use of end-line filters has not been generally adopted in the United Kingdom, partly on the basis of cost and also owing to the absence of good evidence to prove their value. The use of an end-line filter adds an extra junction and point for manipulation into the system, which can act as a potential source of bacterial entry. Perhaps in future their use will increase if they are incorporated into the intravenous administration lines as integrally moulded features; in this situation the problems of disconnection and touch-contamination would be eliminated. A full review of this interesting aspect of intravenous therapy has been provided by Lowe in the *British Journal of Intravenous Therapy* (28). This feature of peripheral and central intravenous catheter care will naturally require scrutiny by individual clinicians and units. At the present time, no firm guidance can be provided.

Summary

The key to the whole question of management of central venous lines from the infection-prevention stand-point is discipline and training. Medical staff must be taught, not only the detailed procedures of how to set up venous lines and how to look after patients with lines in position, but also to question the need for establishing the line in the first place. Nursing staff must be taught in detail how to assist in inserting central venous lines and in their subsequent maintenance. The comprehensive record-keeping required of nursing staff attending to patients with lines, described elsewhere in this volume, must be rigorously followed. The fundamental importance of leaving the line alone except when absolutely necessary must be stressed to all members of the 'caring team'. A close watch must be maintained for signs of possible infective trouble, as described above. This is essentially a nursing and medical responsibility, perhaps assisted by the intravenous infusion team, if this exists locally. These tasks will inevitably fall upon the ward or unit sister, whose experience is often greater than that of the junior medical staff. There is a duty upon the medical and nursing staff to seek expert help from the infection control nurses, the clinical microbiologists and the infection control officer whenever infection supervenes.

By such means, the patient should be enabled to receive the benefits to be expected from the use of central venous catheterization without being exposed to more than minimal infective hazards.

References

1. Paré A.: *Oeuvres Complètes d'Ambroise Paré*, Vol. 2. Paris: Baillière, 1841: 115.
2. Mareschal G.: *Eloge de M. Mareschal: Mémoires de l'Academie Royale de Chirurgie* Vol. 2. Paris: Menard & Desenne, 1819: 23.
3. Cruveilhier J.: Phlebitis: dictionnaire de medicin et de chirurgie pratique. In: Long E. R. (ed.): *Selected nosocomial infection. J. Clin. Eng.* 1979; **4**: 139–45. 1929: 217.
4. Original Article: Thrombophlebitis following intravenous infusions: trial of plastic and red rubber giving sets. Report to Medical Research Council by a

sub-committee of the Council, Blood Transfusion Research Committee. *Lancet* 1957; **1**: 595–7.

5. Colbeck J. C. (ed.): *Control of Infections in Hospitals.* Chicago: American Hospital Association, 1962.

6. Maki D. G., Goldman D. A., Rhame F. S.: Infection control in intravenous therapy. *Ann. Intern. Med.* 1973; **79**: 867.

7. Phillips I., Meers P. D., D'Arcy P.·F.: *Microbiological Hazards of Infusion Therapy.* Lancaster: MTP Press, 1976: 1–177.

8. Powell D. C., Bivins B. A., Bell R. M.: Bacterial endocarditis in the critically ill surgical patient. *Arch. Surg.* 1981; **116**: 311–15.

9. Kennedy R. P., Plorde J. J., Petersdorf, R. G.: Studies on the epidemiology of *E. coli* infections. IV. Evidence for a nosocomial flora. *J. Clin. Invest.* 1965; **44**: 193.

10. Neuhof H., Seley G. P.: Acute suppurative phlebitis complicated by septicaemia. *Surgery* 1947; **21**: 831–42.

11. Moncrieff J. A.: Femoral catheters. *Ann. Surg.* 1958; **147**: 167–72.

12. Bansmer G., Keith D., Tesluk H.: Complications following use of indwelling catheters of inferior vena cava. *JAMA* 1958; **167**: 1606–11.

13. Phillips R. W., Eyre J. D.: Septic thrombophlebitis with septicaemia. *N. Engl. J. Med.* 1958; **259**: 729–31.

14. Crane C.: Venous interruption for septic thrombophlebitis. *N. Engl. J. Med.* 1960; **262**: 947–51.

15. Ashcraft K. W., Leape L. C.: Candida sepsis complicating parenteral feeding. *JAMA* 1970; **212**: 454.

16. Brennan M. F., Goldman M. H., O'Connell R. C. et al.: Prolonged parenteral hyperalimentation: candida growth and the prevention of candidaemia by amphotericin instillation. *Ann. Surg.* 1972; **176**: 265.

17. Curry C. R., Quie P. G.: Fungal septicaemia in patients receiving parenteral hyperalimentation. *N. Engl. J. Med.* 1971; **285**: 1221.

18. Stone H. H., Kolb L. D., Currie C. A. et al.: Candida sepsis; pathogenesis and principles of treatment. *Ann. Surg.* 1974; **179**: 697.

19. Bailey M. J.: Reduction of catheter associated sepsis in parenteral nutrition using low-dose intravenous heparin. *Br. Med. J.* 1979; **1**: 1671–3.

20. Forssmann, W.: Die Sondierung des Rechten Herzens. *Klin. Wochenschr.* 1929; **8**: 2085.

21. Wing E. J., Norden C. W., Shadduck R. K.: Use of quantitative bacteriologic techniques to diagnose catheter-related sepsis. *Arch. Intern. Med.* 1979; **139**: 482.

22. Editorial: Monitoring devices and septicaemia. *Br. Med. J.* 1979; **2**: 1748.

23. Oberhammer E. P.: Contamination of injection ports on intravenous cannulae. *Lancet* 1980; **2**: 1027.

24. McCarthur B., Hargiss C., Schoenknecht F. D.: Stopcock contamination in an I.C.U. *Am. J. Nursing* 1975; **75**: 96–7.

25. Dryden G. E., Brickler J.: Stopcock contamination. *Anaesth. Analg. (Cleve.)* 1979; **58**: 141–2.

26. Ben-Zvi S., Gottlieb W.: Medical instrumentation and nosocomial infection. *J. Clin. Eng.* 1979; **4**: 139–45.

27. National Co-ordinating Committee on Large Volume Parenterals: Recommendations for action on an important problem regarding large volume parenterals. 1979.

28. Lowe G. D.: Filtration in intravenous therapy. A review of clinical and technical aspects of intravenous fluid and blood filtration in four parts. *Br. J. Intravenous Ther.* 1981; **2**(3): 42–52, (4) 37–54.

Chapter 14

The Management of Catheter Embolism

A. C. Edwards

With the increasing use of central venous catheters for prolonged haemodynamic monitoring, drug administration and parenteral nutrition, there has been a steadily increasing frequency in the incidence of catheter embolism, knotting and entrapment reported in the world literature. These complications are potentially serious for the patient who is critically ill.

The possibility that embolism might occur from the shearing of their fine ureteric catheters on the introducing needle was recognized by Cournand and Ranges in 1941 during their earliest investigations. Three years after the introduction of flexible plastic cannulas in 1945, Tuell reported the first fatal case following embolism of an intravenous catheter (1). His 'case' was a dog undergoing a laboratory experiment; he felt that the incident was significant enough to report in the medical literature. He suggested that the three factors which tended to force the catheter along the vein towards the heart in the animal were the blood flow, flexion of joints and the milking action of muscle contraction. Tuell found that even in a dead animal, a catheter could be quickly passed along a limb vein by successive flexion and extension action on the limb.

Incidence

The accidental migration of an intravenous infusion catheter from the arm to the heart was first reported in 1954 by Turner and Sommers, and their patient died (2). Two years later, a case of right ventricular perforation after a catheter embolism occurred (3). Embolism of a catheter fragment to the pulmonary artery was reported by Knutsen and Stenberg in 1959 (4). The first case of catheter embolism from a commercially produced infusion cannula was recorded in 1963 by Taylor and Rutherford (5). Since then, frequent reports have appeared in the world literature, suggesting that this serious complication is more prevalent than first realized and represents the tip of an iceberg. Indeed, a further five cases have just been reported from one centre in Chicago (6). Burri has provided a comprehensive review of the world literature and collected 315 cases up to 1978. He estimates the incidence to be 0·1 per cent of central venous catheters inserted. Moreover, in a confidential survey of German hospitals, he produced at least one case of catheter embolism from each clinic he contacted (7).

The risks to the patient are considerable from this problem. Naturally, there is a great deal of needless anxiety created because the patient knows that a foreign body has been 'lost' into the heart. Although small fragments have been left (especially in the pulmonary artery) without any detrimental effect being noted, this is not the experience from larger series. Early death may occur from arrhythmias, especially if a large fragment or knot lodges in the right ventricle. The late pathological sequelae are real and include pulmonary artery or caval thrombosis and suppuration, bacterial and fungal endocarditis, myocardial damage or perforation with tamponade, coronary artery trauma and pericarditis and, very rarely, paradoxical embolism to distant sites. The reported mortality from such events has varied between 30 and 70 per cent (8, 9). When the fragments have not been retrieved under fluoroscopic control and surgery performed, Burri noted the operative mortality to be 4 per cent.

Aetiology

In his survey, Burri refers to the vague data concerning the precise mechanism by which central catheter fragments embolize. In 49 per cent of his collected case reports, the catheter had sheared on the needle during the insertion procedure. The various reasons why this complication may occur in clinical practice can be predicted, namely:

1. Catheter shearing on an introducing hollow or split needle.
2. Catheter scoring on the needle and subsequent fracture.
3. Kinking and fracture on the body surface.
4. Fracture at the site of retaining sutures.
5. Hub separation from the catheter shaft.
6. Patient interference.
7. Accidental transection of the catheter during suture removal.

Unfortunately, the persistence of the through-needle technique, and the creation of such commercial sets for percutaneous catheterization of subclavian or jugular veins, has been the cause of much morbidity (*Fig.* 14.1). The commonest time of catheter fracture is during percutaneous insertion through a hollow or split bevelled needle, using either a central or peripheral venous approach. Inadvertent withdrawal of the catheter during manipulation, while the needle is still in the vein, can lead to fracture and possible embolism. Catheters inserted via a peripheral vein are prone to kink, especially if there is unrestricted movement of the related joint (e.g. the elbow, for median cubital vein insertion), resulting in fracture of the tubing. Infraclavicular subclavian catheters usually fracture at their venous entry site, either during insertion or on withdrawal, as this is the region of greatest angulation. The fragment may embolize or remain fixed in the vein deep to the skin. On the other hand, the catheter may initially just be 'scored', so that after lying in the bloodstream for a few days, it subsequently fractures and embolizes either spontaneously or on attempted withdrawal. It is also possible for a catheter to be successfully inserted only to be severed once the needle introducer has been withdrawn and is lying externally, as the catheter may still move

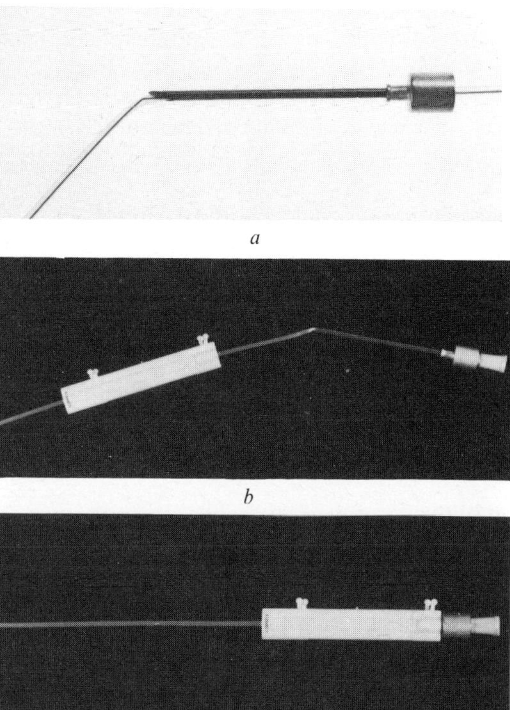

Fig. 14.1. *a*, A through-needle central catheter curving away from the sharp bevel. *b*, The through-needle catheter bending across the sharp bevel where the plastic sheath has been displaced. *c*, The plastic 'protective' sheath in place around the needle.

within the needle and kink over the bevelled edge. Unfortunately, the plastic sleeves and purses do not always adequately immobilize the needle. The use of drum cartridges does not provide protection from the hazard. Even if the clinician has the steadiest of hands, a slight inappropriate movement on the part of the patient is sufficient cause for the needle to be transected and embolize immediately or after a period of time as described above.

Catheters for prolonged intravenous alimentation are often introduced by the percutaneous infraclavicular approach using a needle placement unit. Owing to the acute angle of entry of the catheter into the subclavian vein, catheter fracture or 'scoring' is more likely with this technique than during insertion via the internal jugular or supraclavicular subclavian approaches, both of which follow a more direct line to the central venous system. The use of curved introducing needles created by the surgeon bending the standard equipment will obviously not eradicate this danger (10). Because of the serious nature of this problem, the Department of Health and Social Security in the United Kingdom issued a Hazard Warning Notice recommending that through-needle varieties of central venous catheter should no longer be used (11).

During prolonged placement, polyethylene catheters become brittle and are more likely to fracture if they have an intrinsic defect or have been 'scored' on insertion, especially if they have been used for hypertonic fluid infusion. Catheters are often immobilized by catgut sutures around the vein at the time of cut-down or by silk sutures at the site of skin entry during both percutaneous and venous cut-down insertion. It is important that the sutures are not too tight as they can also lead to fracture of the catheter. A Silastic catheter embolism has been observed in a confused patient who tugged at the catheter, which stretched, snapped at the site of the retaining skin suture and the elastic recoil allowed the intravenous segment to disappear into the circulation (12). Catheter embolism has also been recorded following separation of the catheter shaft from the hub caused by faulty or inadequate bonding (13).

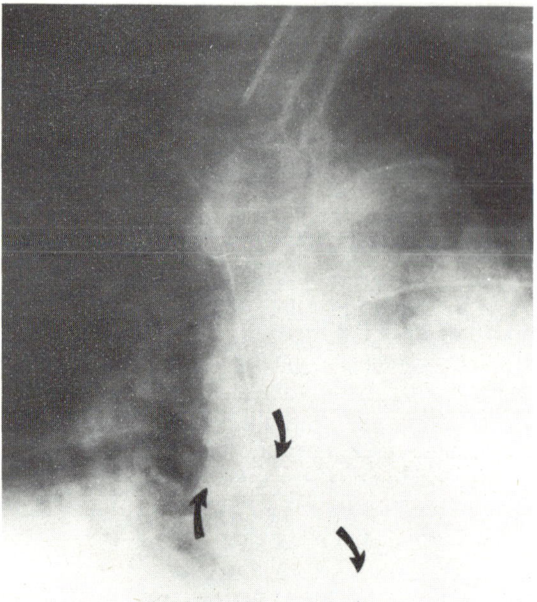

Fig. 14.2. Intra-atrial knotting (shown by the arrows) of a fine-calibre catheter.

time of thoracotomy, with catgut sutures to stabilize them intraoperatively. Attempts at their removal should not be made before the fifth postoperative day if any difficulty is encountered.

Knotting and Entrapment

Catheter knotting has resulted from the presence of redundant loops following too rapid or forceful introduction or has been related to prosthetic valves and intracardiac structures such as papillary muscles (*Fig.* 14.2). It is important that the catheter is introduced gently, slowly and not over-advanced into the heart. This is discussed in Chapter 11. Whenever possible, a check chest X-ray should be performed after the insertion procedure and at intervals during the patient's period of catheterization. There have been cases of accidental snaring of flotation catheters being used for anaesthetic management during open heart surgery by sutures inserted by the surgeon into the atrial wall. These may fracture or damage the heart on attempted forceful withdrawal unless the problem is recognized. Some cardiothoracic surgeons internally fix central venous lines, inserted at the

Detection of Catheter Fragments

Invariably, the clinician inserting a cannula through a needle will have realized that shearing has occurred and an X-ray will detect radio-opaque fragments. Unfortunately, not all catheters are satisfactorily visualized and it is important to take lateral views with the correct degree of penetration (*Fig.* 14.3). The size of the fragment sought can be calculated for the individual catheter if the rest of the device is removed. It is most important, therefore, that the precise type and length of catheter which has been inserted should be recorded. A radiolucent central catheter fragment has been successfully detected in the right ventricle using echocardiography (*Fig.* 14.4) (14). When these techniques fail to detect a foreign body and there is a sufficiently high index of clinical suspicion concerning the possibility of catheter embolism,

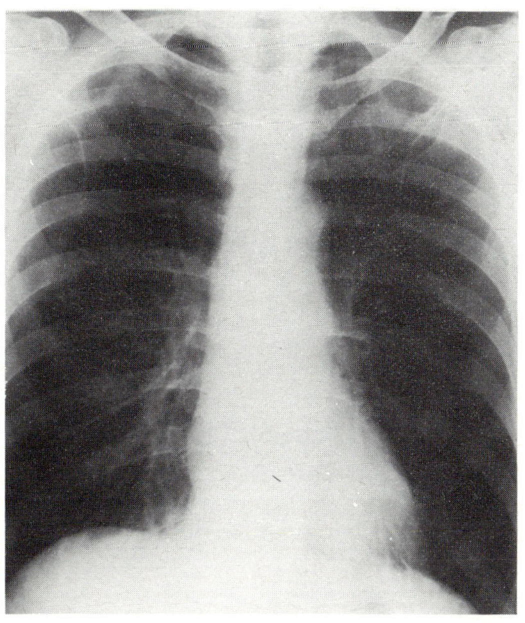
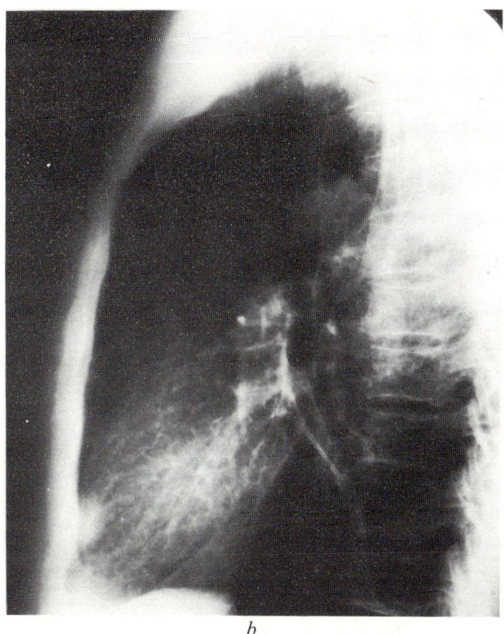

Fig. 14.3. *a*, This shows a catheter embolism fragment in a right lower lobe branch of the pulmonary artery. *b*, A lateral view of the same fragment.

then fluoroscopic angiocardiography should be considered.

Finally, if the fragment is not found local to the site of insertion, in the relevant vein en route to the heart or in the thorax, then serious consideration should be given to the possibility of paradoxical embolism to the arterial side of the circulation via a patent foramen ovale, and appropriate investigations should be instituted (15).

TECHNIQUES OF REMOVAL

Prior to 1967, embolic fragments were either left or removed at thoracotomy; but surgical intervention is potentially dangerous in the ill patients who are usually managed with central venous catheters. Massumi and Ross have been credited as the first to remove catheter fragments successfully using the less invasive percutaneous technique (16). Since then, as Burri has pointed out, numerous reports about percutaneous methods of retrieving catheter fragments have appeared in the literature, and these involve a wide variety of snares, hooks, bronchoscopy and cardiac biopsy forceps and modified ureteric stone baskets (17–21).

If a central venous catheter fractures or becomes disconnected so that there is a risk of embolism, the distal fragment should be immediately grasped, preferably with an instrument such as an artery forceps. If an antecubital fossa catheter is noted to fracture and embolize, an upper arm tourniquet should be applied and an immediate X-ray performed of the chest and arm to localize the catheter. If the proximal aspect of the catheter is still within the venous system of the upper arm, a cut-down procedure and retrieval may be successful.

Bronchoscopy biopsy forceps have been introduced via the internal jugular or femoral vein exposed by a cut-down procedure and this can be useful if there is no free floating end of the embolized fragment over which to place a snare. Their use is limited to the great veins and right atrium owing to their short length, rigidity and requirement for the surgical exposure of a large vein. Cardiac biopsy forceps have been used, but apart from being expensive, these are also relatively rigid. Various modifications of the ureteric or biliary stone basket have been employed for catheter removal. They tend to be too rigid, despite the development of the soft filiform tip, and often require venous cut-down

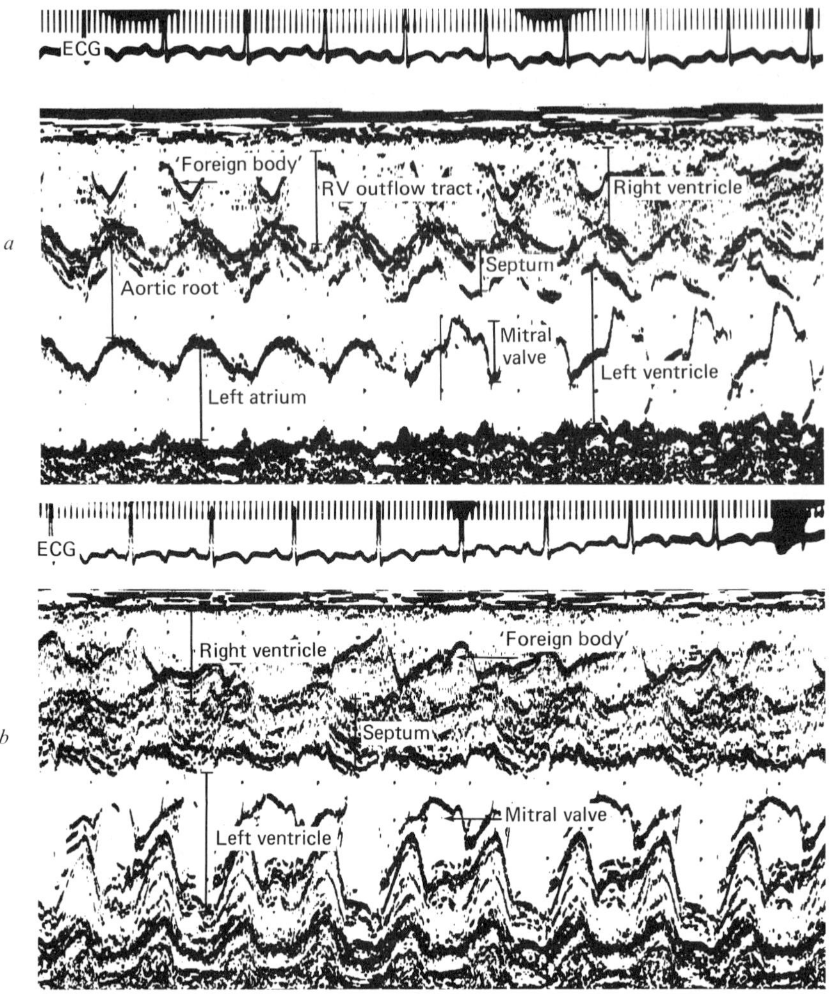

Fig. 14.4. *a*, An echocardiograph 'sweep' from the aortic route to the left ventricle showing continuous bizarre echoes extending from the body of the right ventricle to the right ventricular outflow tract. The echocardiogram is otherwise normal. *b*, An echocardiogram showing continuous bizarre echoes within the body of the right ventricle. (Reproduced by kind permission of Dr J. Davies, MRCP.)

and great care to prevent vascular perforation.

There are now a number of commercial 'intravascular retrieval sets' available which usually consist of unfolding soft helical wire baskets introduced through an 8 F gauge retrieval catheter. These utilize multiple redundant loops and are especially useful for fragments less than 5 cm in length which may be difficult to trap with a single loop snare.

Percutaneous Snare Technique

The percutaneous single snare technique is favoured by the author as it requires equipment that is readily available in most catheterization laboratories, is easy to master, causes minimal discomfort and has a high success rate in the hands of a skilled operator. Some advocate the percutaneous internal jugular approach for catheter fragment removal as it provides a slightly more direct entry to the right heart than the femoral vein approach. Unfortunately, besides being more uncomfortable for the patient, who needs to lie flat and have significant pressure applied to his neck, the effects of a local haematoma are likely to be more serious in the neck. However, the internal jugular vein must be used if there is any history of iliofemoral thrombosis or if pulmonary artery fragments cannot be reached from the femoral approach.

All the surgical and radiographic procedures subsequently described require to be performed using the strictest aseptic technique, adequate draping and the provision of effective infiltration local anaesthesia. A standard Seldinger puncture of the right femoral vein is performed and the venotomy dilated through a 6-mm skin incision using a 9 F gauge dilator. A 9 F gauge grey Kifa catheter (110 cm long, internal diameter 2·8 mm) is then advanced under fluoroscopic control over a Teflon guide wire to the inferior vena cava and right atrial junction. Good fluoroscopy is one of the major requirements for successful removal of embolic fragments, especially when relatively non-radio-opaque tubing is involved. The catheter is manufactured without a tapered tip. A 260-cm long spring safety guide wire (William Cook) (0·025 in, 0·635 mm diameter) is then doubled over and pre-shaped so that, on insertion through the distal end of the catheter, a snare will unfold. The snare is then manipulated over the distal catheter fragment and drawn tight (*Fig.* 14.5). The Kifa catheter, snare and catheter fragment are then withdrawn as a single entity through the skin puncture site. Haemostasis is achieved with direct pressure for 10 minutes.

A modification of this technique is to use a 60 in (152·5 cm) long, 0·021 in (0·53 mm) diameter guide wire with 4/0 silk thread tied near the tip to enable a snare loop to be formed once both are introduced through an 8 F gauge end-hole catheter percutaneously or via peripheral cut-down. It is important using either technique that the loop is positioned over the free floating end of the embolized fragment and that attempts are not made to dislodge the segment of the fragment that has become wedged in the cardiovascular wall. Also, on withdrawal, it is important that the advancing aspect of the snared fragment is a smooth loop and not a hard, pointed end. The femoral vein approach is preferred as a formal cut-down is not usually necessary and the risk of dislodgement at the proximal end of the catheter, if it lies in the right atrium or superior vena cava, is less than when an antecubital or neck vein is used. Subclavian catheters that have fractured and remained fixed at their proximal venous entry site can be removed by cut-down over the vein, but there is always the risk of dislodgement with attendant embolization, arrhythmias or a pneumothorax. Controlled removal by snare technique from the femoral vein is preferred and certainly the upper limb or jugular transvenous approach should not be used.

Removal of Knotted Catheters

Knotted balloon flotation catheters can easily be unknotted using a soft transluminal safety spring guide wire if the problem is quickly

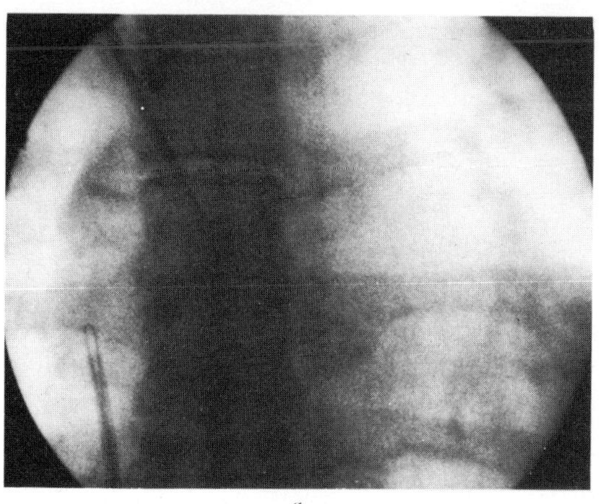
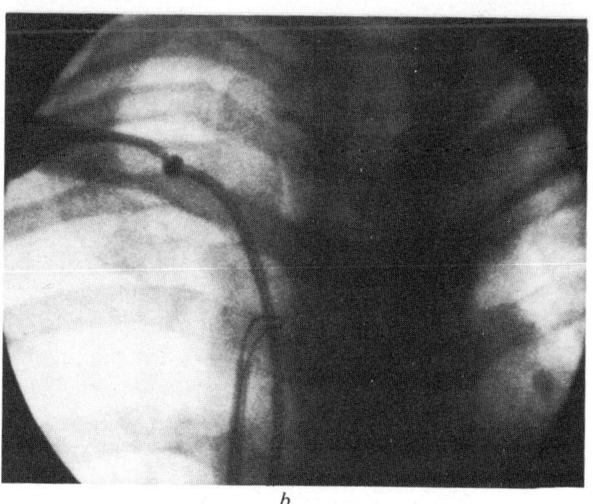

a   b

Fig. 14.5. *a*, A catheter fragment containing a knot being approached by a loop snare introduced from the femoral vein. *b*, The catheter fragment and knotted section have been successfully snared and will then be withdrawn out through the femoral venotomy.

recognized and the knot is not drawn too tight. This should ideally be performed under fluoroscopic control. If this is possible, and the catheter has been inserted by the jugular or subclavian vein, then it should be removed by the femoral vein snare technique. Once the distal segment has been snared, the catheter can be cut off at its proximal skin entry site and, after thorougly cleansing both the skin and catheter shaft with povidone-iodine solution, the assembly may be withdrawn percutaneously from the femoral venotomy. Forceful withdrawal of the knotted segment through a large central vein can create major bleeding. Knotted balloon catheters inserted from an arm vein often cannot be withdrawn through their entry site, but can be removed by gentle withdrawal, also preferably under fluoroscopic control, until a local venous cut-down can be made higher up the arm in order to free the knot. Care must be taken to clamp the distal and the proximal fragments to prevent embolization before the knotted segment is excised after peripheral cut-down.

An alternative technique for use in the removal of knotted catheters which have been inserted through the internal jugular vein is for the catheter hubs to be removed by cutting the catheter. This is then carefully disinfected together with the surrounding skin and the area draped. Simultaneously, the free end of the catheter should be secured with a sterile artery forceps in order to prevent inadvertent air embolization through the catheter lumen and intravascular migration of the device itself. Next a Teflon sheath of suitable calibre (e.g. internal diameter 9 F) is passed over the catheter and rotated into the vein lumen. Many operators prefer to expose the vein by a formal cut-down procedure in order to achieve precise control of the vein in case haemorrhage occurs. The Teflon sheath is advanced to the knot which is gradually tightened and reduced in size by pulling on the catheter. The patient must be kept in a head-down tilt position to stop air entering the circulation between the catheter and the Teflon sheath. The whole assembly is then withdrawn and removed through the venotomy site. Haemorrhage at this point can be considerable, since the minimal size the knot will achieve is 0·75 cm in diameter; it is wise to be prepared to undertake a formal venotomy and for a surgeon quickly to re-suture the vein.

Removal of Entrapped Catheters

When entrapment has occurred, a carefully controlled intravascular 'tug of war' may be necessary. It is best to wait several days for the atrial suture line healing process to become established and the removal operation must be performed with good fluoroscopic control. If the patient is fortunate, the catheter may start to slide free, in which case its passage to the surface can be monitored. The balloon may not escape and it is wise to prepare for this by ensnaring the free end via a femoral venotomy as described. The central catheter may then be cut at the skin and withdrawn back through the femoral venotomy.

If the catheter will not dislodge, then a Teflon sheath inserted via the neck wound may serve to free the device or snap the catheter at the level of the retaining suture. The free fragment can then be snared. However, if no free end is available, the catheter must be pulled free by the use of endocardial biopsy forceps passed through a Teflon sheath introduced percutaneously into the femoral vein using the Seldinger technique (22). All such manipulations carry a serious risk of secondary atrial haemorrhage, and the necessary surgical support must be immediately available.

Summary

Embolization is a serious and increasing complication of central venous catheter insertion. Catheter emboli should be removed as soon as possible by skilled operators and, where transvenous methods fail, direct operative intervention is advised provided that the patient's condition will tolerate further surgical intervention. The following points are provided as a guide for the prevention of catheter fracture and embolism:

1. A standard sterile technique is of paramount importance in the prevention of central venous catheter complications, including embolism.

2. All catheters must be checked for intrinsic defects prior to insertion, the length and shape of the tip should be recorded.

3. Peripheral arm veins should be used unless long term cannulation is required (e.g. parenteral nutrition) or intraoperative monitoring

and drug administration requires that the arms need to be free of catheters.

4. Only radio-opaque catheters should be used for central venous and peripheral venous cannulation.

5. The catheter should have a hub which is permanently fixed to the catheter shaft.

6. The catheter should be inserted through a hollow plastic cannula and *not a hollow or split metal needle*.

7. Sutures fixing the catheter at the site of insertion should not be too tight.

8. The catheter and its related joint should be carefully dressed and immobilized so as to prevent kinking or movement of the catheter at its entry site.

9. The hub and the catheter should be regularly inspected and the integrity of all catheters checked after removal and before the tip is sent for microbiological culture.

10. The integrity of the catheter after removal should be recorded in the patient's notes.

References

1. Tuell, W. S.: In Doering R. B., Stemmer E. A. et al.: Complications of indwelling venous catheters with particular reference to catheter embolus. *Am. J. Surg.* 1967; **114**: 265.
2. Turner D., Sommers S. C.: Accidental passage of a polyethylene catheter from a cubital vein to the right atrium; fatal case. *N. Engl. J. Med.* 1954; **251**: 744–5.
3. Brown C. A., Kent A.: Perforation of the right ventricle by a polyethylene catheter. *South. Med. J.* 1956; **49**: 466–7.
4. Knutsen H., Stenberg K.: Pulmonary embolism after catheter break. *Nord. Med.* 1959; **62**: 1491.
5. Taylor F. W., Rutherford C. E.: Accidental loss of a plastic tube into the venous system. *Arch. Surg.* 1963; **86**: 177–9.
6. Meng R. L., Delaria G. A., Goldin M. D.: Transjugular forceps retrieval of catheter embolus. *Ann. Thorac. Surg.* 1980; **29**: 575–7.
7. Burri C., Ahnefeld F. W. (ed.): *The Caval Catheter*. Berlin: Springer-Verlag, 1978: 53–60.
8. Wellmann K. F., Reinhard A., Salazar E. P.: Polythene catheter embolism. Review of the literature and report of a case with associated fatal tricuspid and systemic candidiasis. *Circulation* 1968; **37**: 380.
9. Fischer R. G., Ferreyro R.: Evaluation of current techniques for non-surgical removal of intravascular iatrogenic foreign bodies. *AJR* 1978; **130**: 541–8.
10. Asimacopoulos P. J., Bagley F. H., McDermott W. V.: A modified technique for subclavian venepuncture. *Surg. Gynecol. Obstet.* 1980; **150**: 240–2.
11. John G. E.: Ds (Supply) Hazard Notice HN (6). London: DHSS, 1972.
12. Edbrook D. L.: Personal communication. 1980.
13. Sprague D. H., Sarwar H.: Catheter embolisation due to faulty bonding of catheter shaft to hub. *Anaesthesiology.* 1978; **49**: 285–6.
14. Davies J., Alvarez R., Allison D. J.: An intracardiac foreign body: diagnosed non-invasively and removed non-surgically. *Brit. J. Radiol.* 1981; **54**: 987–9.
15. Nash G., Moylan J. S.: Paradoxical catheter embolism. *Arch. Surg.* 1971; **102**: 213.
16. Massumi R. A., Ross A. A.: Atraumatic non-surgical technique for removal of broken catheters from cardiac cavities. *N. Engl. J. Med.* 1967; **227**: 195.
17. Dotter C. T., Rosch J., Bilbao M. K.: Transluminal extraction of catheter and guide fragments from the heart and great vessels; 29 collected cases. *AJR* 1971; **111**: 467.
18. Richardson J. D., Grover F. L., Trinkle J. F.: Intravenous catheter emboli. Experience with twenty cases and collective review. *Am. J. Surg.* 1974; **128**: 722.
19. Aldridge H. E., Lee J.: Transvascular removal of catheter fragments from the great vessels and heart. *Can. Med. Assoc. J.* 1977; **117**: 1300.
20. West R. O., Charrette E. J. P., Parker J. O.: Technique for removal of detached polyethylene catheters from intracardiac chambers and great vessels. *Can. Med. J.* 1977; **117**: 1310.
21. Edwards A. C., Sowton, E.: Management of embolised central venous catheters. *Br. Med. J.* 1978; **2**: 669.
22. Block P. C.: Snaring of a Swan–Ganz catheter. *J. Thorac. Cardiovasc. Surg.* 1976; **71**: 917–19.

Chapter 15

Nursing Care

L. T. Sawyer and J. L. Peters

The precise origins of central venous and cardiac catheterization in man are slightly controversial. Benatt, who presented an historical note on the subject to the *Lancet* in 1949, provided an interesting account of the pioneers Forssmann and Bleichroeder (1). Forssmann, in his description of the first experiment upon himself, described how a nurse called Gerda Ditzen assisted him to introduce the catheter (2); nurses have continued to play a key role in this procedure. There can be no doubt that central venous catheterization has become an established procedure within the hospital environment, and now selected patients are being allowed to leave the confines of a medical institution with indwelling central venous lines. Patients can be successfully taught the principles of aseptic technique, catheter maintenance and how to infuse parenteral nutrition solutions. The motivation of such patients on home total parenteral nutrition programmes in the United States of America and Europe has illustrated vividly how the application by the nursing staff of rigid protocols to prevent infection has enabled intravascular devices connected to extracorporeal infusion systems to be used for very long periods of time. Clinical experience has indicated how the same meticulous techniques and maintenance schedules must be instituted for the care of all devices left in communication with the vascular system. There must be no difference between the level of care apportioned to jugular, subclavian, Swan–Ganz or long brachial central venous catheters used for manometry (3–6), and the more sophisticated catheters used for prolonged parenteral feeding or cancer chemotherapy (7). The endless repetition of sound aseptic and catheter care techniques leads to increased safety for the patient (8). In this aspect of patient care there can be no compromises made because the complications already described are so serious.

The precise way in which the patients and their lines can be cared for may vary slightly between institutions in certain details, but the essential principles are the same (9). We would agree with the sentiments expressed by Professor H. A. Lee, of Southampton University, who emphasizes in his lectures on the subject that 'Angio-access obsession leads to perfection and not infection'.

In many establishments within the United Kingdom a team approach is being encouraged for the care of central catheters, particularly when they are used for parenteral nutrition (10). Elsewhere, the emphasis has been on the continuing education of all the involved nursing staff in individual wards and specialized units. The vital importance of a programme of continuing education with respect to central catheters has been highlighted by Colley (11). Each institution, ward or unit should develop its own policy concerning patients with such intravascular devices in place. The protocol should be kept as simple as possible and reviewed at regular intervals with respect to any developments relating to equipment, aseptic technique or dressing procedures. Many units have found posters created by their audiovisual aid department to be an invaluable way of reminding staff, particularly those on duty at night, of current policies in the hospital. In the United Kingdom, the Department of Health and Social Security produces notices concerning hazards and these should be kept on file and policy changes instituted where appropriate. The advisory capacity of the technical departments of the DHSS should play an important role in improving central catheter care throughout the country, since much of the equipment is in widespread use. Furthermore, it is fallacious to assume that because a major technical problem has not been encountered in one's own hospital or unit, it cannot arise.

The nursing and medical literature also provides additional useful educational information for the team. Sporadic case reports concerning unusual events may often serve to effect slight alterations in particular aspects of the patient's central venous infusion system or maintenance programme. An increased vigilance for the unusual event generally leads to an overall improvement in standards. This has been particularly noticeable with the increased use of Swan–Ganz balloon flotation catheters, which have in effect extended the effectiveness of bedside haemodynamic monitoring. The potential hazards of these catheters, with their extra range of penetration into the central circulation, have inevitably materialized. In some respects they are more serious than those problems encountered with standard central catheters, e.g. perforation of the pulmonary artery requiring pneumonectomy, pneumothorax and heart block (12–14). Such events, although uncommon, serve to remind nursing staff of the need to review regularly with their medical staff the necessity for intravascular devices. Most would agree that for long catheters extending through the heart valves and into the pulmonary artery, 3 days should be considered the maximum period of placement of an individual device (unless exceptional circumstances co-exist).

In bedside monitoring and central venous infusion therapy, the sensors and artificial venous conduits need to be safe, applicable to the task, reliable and simple to operate and maintain. Unfortunately, the rigours of clinical practice can lead to insidious equipment failure (15), and it is crucial for the nursing staff to observe the integrity of the apparatus as well as the patient's progress. It may seem unlikely, but accidental micro-shock electrocution can occur; with the fluid pathway of intravenous systems conducting electricity to the patient from faulty bedside electrical equipment (16).

These rather esoteric episodes should not cloud the most important problem that faces nursing staff in central catheter care—*nosocomial infection*. This can arise with such rapidity that it led Altemieir to coin the phrase, 'third-day surgical fever' (17). The prevention of bacterial and fungal colonization of these devices is mandatory. The problem is universal and organisms which in normal circumstances might be considered to be harmless skin commensals, can be pathogenic, e.g. *Staphylococcus epidermis* or *albus* (18). A review of the problem is presented in Chapter 13 and in other texts (19, 20). In the United States of America, where specialist intravenous therapy nursing staff have operated for some time, emphasis has been placed on sound clinical observation and problem-solving. The origins of nosocomial infection arising from peripheral intravenous and central venous catheters can be predicted. All the efforts of intravenous fluid manufacturers and hospital pharmacies in maintaining meticulous techniques and faultless quality assurance are to no avail if the infusion conduit is of poor quality or design, and the nursing care unsatisfactory. The use of stopcocks in central venous systems should be avoided whenever possible, since the nursing profession has recently identified these as being important infection risk factors (21, 22). The valves discovered in the human circulation by Fabricius were designated 'de ostiolis venarum' (little floodgates of the veins); it is tempting to call the current family of plastic stopcocks and side-ports, which are used as convenience accessories to provide circulatory access, 'de ostiolos bacterium'. Walter has already pointed out the ease with which bacteria can colonize hub connector mechanisms (19). It should be understood that 'stopcocks do not stop cocci from entering the circulation, and injection ports provide a fine harbour for micro-organisms' (23).

The aim of this chapter is to provide a perspective and review of the nurse's role in central venous catheter care with reference to:

Patient preparation.
The insertion procedure.
Dressing change procedure.
Infusion line maintenance.
Manometry.
Patient observation.

Heparin-lock procedure.

Removal procedure.

Education of the nursing staff in this field of patient care must start early in their training, with the medical staff setting a good example. Inadvertent lapses of technique are possibly excusable in emergency situations, but 'short-cuts' should *never* be demonstrated to learners. Propagation of the ward or unit protocol should start in the nursing school teaching curriculum and regular up-date tutorials should be incorporated into study days for postgraduate nurses. It is invaluable for close co-operation to be generated with the medical staff concerning all aspects of the patient's extracorporeal infusion line management. This is particularly important in deciding policies concerning the addition of drugs to intravenous infusions (24). Once qualified, nursing staff must apply their own locally organized protocol for intravenous therapy, with the guidelines being provided by a multi-disciplinary group within the hospital or district. The more sophisticated infusion line management of intensive care units or total parenteral nutrition requires additional experience and training. The management of patients with leukaemia and other malignancies using the Hickman variety of catheter has revealed the wide range of drugs and fluids which can be administered into the central circulation (7).

PATIENT PREPARATION

Naturally, in the emergency situation when, for example, an internal jugular, external jugular or brachial vein catheter is being inserted, time is of the essence, and the prolonged discussion of the pros and cons of a procedure would be inappropriate. However, prior to the *elective* insertion of a central venous catheter for parenteral nutrition, an adequate explanation of the procedure should be provided by the medical and nursing staff. The patient may well have anxieties concerning why the procedure is required and may consider that the necessity for the line indicates a deterioration in health rather than a positive step being taken to aid recovery. This may be especially evident when a cut-down operation is planned for the insertion of a feeding line. It is more reassuring for the procedure to be carried out in the operating theatre suite where everything can be prepared before

the patient's arrival, extra staff are available to make the procedure go by more quickly and there is greater space for all concerned. When these operations are carried out in the general ward, the overcrowding of equipment and assistants around the head of the bed can be most alarming. Some units have been able to modify special procedure rooms.

It is a wise precaution for a consent form to be signed by the patient, when the operation is to be carried out electively, either under a general or local anaesthesia in the operating theatre. Unless there are contraindications, a pre-medication should be given 1 hour before the insertion, in order to allay anxiety (e.g. a combination of appropriate doses of pethidine and diazepam). The need for a mask to be worn by the patient should be explained; the benefits are not only in improving the sterility of the procedure, but also the effect of odours from the skin preparation solutions can be diminished. The patient should be forewarned about the degree of head-down tilt they will have to experience and the minor discomfort that will be felt from the local anaesthesia solution being injected. If possible, the Valsalva manoeuvre should be taught, e.g. holding the breath in deep expiration.

The skin should be shaved over a wide area, and this should involve not only the proposed site of insertion, but also the area where any adhesive dressing will be secured and the administration set tubing fixed. This will reduce the patient's discomfort during dressing changes. If the procedure is going to be performed on the ward, the head of the bed must be detached and an adequate head-down tilt must somehow be obtained.

INSERTION PROCEDURE

The nurse must be ready to play an active role throughout this operation, both in assisting the surgeon and comforting the patient. It is valuable for a student nurse to sit at the head end of the bed, trolley or table in order to support the drapes from the face or provide a suitable screen, talk to the patient and observe the various stages:

1. Patient positioning.
2. Skin preparation.
3. Draping procedure.

4. Local anaesthesia.
5. Equipment checks.
6. Percutaneous through-cannula insertion or surgical exposure technique.
7. Catheter fixation.
8. Correct placement checks.
9. Dressing procedure.
10. Post-insertion X-ray.

It always preferable to have gathered all the equipment to hand before the doctor arrives and the procedure commences, so that there is no unnecessary running to and fro. It is useful to place an incontinence pad or similar material behind the head, neck and shoulders or the patient's arm so as to minimize linen changes. In view of the hazard of catheter embolism, through-needle devices, whether dispensed from a sheath or from a drum, should not be used (25). The provision of comprehensive kits by some manufacturers has been a very valuable development with respect to saving nursing time. It is also useful to have a trolley set up with a selection of the preferred gloves, gowns, skin preparation solutions, local anaesthetic agents, syringes, hypodermic needles, suture material and dressings available. Precise instructions should be sought from the medical staff about which intravenous fluid is to be set up, in addition to the make and type of administration set or manometer required. A suitable drip stand should be made ready—this is often the item forgotten by the inexperienced nurse! The *privacy* of the patient should be ensured at all times.

During the various phases of the operation, the nurse should be available to hand the apparatus in an aseptic fashion to the doctor, and anticipate his future technical requirements. Before the procedure commences, the nurse should ensure that all other staff and the patient are wearing a mask. The operator should, by preference, scrub up and don a gown and gloves. The methods have been discussed more fully elsewhere and do not require repetition. However, the nurse can help the patient in several small ways and so minimize the discomfort of the procedure. The patient should be advised to mouth-breathe whilst the skin is being prepared and so avoid some of the noxious odours. These are particularly unpleasant if acetone or similar fluids are used. With the guidance of the doctor, the sterile drapes can be arranged so that there is a free flow of air around the face without obscuring the operative field. Furthermore, the nurse assistant can ensure that an adequate period of time has elapsed after the injection of local anaesthesia, before the insertion procedure commences. Finally, instructions to perform the Valsalva manoeuvre can be passed on to the patient at the time of cannulation and subsequently, whenever the central catheter is left open to the atmosphere.

When the catheter has been successfully placed, secured and the position of its tip checked, it is worth marking the shaft of the catheter and the adjacent skin with indelible ink so that any subsequent movement of the catheter relative to the body surface may be detected at an early stage. If any excess blood has been spilled on the patient's shoulder, neck or arm, this should be cleaned—hydrogen peroxide is the best agent for this. The skin should be cleaned and dried meticulously with sterile gauzes before an Op-Site dressing (Smith & Nephew) is applied. A small square of gauze or 'Lyofoam' fashioned with a slit should be placed around the entry site prior to the application of the dressing. The practical result of this is that the wound can be inspected regularly through the transparent dressing without incurring an increased risk of nosocomial infection. The date of insertion should be printed on the dressing in indelible ink and all the junctions in the system checked. Many institutions now advise wrapping the connection with adhesive tape. A full note of the surgeon, time of the procedure, catheter type, length and other relevant details should be made in the nursing report and a similar record should be entered by the doctor involved into the clinical notes.

The patient should be brought out of the head-down tilt position, made comfortable in bed and allowed to rest. The infusion system should be checked to ensure that the fluid is running and flowing at the correct rate. If the line is to be used for manometry, then the nurse may take the first base-line reading. The position of the infusion line on the chest wall should be arranged so that no sharp kinks are created. (*Fig.* 15.1)—angulation-obstruction. The line should be secured with hypoallergenic tape, e.g. Op-Site, and this can be accomplished by cutting a large sheet up into 5-cm wide strips. It is unusual for patients to experience tape-sensitivity to this material.

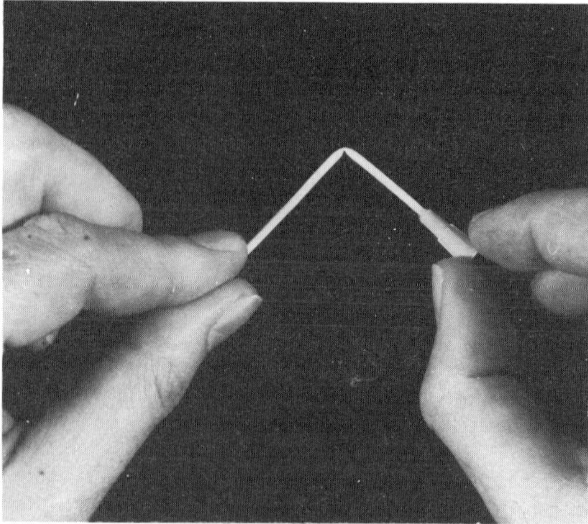

Fig. 15.1. Angulation-obstruction of a central venous catheter lumen can occur easily unless the device is carefully fixed to the skin surface. This simple problem will impede the progress of any intravenous infusion, impair the ability to make accurate CVP recordings and lead to eventual catheter thrombosis, stress fracturing and leakage.

DRESSING CHANGE PROCEDURE

A standardized dressing change procedure should be established as an integral part of hospital policy for central venous catheters. Many institutions now adopt a Monday–Wednesday–Friday programme for dressing changes, although there is no good evidence as to exactly which schedule is the most satisfactory. The aim should be to keep the catheter entry site clean, dry and covered by a membrane which will prevent spillage of saliva, nasogastric aspirate etc. from reaching the dressing. The aphorism 'nothing will grow in a desert' is particularly apt in this respect. The trend in recent years has been away from the routine use of antibiotic ointments applied to the catheter entry site. The application of povidone-iodine or similar antimicrobial compounds is effective in providing a hostile environment for both bacteria and fungi. Povidone-iodine can be applied as a dry spray (e.g. Disadine, Stuart Pharmaceuticals), or formulations of this compound as an ointment and quick-drying paint are also available.

In patients with burn injuries who have central catheters, the dressings may require to be changed more frequently. Similarly, the presence of a tracheostomy creates problems in managing the catheter site, especially if a tunnel has not been created. If the dressing looks wet and soggy from external contamination by whatever cause, it must be changed immediately and always using a full aseptic technique. Junior medical staff should be discouraged from poking about under the edges of the dressing 'just to have a look', in case the line is the possible source of a post-operative fever. Any manipulation should be performed correctly. For the procedure to be carried out without a mask, using unwashed hands and no sterile instruments, simply lends credence to the catch-phrase 'inspection means infection'. Such transgressions of accepted technique should not happen in the nineteen-eighties.

The patient should understand that only the dressing is to be changed and not the whole central venous catheter. The procedure should be performed by a trained member of staff and preferably assisted by a junior nurse learning the technique. The patient and staff should wear sterile masks and, in situations where the patient suffers from severe immunosuppression, e.g. in leukaemia or oncology units, the nurse carrying out the procedure should also wear a sterile gown. If commercially created kits are not available, a small dressing pack will suffice. Thus, the requirements will be:

> Trolley
> Small sterile dressing pack containing:
>> Galley pots
>> Sterile gauze
>> Cotton wool or sponges
>> Forceps × 3
>> Scissors
> Skin cleansing agents:
>> 3 per cent hydrogen peroxide
>> Povidone-iodine
>> Chlorhexidine
> Op-Site

The nurse and assistant should both carefully wash their hands and the person carrying out the procedure must don comfortable sterile gloves. The aim should be to employ a no-touch technique using the instruments for the fine work around the catheter entry site. After making the patient comfortable with pillows, the old dressing should be loosened and removed, preferably by the assistant under supervision. It is critical that this manoeuvre should be done slowly and carefully so that the catheter is not inadvertently dislodged. The position of the catheter should be examined to see if there has been any dislocation into or out of the patient. The indelible ink marks previously mentioned under the insertion procedure are an invaluable aid in this respect. Dislodgement or dislocation can easily occur if a suture has not been used because of the pull of the relatively heavy infusion line or a sudden movement on the part of the patient (*Fig.* 15.2). It is a wise precaution

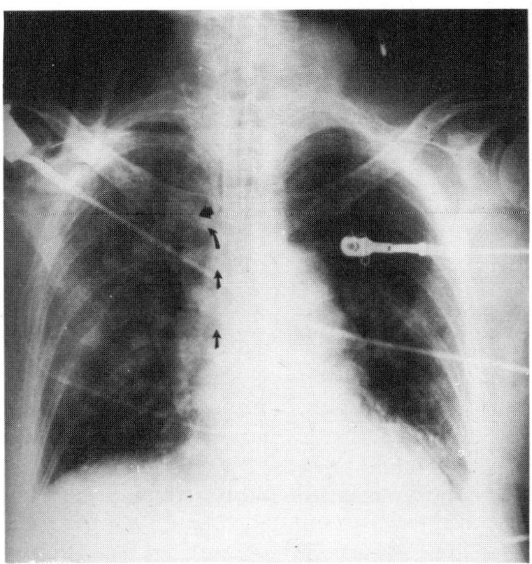

Fig. 15.2. Failure to provide adequate anchorage to this catheter caused the device to slowly dislocate out from its original position in the superior vena cava (narrow arrows) to a point in the subclavian vein (broad arrow). This problem occurred as a result of the patient's movement and the weight of the infusion lines.

to place a small, separate 5-cm wide strip of Op-Site between the insertion site dressing and the catheter hub mechanism in order to anchor the catheter shaft to the skin (*Fig.* 15.3). The nurse should then check for:

1. Pathology in the plastic—kinks or stress fractures.

2. Pathology in the patient—the development of erythema, flare or cellulitis, pus or crusting at the insertion and adjacent suture site.

A sterile towel should be arranged around the site after the wound has been cleaned with 3 per cent hydrogen peroxide, saline or povidone-iodine solution. Some centres prefer to use agents which defat the skin, e.g. acetone. The entry site should be left absolutely dry by gently

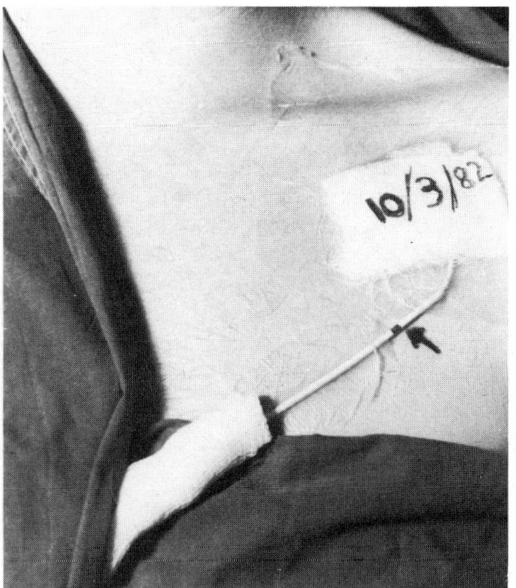

Fig. 15.3. A separate adhesive Op-Site dressing has been placed over the catheter shaft between the hub mechanism and the exit site dressing in order to provide more secure anchorage and prevent angulation-obstruction from occurring.

swabbing with sterile gauze, and then treated with dry povidone-iodine spray (e.g. Disadine). This should be restricted only to the area immediately around the catheter entry site for a radius of perhaps 2 cm. If povidone-iodine is sprayed over too wide an area, some adhesive dressings will fail to stick adequately to the patient. A small square of sterile gauze or 'Lyofoam' should be fashioned using scissors so that a small slit extending to the centre of the gauze is created, enabling it to be slipped around the catheter shaft next to the skin. This gauze should also be treated with povidone-iodine spray and then an additional slightly larger square of sterile gauze placed over the first dressing (*Fig.* 15.4). The skin around the gauze should be gently dried and a strip or sheet of Op-Site of the appropriate size carefully laid over and around the dressing. When the line is situated in the neck or subclavian region, it is best to apply the Op-Site by working from the most posterior aspect of the patient towards the front, keeping the sheet of film on a slight stretch to avoid wrinkles, and simultaneously peeling the protective backing off the material in small stages. With a little practice beforehand, the art of handling this dressing can be readily mastered

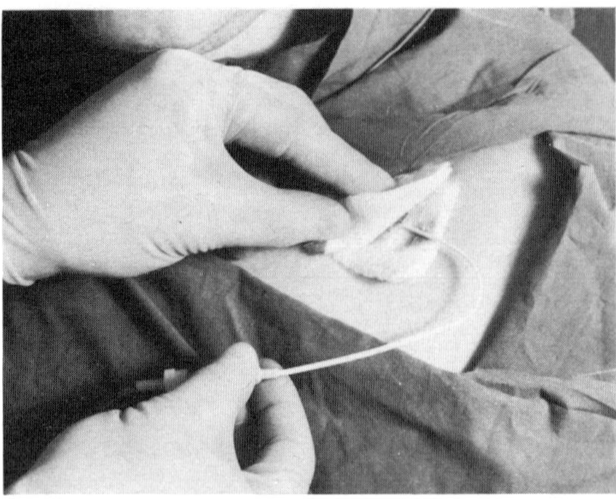

Fig. 15.4. Sterile gauze squares with a central slit being placed around the catheter shaft at the exit site, treated with povidone-iodine aerosol spray and being covered with a further sterile gauze.

and most manoeuvres accomplished single-handed. It is vital that when scissors are being used in the vicinity of the catheter, it is not accidentally snicked in the dressing procedure. A note of the date on which the dressing was changed can be made in indelible ink on the Op-Site and should also be recorded in the nursing report (*Fig.* 15.5).

INFUSION LINE MAINTENANCE

A qualified registered nurse has an extremely responsible and primary role to play in the management of central intravenous infusion systems. In the United Kingdom, the Breckenridge Report of 1977 (24) determined that the nurse's responsibility would continue to include:

1. Checking that the container and fluid show no obvious faults or contamination.

2. Checking that the prescribed fluid is administered to the right patient.

3. Observing whether the intravenous line remains patent.

4. Inspecting the site of injection and reporting any abnormality.

5. Controlling the flow at the prescribed rate.

6. Observing and reporting on the condition of the patient.

7. Maintaining all the necessary records.

Any drugs, or additions to the infusion, can only be given when the prescription is clearly written, providing the precise dosage, the method of administration, rate, date, and time and is duly signed by the doctor. If there are reasonable grounds to question the accuracy or completeness of a prescription, the nurse has a duty to do so. The formulation of large 3-litre bags of total parenteral nutrition under laminar flow conditions considerably reduces the workload of the nurse in the ward area; nevertheless, the container must still be checked for faults and evidence of incompatibility (e.g. precipitation) if drug additions have been made.

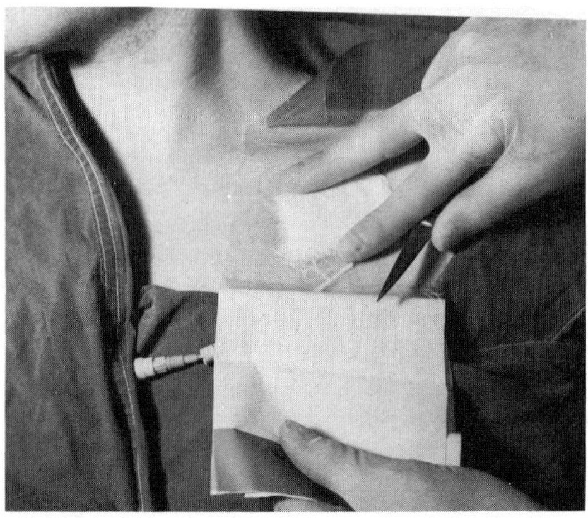

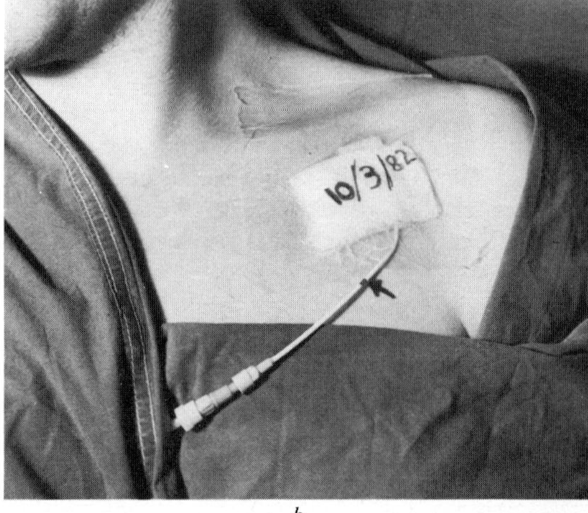

a   b

Fig. 15.5. Note the way in which the adhesive Op-Site film dressing is being slowly applied to the skin without wrinkling by working from above downwards (*a*). Afterwards the date of dressing change is marked and the indelible ink check mark against catheter dislocation can be seen (*b*).

Integrity of the Infusion Line

Whilst there is no doubt that high standards of quality assurance are applied by the manufacturers of administration sets, central catheters and accessory equipment, once the line is subject to the clinical environment where there is an inherent potential for human error to occur, serious faults may develop. The main problems encountered are:

1. Disconnection of a catheter hub–infusion line junction.
2. Junction or stopcock separation.
3. Hub separation from the catheter shaft.
4. Catheter shaft fracture or trauma.
5. Embolization of catheter fragments.
6. Disruption of three-way stopcocks and manometers.

The first four of these events can lead to the extremely serious sequelae of air embolism, cardio respiratory collapse, neurological damage or death. Catheter shaft fracture and disconnection problems, in addition to allowing air into the circulation, invariably cause leakage of fluid; the entry of bacteria and fungi is facilitated and the central catheter will have to be removed. Examples of these problems are illustrated in *Figs.* 15.6 and 15.7. The nurse has to be particularly wary since some of these events can occur under the dressing. The need to protect the lumen of the line from contact with the atmosphere is obvious, and this is why the incorporation of three-way stopcocks is undesirable. It is an easy matter for a confused patient to twiddle with such devices on the body surface and turn the tap to an open port, or conversely, a busy nurse can administer a bolus injection through the tap and leave it in the open position if called to another emergency on the ward or unit. Problems with the infusion administration sets are more uncommon, since they are made of more durable plastic and are not subjected to the same degree of movement from the patient's body as the slender central catheter. Furthermore, the administration set is changed every day whilst the central catheter remains in place for more prolonged periods of time.

Careful observation of all the components of this plastic conduit is necessary if it is to maintain the proper function of a 'life-line'. The detection of any major defect requires the removal of the line if it is made of FEP, polyethy-

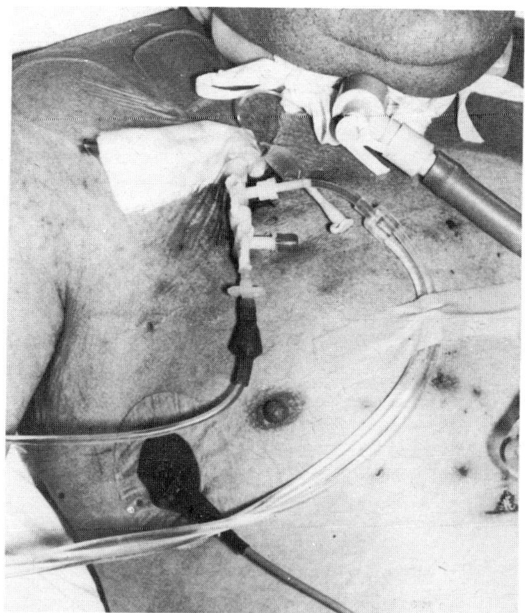

Fig. 15.6. *Stopcocks do not stop cocci from entering the circulation*—the undesirable features of using three-way stopcocks attached to central venous catheters are shown in this illustration. First, the assembly is close to a tracheostomy tube. Secondly, two stopcocks have been used in series and these were able to rotate, one on the other, with movement of the underlying pectoral muscles of the anterior chest wall. Thirdly, a spare and superfluous side-port has been provided as a harbour for micro-organisms, even though it is capped.

lene, PVC or polyurethane. If there is particular difficulty with gaining access to an individual patient's venous system, then it is probably safer to employ a re-insertion technique using a guidewire method (26, 27). Recently, the manufacturers of the Hickman and Broviac family of catheters (Evermed), have supplied repair kits for these silicone rubber devices. Splitting of the silicone close to the hub may occur and patients or staff have accidentally injured the line. Following the early detection of a such a fault, the line should be clamped proximal to the defect after filling the dead space of the catheter with heparin (*see* Heparin-lock technique). The region of the defect should be wrapped in a povidone-iodine soaked swab until a full aseptic technique can be instituted for the elective repair of the line. This procedure is invaluable for patients who are in the middle of a chemotherapy regime in whom further surgical intervention would be contraindicated. A particu-

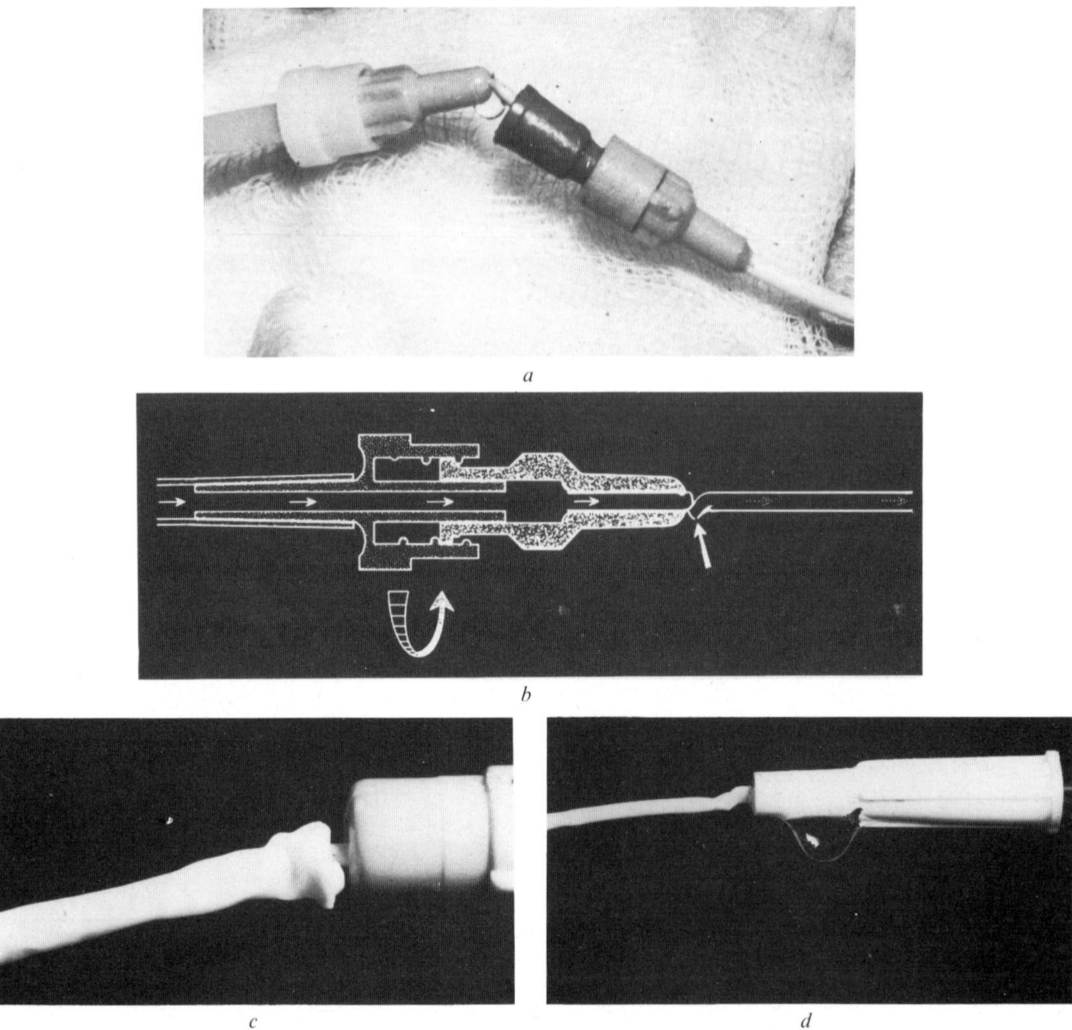

Fig. 15.7. Reveals a complication of fixed-collar Luer-lock mechanisms on administration sets. When these are screwed on to the catheter hub through 360°, the hub–shaft junction twists, and over the course of several days this site will eventually develop a minute stress crack and commence leaking. Alternatively, the entry of air or micro-organisms will take place. This problem is demonstrated in (*a*) and the aetiology shown in (*b*), (*c*) and (*d*).

larly fine example of human error is shown in *Fig.* 15.8: a houseman had unwittingly used the shaft of a Hickman catheter to administer bolus injections! Silicone tubing is not self-sealing and consequently irreparable physical damage was done to the line in this particular case and infection introduced.

The nursing profession must also recognize that a technique used with a particular catheter cannot be adapted for universal application. An example of this is the use of rubber-shod artery forceps and similar plastic tubing clamps, which can be used with care on infusion administration sets, extension tubes and wide-bore silicone catheters (e.g. Hickman) during the line change procedure. However, such clamps must not be used on other types of plastic central venous catheter. Minute splits can be induced and allow the leakage of fluid or entry of micro-organisms and air (*Fig.* 15.9).

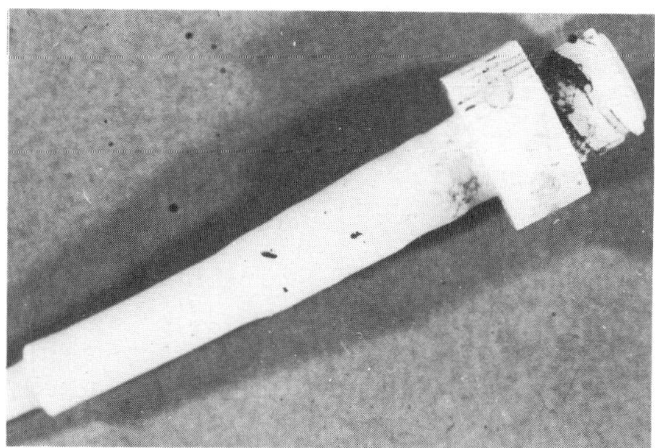

Fig. 15.8. Human error and infusion line maintenance. The shaft of a Hickman catheter has been used to administer bolus injections. This practice should *never* be employed. In this case the line became contaminated and had to be removed prematurely.

ADMINISTRATION SET CHANGING PROCEDURE

It is generally accepted that administration and manometer sets should be changed daily. Also, the infusion line should be replaced after Intralipid has been given. In patients who are receiving blood products through wide-bore silicone central catheters, it is recommended that a line change should be instituted after this form of therapy. If stopcocks have been included for important over-riding clinical considerations, these should also be replaced with new sterile units.

The need for a meticulous no-touch technique in this procedure is highlighted by the vivid demonstration of Walter (19) that bacteria can

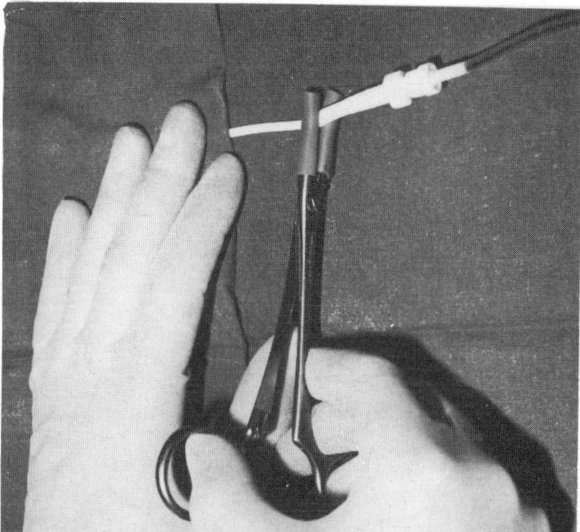

a

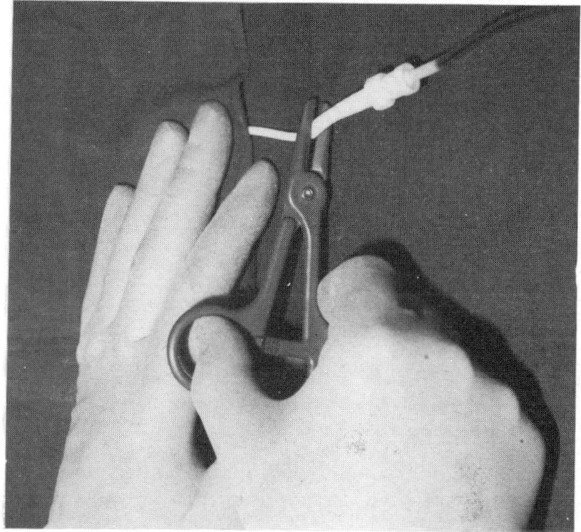

b

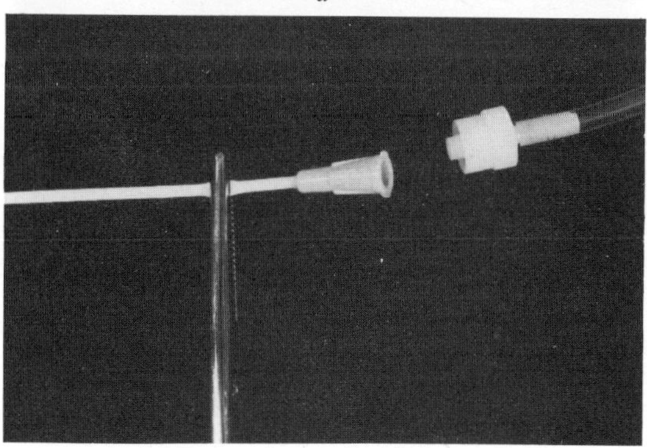

c

Fig. 15.9. A Hickman catheter being safely clamped using rubber-shod forceps (*a*) and plastic clamping forceps (*b*). However, artery forceps should *never* be used to clamp other non-silicone central venous catheters (*c*).

be introduced to the Luer connector from a contaminated thumb. The same scrupulous care must be used to avoid touching the spike of the set which is inserted into the bag or bottle of infusate. The Luer connector of the administration set must be kept protected by the sterile cap as soon as the priming procedure has been performed. The importance of the Luer junctions cannot be over-emphasized. Walter has stressed that contact contamination of the Luer hub is the likely cause of the confusing and contradictory results described in the literature. Blood or infusion fluid accumulates in the interstices of the mechanism and can act as a nidus for bacterial colonization. If the thread of the fixed Luer-lock collar does not allow the male

Luer plug to fit home into the female half of the connector, then in effect there is a potential sinuous connection between the inside and outside of the Luer-lock mechanism. The internal aspect of the Luer joint can be considered to be a small cavity which can harbour bacteria (19).

This background has led to the adoption during the past year of a more rigorous attention to detail during the line-change procedure with respect to the central venous catheter hub and Luer-lock mechanism. In Sweden, the importance of the hub as a factor in causing infection has been recognized by Holm and his colleagues. They have been flaming the metal hubs of their central lines using a small methylated spirit lamp in an effort to overcome the problem (28). At University College Hospital, London, the infusion-line change procedure for central venous catheters is treated as a formal sterile procedure. The new line should be prepared and primed in advance and delivered to the bedside before the old infusion has finally run through. The system should *not* be stopped for prolonged periods since intraluminal thrombotic occlusion of the catheter will surely occur. The patient and nurse who performs the line change procedure should wear a mask and, in addition, the nurse should scrub, dry her hands and don sterile gloves. In the leukaemia unit, a sterile gown is also worn. The patient should be made comfortable, preferably in the supine position; if this is impossible, then the Valsalva manoeuvre should be requested at the appropriate point in the procedure. The equipment required will be:

Trolley
Small sterile dressing pack
Povidone-iodine spray (Disadine, Stuart
    Pharmaceuticals)
Heparinized saline, 5 ml 10 i.u./ml (Hepsal,
    Weddell Pharmaceuticals)
5 ml syringe
Op-Site dressing (Smith & Nephew)

The old dressing surrounding the catheter to administration set junction should be removed by the nurse's assistant and discarded, whilst the line is simultaneously supported clear of the patient's skin. A sterile sheet or towel must then be placed between the line and the patient before the hub connection is liberally sprayed with povidone-iodine around its circumference. After a period of 2 or 3 minutes, the nurse may then prepare to change the line. A 5 ml syringe should be filled with sterile Hepsal in an aseptic fashion. The flow control valve of the old administration set should be closed off. The line may be quickly released by the nurse and removed by her assistant, whilst simultaneously the syringe is inserted into the central catheter hub. The catheter should be gently flushed with the solution and the new set held in readiness by the assistant for immediate fixation. As soon as the heparin injection has been completed, the assistant can remove the syringe and the nurse performing the procedure should rapidly and gently attach the new administration set to the central catheter hub. Whenever such disconnections are being performed, the patient should be instructed to hold his breath in deep expiration to prevent the influx of air. As long as there is no delay and these procedures only take a fraction of a second to accomplish, there is no danger of any significant air embolism occurring. When a patient has a FEP, PVC, polyurethane or polyethylene catheter in place, it must *not* be clamped, kinked or occluded by a finger (*Fig.* 15.10; *see also Figs.*

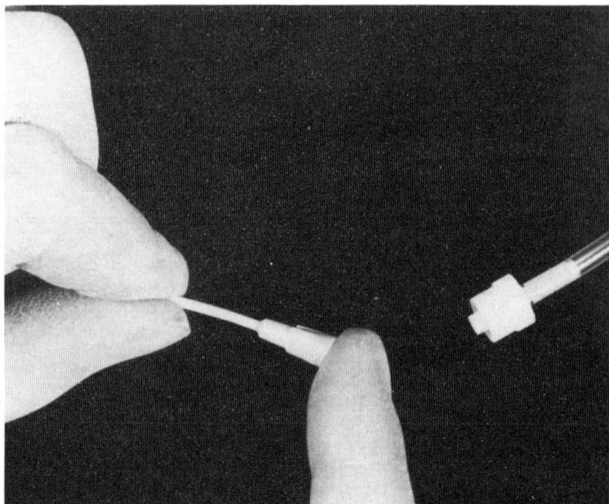

Fig. 15.10. A finger should *not* be used to occlude the catheter hub.

15.1 and 15.9*c*). Such activities will simply injure the catheter shaft. However, soft rubber-shod clamps and purpose-built plastic clamps may be used on the softer silicone Hickman and Broviac catheters. It is important that these devices are not applied too close to the hub since they will force the silicone against the internal spline of the plastic hub mould, causing it to split and the catheter will subsequently leak.

Once the old set has been passed to the assistant, and the new Luer-lock connected, this should be gently slipped on and carefully fixed. It is important that the lock is wound around to a firm closed position. The new assembly should again be liberally sprayed with povidone-iodine, and then wrapped in an onion-skin fashion with sterile gauze. The inside layer of this should be further sprayed with povidone-iodine and the 'junction dressing' secured to the patient with a sheet of Op-Site (*Fig.* 15.11). Finally, the administration tube should be carefully secured so that it does not drag. The infusion should be restarted at the correct rate. If a 3-litre bag system is being used for parenteral nutrition, or a single infusion line is required, it is very useful to use a Continu-Flow set (Travenol) since this enables regular intermittent low-dose heparin therapy to be administered three or four times per day, e.g. Hepsal, 5 ml 10 i.u./ml. There is evidence that this is beneficial in reducing the fibrin formation on the internal catheter lumen and hence catheter sepsis (29). The use of heparin in this low concentration also produces the minimum effect on free fatty acid levels caused by its ability to increase lipoprotein lipase activity. This effect can result in a reduction in the plasma protein binding of a number of drugs and hence an increase in the pharmacological effects of concurrent therapy (30).

INFUSION FLOW CONTROL

Maintaining a satisfactory flow rate prescribed by the doctor will only be ensured by diligent nursing care and regular inspection of the line. This aspect of catheter care is assuming a steadily greater importance in hospital practice. There are now numerous volumetric pumps available which can safely propel fluid in standard aliquots into the venous system. They possess the advantage that small variations of the patient's venous pressure do not impede the influx of fluid. The accuracy achieved is undoubtedly superior when compared to that obtained by the clamps of gravity-fed administration sets. Furthermore, the amount of nursing time spent attending to the patient's infusion is greatly diminished (31). As with all such devices, accidents have occurred. It is essential in central venous infusions that the catheter is in a satisfactory intravascular situation, since disaster can occur if the line has eroded through to the mediastinum or the tip has achieved an extravascular site at the time of insertion (32). The steady instillation of fluid will carry on with a pump. Sudden surges of syringe pumps can occur if the device is tampered with, or the electrical circuit becomes faulty for any reason. In a recent incident, for example, a patient suffered a respiratory arrest following sudden over-infusion of buprenorphine (33).

The introduction of plastic flow control devices which are interposed into the intravenous infusion system has been advocated for use during parenteral nutrition where 3-litre bag systems are in operation (34). However, devices such as the Dial-a-Flo (Abbott Laboratories)

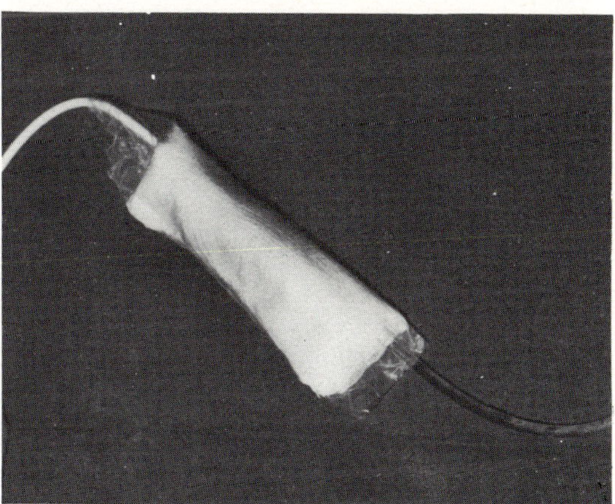

<table><tr><td align="center">a</td><td align="center">b</td></tr></table>

Fig. 15.11. The application of a catheter hub-administration set 'junction dressing' (povidone-iodine). This forms an onion-skin or sterile envelope around this important region (*a*). It may be stored in an envelope of Op-Site (*b*).

and Helix (Van Leer Medical) are inaccurate at low flow rates and are affected by variations in venous pressure (35). Furthermore, the use of these devices adds extra unprotected joints into the system, since they do not possess Luer-lock mechanisms and these can be potential sources of bacterial or air entry. When single large volumes of fluid are being administered or potent drugs infused (e.g. potassium chloride) under the influence of gravity alone, it is wise to use a Dial-a-Flo or apply a second metal gate clamp to ensure against a sudden influx of fluid or drug into the patient.

The major factor influencing drip rate during infusion is the variations which occur in the central venous pressure of the patient (36). This can cause minor fluxes of blood to occur in a retrograde fashion into the tip of the central line. Consequently, if the flow is interrupted for any reason, a firm and sizeable thrombus can occlude the catheter lumen. If this is neglected, then bacterial colonization of the catheter tip will follow.

Clearance of Catheter Thrombus

Gilligan and co-workers introduced the technique of rapidly clearing such aggregates by using a small dose of streptokinase (Kabi-Vitrum), in patients fitted with Hickman catheters (37). They injected a dilute mixture of streptokinase (2000 i.u./ml in 0·9 per cent sodium chloride) into the dead space of the catheter. This manoeuvre can be accomplished, for example, using a Continu-Flo set, by clamping the infusion line close to the proximal injection port; after cleansing the injection membrane, the streptokinase is inserted and left for an hour. The clamp is then released and the infusion recommenced. Alternatively, a syringe containing a small dose of streptokinase or urokinase, e.g. 10 000 i.u., can be placed in the hub of the catheter using a strict aseptic technique and left for 1–4 hours. This invariably frees the lumen and the catheter can be further cleared by gently flushing with 10 ml of Hepsal. Forceful injections should be avoided since the catheter tip may have become adherent to or partially penetrated the wall of a great vein or the heart. Gilligan and co-workers did not detect any adverse allergic or haemorrhagic reactions in their initial patients.

Fault Finding

When an infusion starts to slow or stops, the cause must be found and remedied without delay. The following situations may have developed:

The intravenous bottle or bag
1. Empty.
2. The administration set spike is blocked by a fragment from the bag or bottle seal.
3. The airway in the i.v. bottle or burette has become occluded.
4. The airway has been omitted.

Infusion line, drip chamber and burette
5. Flap valve of burette stuck in the down position.
6. Faulty air vent in burette.
7. Filter mesh occluded by debris from previous blood transfusion.
8. Tube clamp turned off.
9. Intravenous tubing is kinked.

Central catheter problems
10. Angulation-obstruction of the catheter.
11. Twist occlusion of the catheter shaft (*see Fig.* 15.7).
12. Thrombotic catheter occlusion.
13. Superior vena cava occluded by thrombus.
14. Intravascular looping, knots or kinks.
15. Dislocation of catheter into extravascular position.
16. Catheter tip impacted in the vessel or heart wall.

Whilst the first few causes are easily remedied and detected by examining whether or not the drip chamber is collapsed or a flow can be achieved from the infusion administration set; those problems associated with the central catheter itself can be more sinister, and the nursing staff should exercise a high level of suspicion when dealing with this problem. A careful examination of the whole system should be made and recent chest X-rays consulted with the medical staff to see whether malposition has occurred. It may be necessary to perform a chest X-ray after the injection of radiographic contrast medium, e.g. Conray 280. The multiplicity of causes presenting as cessation of flow re-inforces the message expressed in a recent *Lancet* Editorial that 'care and observation of drips is a job for nurses who understand the implications of inattention. It may be cheaper to employ the right staff than to settle an action of negligence' (38).

MANOMETRY

The majority of central venous catheters inserted for pressure measurement are left with their tips situated in the superior vena cava or brachiocephalic veins and linked to a simple saline manometer system. The manometer system is usually mounted upon an intravenous stand by the bedside and calibrated with a simple adhesive tape measure or clipped on to a purpose-made ruler equipped with an extending telescopic spirit level (*Fig*. 15.12). The manometer system is fitted with a three-way tap as shown and this enables:

1. The manometer arm to be in communication with the intravenous infusion bottle or bag for priming purposes. When the nurse carries out this manoeuvre it is essential to ensure that excess fluid does not overshoot out of the manometer arm. Some tubes are fitted

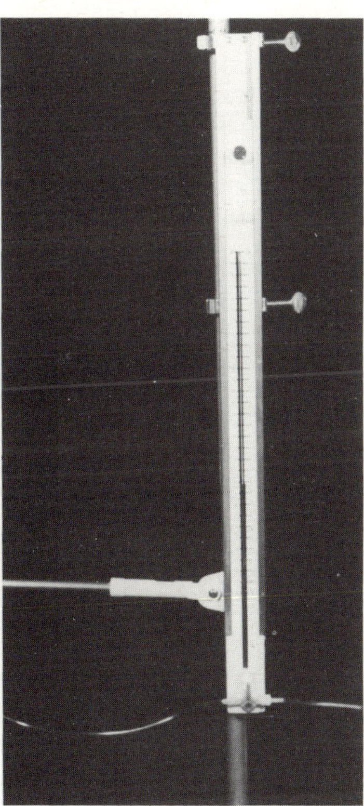

Fig. 15.12. A telescopic spirit level and central venous manometer scale.

with a small plug of sterile cotton wool, and if this becomes wet, pressures cannot be accurately recorded and may be falsely high.

2. The manometer to be in communication with the central venous catheter and the venous circulation. Falsely high readings may be obtained if the catheter is occluded or malfunctioning for any of the reasons previously described. It is important that the manometer arm is re-primed and closed off from the circulation after each reading, since if it is left open, air can enter the circulation in patients who are either hypovolaemic, tachypnoeic or on a ventilator.

3. The central venous catheter can remain in direct communication with the intravenous infusion bag. The pressure (CVP) may be recorded intermittently and in each case a small volume of fluid must naturally enter the patient as the level of fluid in the manometer arm falls in synchrony with respiration and the fluctuations of the right atrial pressure. These aliquots of fluid can assume importance in the fluid balance of children and some adults. The volume given in this way should be incorporated into the fluid regimen.

The sequence of events during CVP measurement should be (*a*) establish the zero reference level (*see below*); (*b*) prime the manometer arm; (*c*) read the pressure with reference to the zero level; and (*d*) return the tap and re-set the i.v. control clamp to allow a slow infusion from the bottle or bag into the central catheter and patient.

A further variation of the manometer principle is illustrated in *Fig*. 15.13. Placement of the tap in the position shown allows the fluid to run down the manometer arm past the small vent in the top of the tubing. The zero-reference level must be marked as described in Chapter 3 by drawing an imaginary line from the fourth intercostal space at the sternum around the side of the chest and bisecting this line with another line drawn from the axilla downwards. Where these lines cross, mid-way between the anterior and posterior chest, is the place at which the zero-point should be marked. This is sufficient for most clinical purposes. Readings will be accurate for patients lying flat and those sitting up to an angle of 45°; falsely low readings may be obtained if the patient sits up to 90° or has his legs dangling. The central catheter can be connected directly to a transducer and oscilloscope, which will also require to be calibrated against the zero reference level. Patency of the line must be ensured by incorporating, for example, an Intraflow device (Sorenson Research and Abbott Laboratories) which will deliver a continuous flush of heparinized saline at 3 ml/h (5000 units of heparin per 1000 ml of 5 per cent dextrose). Swan–Ganz catheters will also require to be linked by such devices at both the pulmonary artery port and the CVP port. It is important that these connections are kept clean, sprayed and taped at all times. There have recently been suggestions towards simplifying the complexity of this apparatus (39).

PATIENT OBSERVATION

The spectrum of complications that can arise has been fully discussed in Chapter 12. The nurse and supervising medical staff must incorporate an inspection of the infusion system as a part of the regular daily history taking and examination of the patient. The more important symptoms and signs to be aware of and looked for with respect to the catheter include:

1. *Fever, rigors and confusion*
   Catheter sepsis (or unrelated focus of infection)
2. *Superficial thrombophlebitis*
   Brachial vein catheter infection
3. *Swelling in the arm*
   Axillary or subclavian vein thrombosis
4. *Oedema of supraclavicular fossa*
   Subclavian vein thrombosis
5. *Oedema of the face*
   Subclavian, jugular or innominate vein thrombosis
6. *Chest pain*
   Air embolism from catheter disconnection
   Catheter embolism
   Pulmonary embolism
   Pneumothorax
   Pericardial tamponade
   Cardiac perforation
7. *Breathlessness and hypotensive collapse*
   Fluid overload
   Pneumo-, hydro- or haemothorax
   Pericardial tamponade
   Hydromediastinum
   Arterial haemorrhage
   Air, pulmonary or catheter embolism
   Pneumomediastinum
   Pulmonary arterial haemorrhage

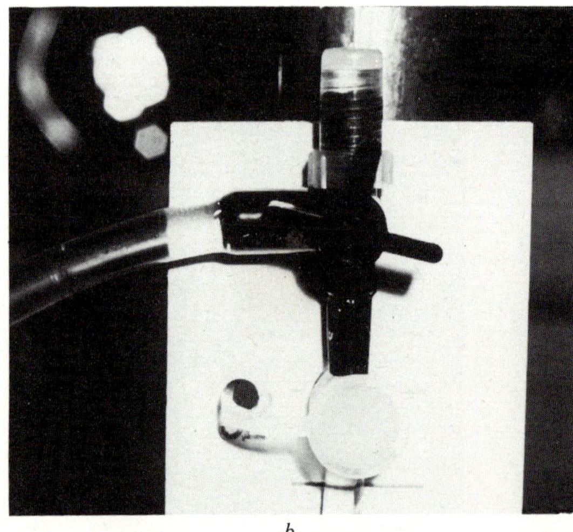

a   *b*

Fig. 15.13. A further variation on the central venous manometer design with a side-arm for calibrating the zero reference level (*a*). The three-way stopcock is situated in a different position at the top of the manometer column. (Reproduced by kind permission of Dr M. Schleusing, Altenburg, Germany.)

The more serious complications require rapid evaluation, with chest X-rays and contrast radiography being performed where appropriate. Sometimes the more spectacular of these complications can develop rapidly in the post-operative course, even before the patient has recovered consciousness. This is particularly the case when the patient has been on heparin therapy, e.g. during open-heart bypass surgery. In these dangerous circumstances, it is often difficult to differentiate these complications from other postoperative events.

HEPARIN-LOCK TECHNIQUE

In patients with Broviac or Hickman catheters inserted for prolonged parenteral nutrition or chemotherapy, it is possible to fill the catheter with heparin solution and close the lumen off from the atmosphere using a small cap component provided by the manufacturers (Evermed). A sterile supply of these must be obtained for each individual. As with all manipulations of central catheter hubs, a meticulous technique has to be adopted. Many patients have now managed to accomplish this, being able to go to work and recommence their infusion of nutrition each evening. The manoeuvre is essentially the same for both nurse or patient. The persons involved should wear masks and wash their hands after assembling the equipment. This should comprise:

Alcohol medical wipes (e.g. Medi-swab)
Small dressing pack
Sterile rubber-shod artery forceps
Heparin: 2 ml of 1000 i.u./ml
Heparinized saline: 5 ml of 10 i.u./ml
    (Hepsal, Weddel Pharmaceuticals)
5 ml syringe
2 ml syringe
Hypodermic needles
Luer-locking cap

A drape should be placed on the patient's chest and, if working without assistance, two pairs of sterile gloves should be worn. This enables the complete procedure to be performed using an essentially no-touch technique. This is illustrated throughout *Figs.* 15.14*a–g*. The Luer-lock cap should be placed face-upwards on a sterile gauze. The syringes can then be loaded with 2 ml of heparin (1000 i.u./ml) and 5 ml of Hepsal, respectively, after the routine checking

of the ampoules has been performed. All air should be expressed from each syringe. Their different sizes ensures there is no mistake during the procedure. The Luer-lock cap should then be filled with Hepsal in order to displace air when it is attached to the catheter.

The catheter connection dressing should then be removed and discarded whilst the junction is liberally treated with povidone-iodine. The catheter should next be clamped with the sterile rubber-shod forceps and 2 or 3 minutes allowed to elapse before wiping off the excess povidone-iodine with a sterile gauze swab. The administration set can be closed off and then removed from the hub. At this point the catheter should be held clear of the drape and the 2 ml heparin syringe (1000 units/ml) should be inserted into the catheter hub without touching the junction. The syringe should be re-checked to ensure that there is no air present. The rubber-shod clamp should then be slowly released and simultaneously approximately 1·5 ml of the heparin solution injected before the clamp is gently re-applied. This re-clamping action should be carried out whilst the injection is still in progress and near the 2 ml mark. This prevents the undesirable reflux of blood into the catheter tip. The central catheter hub must now be rested upon an unfolded sterile gauze and the outer layer of gloves taken off. The central catheter hub should then be lifted up free of the gauze on which it has been placed, and the catheter cap held face-upwards so that the Hepsal does not spill. The central catheter hub with its meniscus of heparin should then be placed downwards on to the locking cap and the assembly screwed together, so displacing any air. The capped hub should next be treated with povidone-iodine solution, dried off after a short interval and the junction secured with sterile adhesive tape, e.g. Op-Site, using a no-touch technique. Although by tradition the stronger concentrations of heparin have been used for the purpose, it may be possible to accomplish this method using the lower dose of heparin found in Hepsal (41).

New Alternative Technique

The difficulties encountered priming the locking cap can be overcome by using a Luer-locking cap possessing a firm latex diaphragm; this can be screwed in place using a non-touch technique

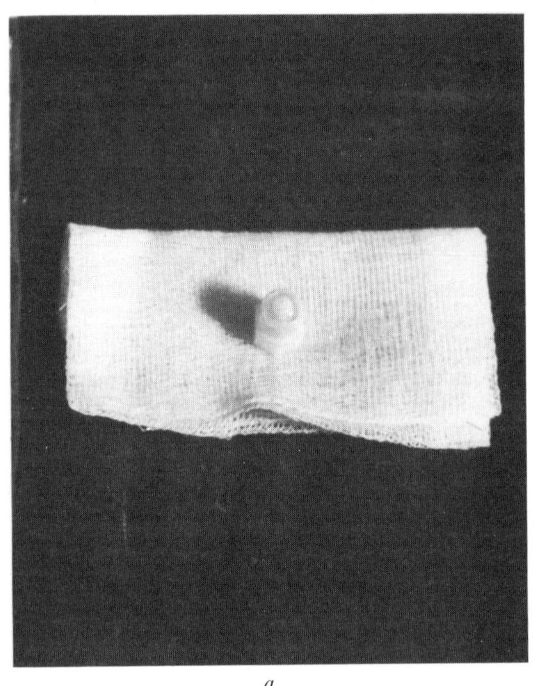

a

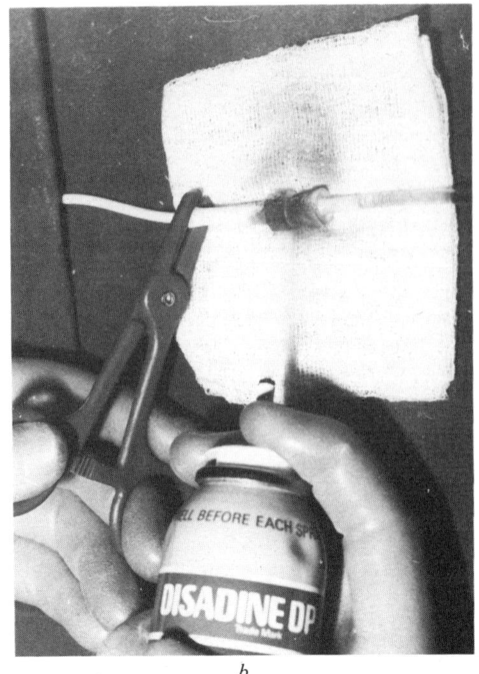

b

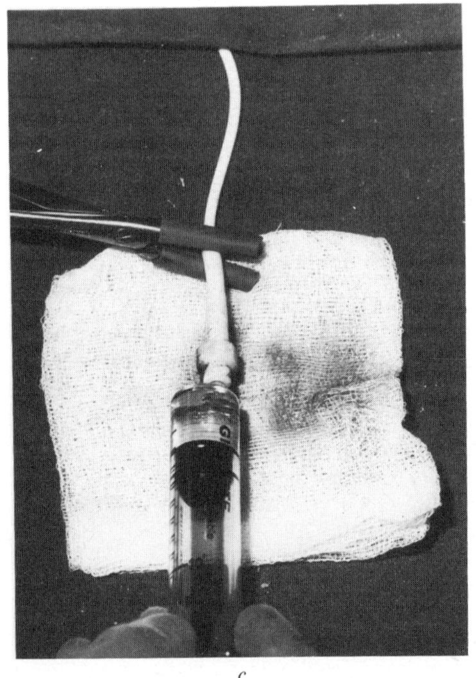

c

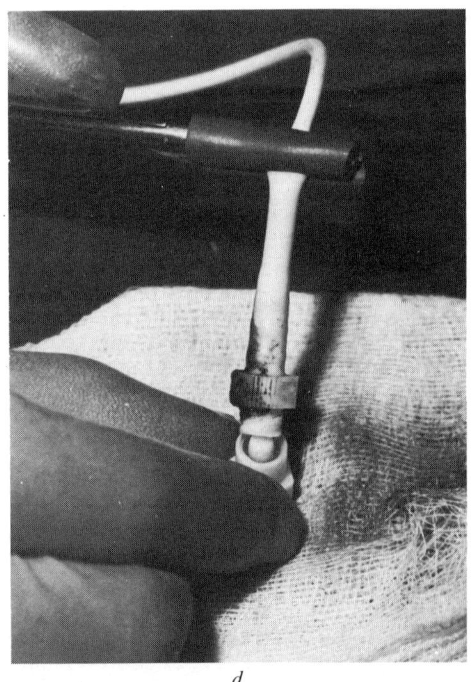

d

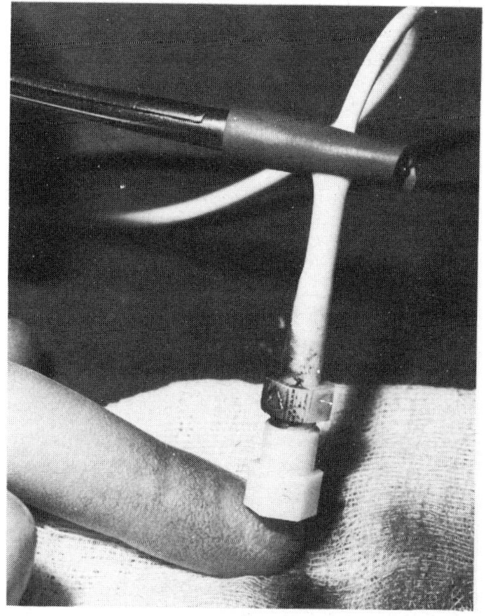

e

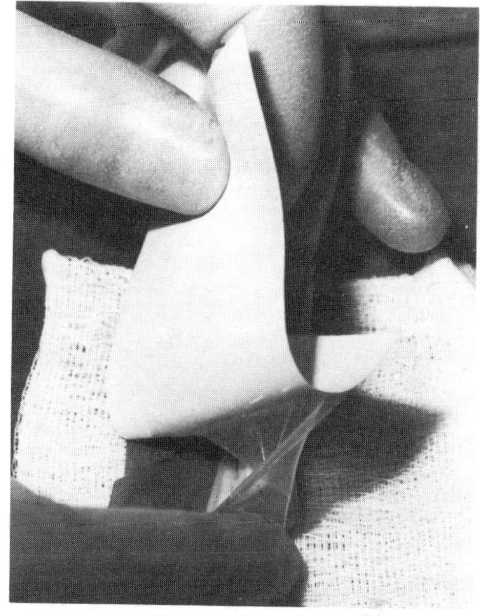

f

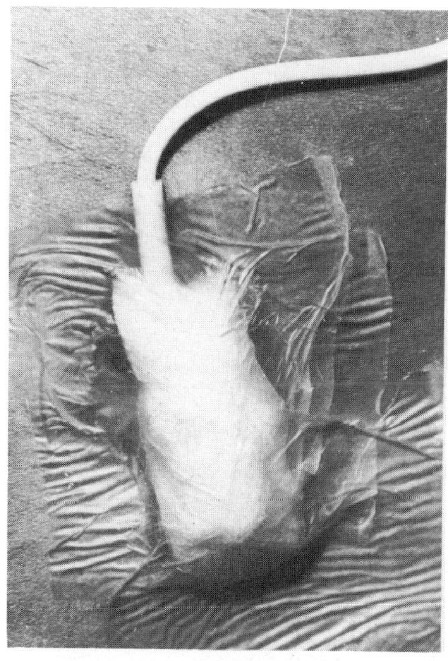

g

Fig. 15.14. *a*, The sterile cap, filled with heparinized saline is placed on sterile gauze. *b*, The catheter dressing has been removed, the catheter hub–administration set junction sprayed with povidone-iodine and gently clamped with sterile rubber-shod or plastic forceps. *c*, After removal of the administration set connection, the catheter is now primed with heparin (1000 i.u./ml) with the rubber-shod forceps being released and re-applied as 1·5 ml of the heparin solution is injected into the catheter lumen. *d*, The exposed hub is rested upon a sterile gauze whilst the cap (filled with heparinized saline) is brought to the hub. *e*, The catheter hub is placed downwards on to the cap and the components are screwed together. *f*, The capped line is sprayed with povidone-iodine, dried and taped with sterile Op-Site intravenous dressing (6 × 8·5 cm). *g*, The taped hub should then be placed in a sterile gauze envelope and fixed to the skin.

(H. G. Weller & Co. Ltd). The derived concentration and volume of heparin solution may then be projected through the latex using a sterile needle.

Blood Sampling from Central Catheters

This procedure was first suggested by Forssmann after his original experiment. It has not been generally recommended for routine use because of the possibility of depositing a fine layer of fibrin along the internal wall of the central catheter which could act as a focus for bacterial colonization. Furthermore, it encourages unnecessary manipulation of the catheter infusion system. There is a place for central venepuncture in patients with very poor peripheral veins and in those who are suffering from severe disorders such as leukaemia which demand multiple blood sampling procedures to be performed. Peripheral venepuncture in such patients can be associated with severe subcutaneous bruising or haematoma formation; these wounds can themselves be the source of systemic infection.

Hickman and his colleagues have been able to accomplish central venous blood sampling without detriment in immunosuppressed patients by adopting a meticulous aseptic technique (7). The procedure should only be carried out by a member of the medical staff, and a mask and gloves should be worn. It may be incorporated with the infusion line change procedure and a strict no-touch technique must be adopted. The hub dressing should be removed and this area carefully cleaned with povidone-iodine solution for 2 minutes. Next, the administration set should be turned off, the Hickman catheter clamped and the tubing disconnected. A sterile syringe may then be quickly linked to the central catheter hub without touching these points and the appropriate volume of blood aspirated.

During the first phase of this procedure the blood should be refluxed back and forth in the syringe to allow adequate mixing to occur before the desired volume is finally removed. Some may prefer first to aspirate a small quantity of blood and then change to a fresh syringe. After the sampling has been completed, the line should be flushed with 5 ml of heparinized saline, e.g. Hepsal 10 i.u./ml (*Fig.* 15.15). Recently, at University College Hospital, London, a slight variation of this technique has been used, which obviates the need to disconnect the line. The administration set (Continu-Flo, Travenol Laboratories) is clamped just distal to the injection port nearest to the central catheter hub. The tubing and injection port are carefully cleaned in the usual manner and surrounded by sterile drape. Using a no-touch technique, a sterile needle mounted upon an empty syringe is passed into the Y-piece of the port through the membrane and blood aspirated back up the line into the administration tubing. The first sample can be discarded as discussed above and the definitive sample taken with a clean syringe. The catheter should be flushed with a 5 ml dose of Hepsal and the infusion simultaneously com-

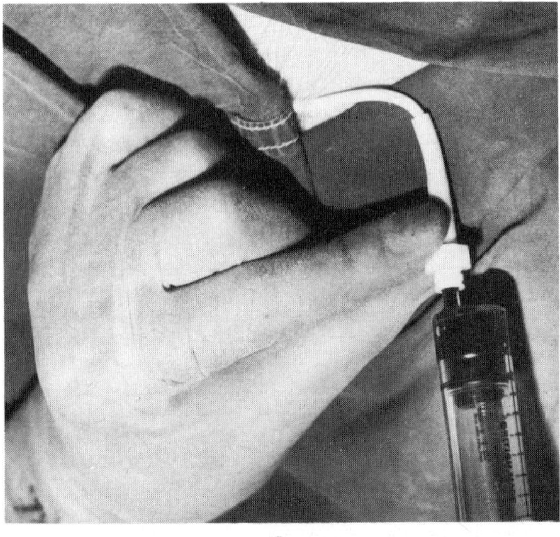

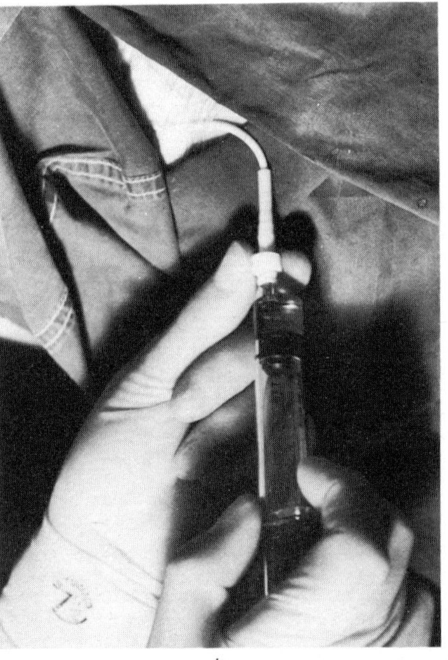

a　　　　　　　　b

Fig. 15.15. Using a no-touch technique, blood may be aspirated from silicone right atrial catheters (*a*), and the catheter flushed through with heparinized saline after the procedure (*b*).

menced. The needle can then be withdrawn and the injection port sprayed with povidone-iodine (*Fig.* 15.16).

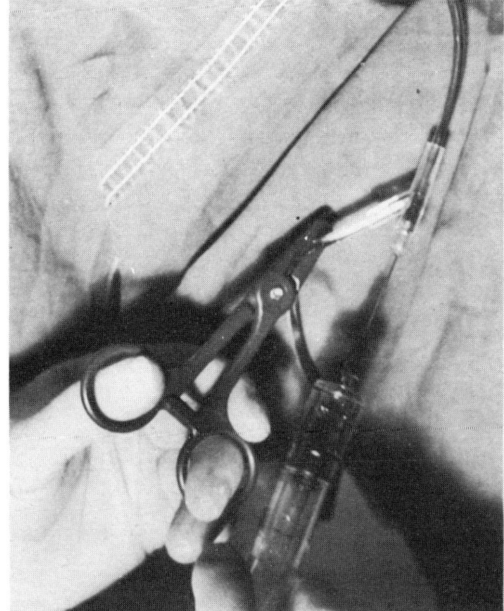

Fig. 15.16. An alternative technique which does not involve disconnection of the catheter–administration set junction. After carefully cleansing the proximal injection port and closing off the administration line with sterile rubber-shod forceps as shown, blood may be aspirated back down the line by using a needle mounted upon a syringe. Variations in the technique are also shown. Note the sterile drapes and strict aseptic protocol. The line must be carefully flushed with heparinized saline after the procedure.

REMOVAL PROCEDURE

When a catheter has been used for parenteral nutrition, the regimen may need to be gradually reduced in concentration and the patient weaned off intravenous feeding on to oral or enteral nutrition. Once the decision has been taken to remove a central catheter, the patient should be informed. Removal should also be treated as a sterile procedure since valuable microbiological information can be gained from the device. Conventional jugular, subclavian and brachial vein catheters are easy to remove. The Hickman and Broviac catheters may require a formal minor operation in order to release the device safely because of the growth of fibrous tissue into the Dacron cuff.

The patient should be placed in the supine position and the nurse should prepare in the way previously described for other central catheter procedures. A sterile drape should be placed on the patient's chest and the dressing taken down by an assistant. The area of skin around the entry site must be cleaned with hydrogen peroxide and povidone-iodine before being left for several minutes. Any retaining suture should then be carefully divided without cutting the catheter, which could be disastrous. If such an untoward event occurs, the portion of the catheter in the skin must be grasped immediately with forceps and retrieved. If the proximal portion retracts beneath the skin, then the patient should be instructed to lie still and a member of the medical staff called immediately. It may be possible to retrieve the catheter from within the subcutaneous tissues before embolization occurs.

Where no untoward episode has occurred, the catheter shaft should be clamped by a forceps whilst the administration set is turned off and detached by an assistant. The central catheter should next be gently and quickly removed through the puncture site and a piece of sterile gauze pressed onto this wound. The catheter must be checked to ensure that it has been completely retrieved and no fragments have been lost. The terminal 2 cm should be snipped off with sterile scissors and placed in a microbiological transport culture medium using sterile forceps. The remainder of the catheter should also be placed in a sterile specimen pot and sent so that further microbiological analysis can be performed if necessary. The puncture site should be covered by a small occlusive Op-Site dressing since a case of air embolism via the removal track has been recorded (42). The patient can then be returned to a more comfortable position and should be kept under observation for a period of 24 hours, since pulmonary emboli have been known to occur from the fibrin sleeve which forms around catheters. In addition, this final manipulation of an infected catheter can trigger off an episode of septicaemia.

Removal of Tunnelled Catheters

Removal of this type of catheter is best performed in a specialized procedure room, and should be treated with respect, since the catheter will the catheter's Dacron cuff be embedded in the subcutaneous fat, but there will also be a suture securing the line to either the cephalic or external jugular vein. Furthermore, the natural elasticity of the material allows it to stretch at these points of anchorage and the device has been known to snap, with embolization of the fragment which recoils into the circulation.

The procedure should be carried out by a doctor with a nurse in attendance to assist. As well as a routine dressing pack, extra drapes should be available and also a small cut-down set of instruments. The patient should be given a premedication, since the procedure is never comfortable. It is also valuable to infuse a small dose of diazepam through an injection port on the administration set. The operation should take place with the patient lying flat and wearing a mask. It is also a wise precaution to have the upper half of the body stripped and the patient lying on an incontinence pad. This latter precaution helps to protect the bed linen from staining with povidone-iodine. Syringes, needles and local anaesthetic solution should be available to infiltrate into the subcutaneous tissues and track of the catheter if the need arises. The doctor should scrub-up and don gown, mask and gloves. The area of the catheter track and exit site should be generously cleaned with povidone-iodine solution. The chest and abdomen should be covered with surgical drapes and the instruments opened. Any retaining suture should be carefully released and the catheter can be clamped using an artery forceps. Next, the catheter should be gently and firmly pulled in the line at which the catheter leaves the chest wall, i.e. horizontal. The catheter should simultaneously be palpated with the free hand in order to detect whether or not the Dacron cuff moves. Usually, this works free and the catheter can be wound around the artery forceps or index finger like a rope around a windlass. The pull exerted should be steady and sustained until the cuff and tip are free and on to the sterile towel. Gentle pressure with a sterile gauze should be exerted by the assistant beneath the drapes over the site of the cephalic or external jugular vein for *at least* 10 minutes. The operator should then despatch the tip of the catheter in an aseptic fashion into a sterile pot for immediate culture and check that the full length of the device has been removed. This is best done by having made

a note of the segment inserted and the piece trimmed off at the original operation.

If any difficulty should arise, then the skin overlying the site of the Dacron cuff should be infiltrated with local anaesthesia and a cut-down performed to the catheter. This should be mobilized by blunt dissection and then gently elevated out of the wound, clamped both proximal and distal to the cuff before this is excised. The distal segment will then slide out freely through the exit site. The proximal or venous site of the catheter can then be further mobilized and the device pulled gently out of the vein before pressure is applied by the assistant whilst the wound is closed. It is a useful manoeuvre to try to dissect out as much of the sinus track as possible. The catheter should be sent for culture as previously described and a sterile occlusive dressing placed on the wound. The authors have found it useful to lay a 1 litre intravenous fluid bag over the track and either strap it down in place with a shoulder spica of crêpe bandage or ask the patient to stay lying down and apply pressure with this hydraulic pack for about half-an-hour. This manoeuvre is particularly useful if extra dissection has been required.

Conclusion

The importance of nursing care to every aspect of the central venous catheterization procedure has been emphasized. Meticulous attention to each detail has resulted in the steady decline of infection and complication rates reported from major institutions where audits have been performed, which attests to the efficacy of proficient nursing care. The guard against infection can never be diminished, as Mehtar and Taylor recently emphasized when they detected episodes of staphylococcal cross-infection arising from a bandaged splint used for supporting arms during intravenous therapy (43). The discoveries of Ignatz Semmelweis and Joseph Lister in the last century, which led to the current foundations of surgical hygiene, still hold good more than a hundred years later.

References

1. Benatt: A. J.: Cardiac catheterisation. A historical note. *Lancet* 1949; **1**: 746–7.
2. Forssmann W.: *Experiments on Myself.* New York: St Martin's Press, 1974: 85.

3. Latimer R. D., Marcuson R. W.: Central venous catheterisation. *Nursing Times.* 1972; Sept. 7: 1124–6.
4. Haughey B.: C. V. P. lines: monitoring and maintaining. *Am. J. Nursing* 1979; **79**: 635–8.
5. Woods S. L.: Monitoring pulmonary artery pressures. *Am. J. Nursing* 1976; **76**: 1765–71.
6. Graham E.: Central venous pressure. *Nursing Mirror* 1977; Dec. 15: 22
7. Bjeletich J., Hickman R. O.: The Hickman indwelling catheter. *Am. J. Nursing* 1980; **80**: 62–5.
8. Englert De A.: The role of the nurse in intravenous hyperalimentation in the United States. In: Proceedings of the 2nd European Symposium on Parenteral and Enteral Nutrition, Newcastle, September 1980. *Acta Chir. Scand.* 1980; Suppl. 507: 298.
9. Phillips K. J.: Nursing care in parenteral nutrition. In: Fischer J. E. (ed.): *Total Parenteral Nutrition.* Boston, Mass.: Little, Brown, 1976: 101–10.
10. Powell-Tuck J., Farwell J. A., Nielsan, T. et al.: A team approach to long-term intravenous feeding in patients with gastro-intestinal disorders. *Lancet* 1978; **2**: 825–8
11. Colley R.: Education of the hospital staff. In: Fischer J. E. (ed.): *Total Parenteral Nutrition.* Boston Mass.: Little, Brown, 1976: 111–25.
12. Farber D. L., Rose M., Bassel J. et al.: Haemoptysis and pneumothorax after removal of a persistently wedged pulmonary artery catheter. *Crit. Care Med.* 1981; **9**: 494–5.
13. Deren M. M., Barash P. G., Hammond G. L. et al.: Perforation of the pulmonary artery requiring pneumonectomy after the use of a flow-directed (Swan–Ganz) catheter. *Thorax* 1979; **34**: 550–3.
14. Thomson I. R., Dalton B. C., Lappas D. G. et al.: Right bundle-branch block and complete heart block caused by the Swan–Ganz catheter. *Anaesthesiology* 1979; **51**: 359–62.
15. Guntupalli R. M.: Mechanical aberrations with pulmonary-artery catheters. *Anaesthesiology* 1979; **50**: 374.
16. Bjoraker D. G.: Blood warmers as a source of solution-conducted leakage currents. *Anaesthesiology* 1978; **49**: 286–8.
17. Altemieir W. A., McDonough J. J., Fullen W. D.: Third-day surgical fever. *Arch. Surg.* 1971; **103**: 158.
18. Sitges-Serra A., Puig P., Jaurrieta E. et al.: Catheter sepsis due to *Staphylococcus epidermidis* during parenteral nutrition. *Surg. Gynecol. Obstet.* 1980; **151**: 481–3.
19. Walter C. W.: Bacterial contamination of intravenous infusion due to faulty technique. In: Johnston I. D. A. (ed.): *Advances in Total Parenteral Nutrition.* Lancaster: MTP Press, 1978: 325–38.
20. Allen J. R.: Prevention of infection in patients receiving total parenteral nutrition. In: Proceedings of the 2nd Congress of European Society of Parenteral and Enteral Nutrition. Newcastle, September 1980. *Acta Chir. Scand.* 1980; Suppl. 507: 405–18.
21. McArthur B. J. Hargiss C., Schoenknecht F. D: Stopcock contamination in an I.C.U. *Am. J. Nursing* 1975; **75**: 96–7.
22. Dryden G. E., Brickler J.: Stopcock contamination. *Anaesth. Analg.* 1979; **58**: 141–2.
23. Peters J. L., Fisher C., Mehtar S.: Risks from cannulae used to maintain intravenous access. *Br. Med. J.* 1981; **282**: 222–3.
24. Breckenridge A. M.: Responsibility of nurses. In: Report of the Working Party on the Addition of Drugs to Intravenous Infusion Fluids. London: Department of Health and Social Security, 1977: ch. 9, 7–9.
25. John G. E.: D.S. (Supply) Hazard Notice H.N. (6). London: DHSS, 1972.
26. Blewitt J. H., Kyger E. R., Patterson L. T.: Subclavian vein catheter replacement without venepuncture. *Arch. Surg.* 1974; **108**: 241.
27. Brotman S., Wiles C. E., Cowley R. A.: Method for reintroduction of Swan–Ganz catheter. *Arch. Surg.* 1981; **116**: 483.
28. Holm I.: Parenteral nutrition in surgical and medical gastroenterology. *Acta Chir. Scand.* 1977; **143**: 297–305.
29. Bailey M. J.: Reduction of catheter associated sepsis in parenteral nutrition using low-dose intravenous heparin. *Br. Med. J.* 1979; **1**: 1671–3.
30. Wood M., Wood A. J. J.: Reduction of catheter-associated sepsis in parenteral nutrition using heparin. *Br. Med. J.* 1979; **2**: 611.
31. Poston J. W., Parish P. A.: Clamps and electronic gravity-fed controllers in controlling flow-rates in patients. *Br. J. Intravenous Ther.* 1980; **1**: 8–11.
32. Ayalon A., Anner H., Berkatzky Y. et al.: A life-threatening complication of the infusion pump. *Lancet* 1978; **1**: 853.
33. Chow A. E.: Syringe pump malfunction. *Anaesthesia* 1981; **36**: 523–5.
34. Mitchell A., Draper C., Lee D. R. et al.: A simple system for parenteral nutrition. *Ann. R. Coll. Surg. Engl.* 1981; **63**: 173–7.
35. Rothalia S. V. S., Tinker J.: Recent developments in infusion devices. *Br. J. Hosp. Med.* 1981; Jan.: 69–75.
36. Flack F. C., Whyte T. D.: Behaviour of the standard gravity-fed administration sets used for intravenous infusion. *Br. Med. J.* 1974; **3**: 439–43.
37. Gilligan J. E., Phillips P. J., Wong C. H. et al.: Streptokinase and blocked central venous catheter. *Lancet* 1979; **2**: 1189.
38. Maki D. G., Goldman D. A.: Dangerous drips. *Lancet* 1976; **1**: 291.
39. Gardner R. M., Parker J.: Simplified pulmonary artery/right atrial pressure monitoring system. *Anaesthesiology* 1981; **54**: 353–4.
40. Morgan R. N. W., Morrell D. F.: Internal jugular catheterisation. A review of a potentially lethal hazard. *Anaesthesia* 1981; **36**: 512–17.
41. Hanson R. L., Grant A. M., Majors K. R.: Heparin-lock maintenance with ten units of sodium heparin in one millilitre of normal saline solution. *Surg. Gynecol Obstet.* 1976; **142**: 373–6.
42. Paskin D. L., Hoffran W. S., Tuddenham W. J.: A new complication of subclavian vein catheterisation. *Ann. Surg.* 1974; **179**: 266.
43. Mehtar S., Taylor T.: A review of bacteriological observation in the care of i.v. cannulae. *Br. J. Intravenous Ther.* 1981; **2**: 16–22.

II Central Venous Catheters and Parenteral Nutrition

Chapter 16

A Primer in Metabolism with Reference to the Care of Surgical Patients

M. J. Rennie

The aim of this chapter is to provide basic information for those interested in the metabolic changes that occur during the care of patients in the surgical ward. I hope that it will provide a background of information of sufficient depth to allow the interested house surgeon to understand the changes that occur as a result of malnutrition, stress, surgical trauma and infection in patients under his care and also to provide him with a basis for the rational criticism of new theories, techniques and treatment regimens as they are reported in the literature and to decide how important and appropriate they may be for patient care.

The processes that comprise the metabolic economy of the body may be conveniently listed and detailed according to the type of substrate dealt with; thus, major headings of fat, carbohydrate and protein metabolism are likely to be a feature of any textbook on nutrition. This is not quite the approach I am going to use here; instead, the underlying interrelationships between the various branches of metabolism will be emphasized by regarding nutritional processes from a functional point of view, stressing metabolic control, contributions of fuel supply, maintenance of the body mass and growth and repair in response to injury.

GENERAL PRINCIPLES OF METABOLIC CONTROL WITHIN THE BODY

The detailed work of many academic and clinical scientists has led to the piecemeal building-up of an edifice, the overall structure of which can now be discerned. For any metabolic pathway that has major functional significance, there will be a number of common control features. Control in pathways will be exercised by regulation of the activity (*a*) of enzymes which catalyse particular reactions and (*b*) of transport systems for blood-borne metabolites. Much more is known about regulation of metabolic pathways in carbohydrate and fat metabolism than in protein metabolism, although the same principles are likely to apply.

The tactics of metabolic control appear to be universal, i.e. to place regulatory steps at the beginning and end of metabolic pathways (or important sub-sections of them), and also at pathway branch-points. The pathway's products often inhibit the activity of the initial steps, i.e. there is feedback control. Regulatory steps are usually catalysed by enzymes which have a *low activity* compared to the other enzymes of the pathway (i.e. they are rate-limiting 'bottlenecks') and they proceed effectively in one direction only. Non-regulatory enzymes, which form the pathway between the regulatory enzymes, catalyse reactions occurring with equal facility forwards or backwards.

In general, control of the regulatory enzymes may occur in four different ways. First, there may be changes in enzyme concentration of a tissue, either *generally* during its growth or wasting (as observed in the gut and heart in response to change in 'work load') or *specifically* as an increase or decrease of a particular enzyme by a specialized mechanism of induction or repression (as occurs in liver in response to a drug or an increase in dietary protein). Both mechanisms appear to have clinical significance.

Secondly, there may be regulation by the

amount of the substrate dealt with by the enzyme. This is usually most important for processes which can proceed in either direction and the control of the level of the substrate is usually under the control of the rate-limiting enzyme that produces the substrate. A good example of this is given by consideration of the metabolism of glucose in peripheral tissues. The flux of substrate through hexokinase (which phosphorylates glucose) depends to a large extent on the delivery of glucose to the tissue and so is controlled by the provision of glucose via the blood, which is in turn regulated by the rate-limited production of glucose by the liver and not in the muscle at all! The passage of material through sequences of steps which are reversible simply depends on the relative concentrations of reactants and products amongst the various steps. The nature of the enzymes catalysing them will ensure the even distribution of material between the various steps of the pathway. The *overall* magnitude of the flux through the pathway will be controlled by the bottleneck enzymes of the initial regulatory step.

The third method of control is through the modification of the activity of the regulatory enzymes by small molecules (such as ATP or NADH) which act by binding to the enzyme to alter its catalytic activity. These so-called allosteric effectors, which act at sites distinct from the catalytic site, may change either the maximum rate of the enzyme or its affinity for a substrate. This type of regulation has been most convincingly worked out for control of glucose breakdown, in particular for phosphofructokinase.

The final major regulatory mechanism of metabolic pathways is through the modification of the structure of regulatory enzymes, usually by the addition or removal of phosphate groups from their protein backbones. Enzymes of glycogen, glucose, pyruvate and fat metabolism can exist in phosphorylated and dephosphorylated forms which are interconvertible by enzymes adding and removing phosphate groups. The modifying enzymes themselves are often found to be modulated by allosteric effectors.

Overlying all of these controls, which operate at the intracellular level, are controls which are exercised by nervous and hormonal mechanisms. The release of acetylcholine and noradrenaline from nerve endings causes acute changes which ultimately rely on intracellular allosteric or phosphorylation/dephosphorylation mechanisms; there may also be long term changes in response to neural activity which result in the growth or transformation of a tissue, for example in response to an altered pattern of muscle stimulation. Hormones also have acute and long term effects, many of the acute effects being modulated by the control of enzymes involved in the regulation of phosphorylation and dephosphorylation. In the heart, for example, adrenaline and insulin have opposite effects in changing the intracellular concentrations of cyclic AMP, a small molecular weight effector which stimulates the phosphorylation of regulatory enzymes. The long term effects may be the result of changes in the protein synthesis capacity of cells as in the case of the effect of thyroid hormones on muscle.

CONTROL POINTS OF CARBOHYDRATE, FAT AND AMINO ACID METABOLISM

Carbohydrate Metabolism

Regulation of whole pathways is best localized at the rate-limiting steps of pathways, and it is therefore apparent that for carbohydrate metabolism the breakdown of glycogen, both in muscle and liver, the process of glucose transport into cells and its phosphorylation are likely to be controlled steps. Indeed all of these can be influenced by small molecular weight effectors—end products of either their own reactions or of the whole pathway—and by hormones.

So far as the breakdown of the glycosyl units provided by the processes of glycogenolysis and glucose transport are concerned (glycolysis), the major regulatory step is the formation of fructose 1,6 bisphosphate by phosphofructokinase, an enzyme that is under extensive metabolic control by intracellular concentrations of ATP, ADP, AMP and inorganic phosphate, and also of its substrate, its product and by citrate (not quite an end product of the pathway but a metabolite, the level of which seems to reflect the extent of activity of fatty acid oxidation (*Fig.* 16.1).

The control of glucose oxidation is by and large the control pyruvate oxidation, and this

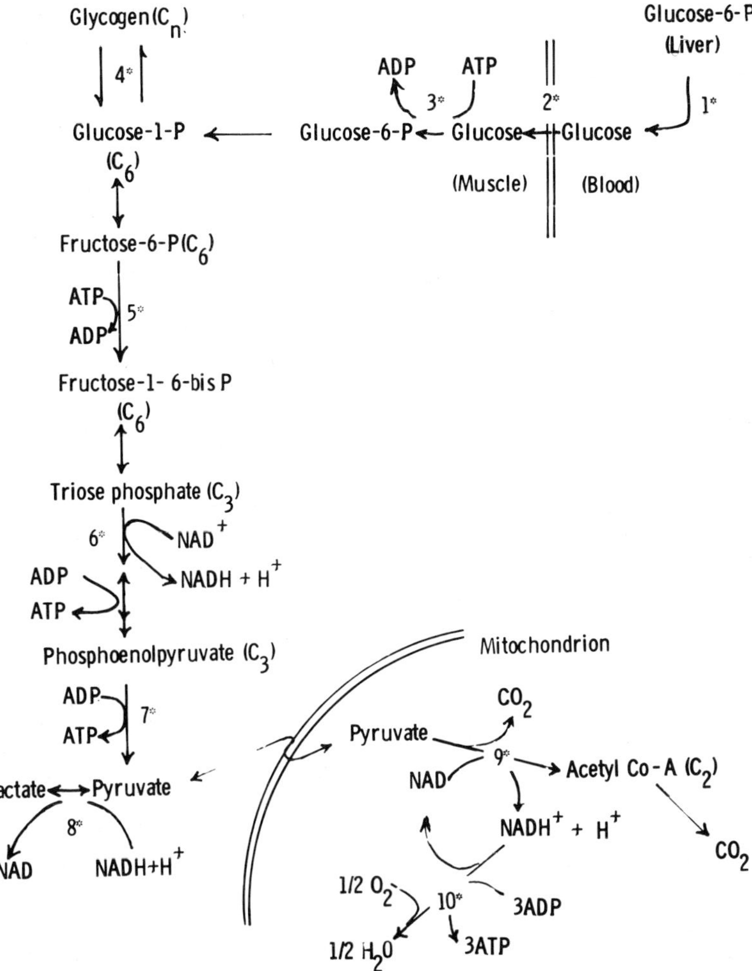

Fig. 16.1. A scheme of carbohydrate metabolism, showing control points with examples of all major forms of control.

1*, Release of glucose into blood by *glucose-6-phosphatase* in the liver—the flux-generating step.

2*, Glucose penetration of muscle membrane—a carrier-mediated step whose control is still largely unexplored except for the recognition of insulin stimulation of its maximum rate.

3*, Glucose phosphorylation by *hexokinase* feedback—inhibited by glucose-6-phosphate and dependent on ATP. Steps 2* and 3* comprise 'glucose uptake'.

4*, Enzymes interconverting glycogen and glucose-1-phosphate-glycogen phosphorylase (degrading) and glycogen synthetase. Enzymes are under many layers of control via allosteric, phosphorylation/dephosphorylation, hormonal (via cyclic AMP) and nervous control (via Ca^{2+}), as well as product and substrate interactions (*see* Rennie and Edwards, 1981).

5*, Formation of fructose-1-6-bisphosphate by *phosphofructokinase*, an irreversible enzyme allosterically contracted by ATP, citrate, H^+ and F-1-6-P (inhibiting) and AMP, ADP, F-6-P and NH_4^+ (activating).

6*, Oxidation of three-carbon phosphate to reduce NAD (reducing carrier); chemical potential of oxidized product used to drive phosphorylation of ADP.

7*, Production of second ATP per triose residue using chemical potential of phosphoenol pyruvate. NB: Since two C3 units each give 2 ATPs, each C6 unit gives 4 ATPs minus 'priming' ATPs at steps 3* and 5*, i.e. net 2 ATPs per C6 unit.

8*, *Lactate dehydrogenase* reaction—reversible and occurs if (*a*) reaction 9* is blocked or too slow, or reaction 10* impossible through lack of oxygen. Reaction 8* regenerates NAD^+ for reaction 6* and therefore allows continued ATP production by glycolysis without pyruvate oxidation.

9*, Decarboxylation and oxidation of pyruvate by *pyruvate dehydrogenase*. Reducing equivalents trapped by NAD^+ and fed into electron transport chain (10*) to power phosphorylation of ATP. Pyruvate dehydrogenase controlled by substrate (activates) and product (inhibits) by allosteric inhibition and activation (ATP, NADH) and by phosphorylation and dephosphorylation.

10*, Oxidative phosphorylation controlled by availability of NADH and ADP (and probably O_2 delivery to some extent).

is effected almost entirely by the regulation of pyruvate dehydrogenase, through which all carbohydrate moieties entering the oxidative processes of the Krebs cycle and the electron transport chain must pass. The oxidation of pyruvate to acetyl CoA, the only substance actually oxidized within the Krebs cycle (tricarboxylic acid cycle), occurs within the mitochondrion. The action of the enzyme (activating a complex of three separate enzymes) is irreversible—a major qualification for its consideration as a regulatory enzyme. In heart and in skeletal muscle the enzyme is pivotal in the control of energy metabolism, although in the liver and in adipose tissue it is also important in controlling the proportions of carbohydrate catabolized or used for fat biosynthesis. Conditions associated with an increase in circulating free fatty acids and the formation of ketone bodies, such as diabetes, starvation and the response to trauma, result in an inhibition of pyruvate dehydrogenase. Within the tricarboxylic acid cycle itself it is likely that the regulatory enzyme is 2-oxoglutarate dehydrogenase, which is a multi-enzyme complex with a similar sequence of reaction steps to those of pyruvate dehydrogenase. It is regulated by its own substrate and products, but unlike pyruvate dehydrogenase does not appear to be regulated by phosphorylation/dephosphorylation. It is the inhibition of this enzyme by increased concentrations of its product and substrate which is the major factor causing the accumulation of citrate during the switch to oxidation of fatty acids and ketone bodies from pyruvate.

Regulation of Lipid Metabolism

Lipid fuels are supplied to mitochondria, the organelles of their oxidation, from two sources; free fatty acids may be liberated from triglyceride stored either intracellularly within the tissue of their catabolism or stored in adipose tissue. In each case the net concentration of free fatty acid appears to be controlled by the balance between reactions synthesizing triglycerides and those breaking them down by lipolysis. Both the synthesizing and lipolysing reactions appear to be under control by small molecular weight effectors, product inhibition and also by phosphorylation/dephosphorylation. For fatty acids traversing the blood-

stream from fat depots to tissues where they may be oxidized, there are two important considerations for control of their utilization. Fatty acids transported as lipoprotein triglycerides can only be taken up by tissues following lipolysis, usually carried out by lipoprotein lipase adsorbed to the capillary wall, particularly in muscle tissues. On lipolysis these free fatty acids join the pool of free acids circulating in the plasma, which are mainly bound to albumin. Uptake of free fatty acids is not a saturable process and appears to depend solely on the concentration of free fatty acids in the plasma. The availability of free fatty acids can vary over a fourfold range, being increased in, for example, trauma, starvation and diabetes. The fact that fatty acid uptake is linearly related to the plasma fatty acid concentration over a wide range distinguishes fatty acid uptake from the uptake of glucose, which can be saturated at concentrations of about 10–15 mmol in the presence or absence of insulin. Therefore, hyperglycaemia does not necessarily result in increased glucose uptake. This means that, because fatty acids tend to be taken up by muscles as available, and because their metabolism results in the accumulation of citrate which inhibits glucose uptake, fat metabolism can 'crowd out' glucose metabolism.

The uptake of fatty acids in mitochondria involves a pair of exchange enzymes which shuttle the fatty acid across the inner mitochondrial membrane into the mitochondria after chemically joining it to carnitine, a substance which may limit fatty acid oxidation if it is not present in sufficient amounts. Such a circumstance occurs in renal failure, when for an unknown reason the muscle concentration of carnitine falls, probably resulting in decreased fatty acid oxidation and being to some extent responsible for the rise in plasma triglycerides.

The rate-limiting processes of fatty acid oxidation are much less well understood than those of carbohydrate breakdown or pyruvate oxidation. No single rate-limiting step has been identified, although since none of the isolated enzymes of the β-oxidation of fatty acids fulfil the obvious requirements, it seems more likely that the enzymes are all freely reversible and that control is exercised by means of the supply of the substrates for the various interactions, namely acetyl CoA, acceptors of reducing equivalents such as oxidized NAD and flavine mononucleotides and free co-enzyme A.

The oxidation rate of all fuels, including glucose, depends upon the oxidation/reduction state of the electron transport chain (i.e. the NADH/NAD ratio), which is in equilibrium with the cellular ADP/ATP ratio. In this way, increased energy demand (i.e. increased ATP use) causes increased respiration. Fatty acid oxidation has an advantage over pyruvate oxidation in this respect: from an energetic point of view it is less efficient since it involves the production of only two molecules of ATP per molecule of oxygen taken up instead of three for pyruvate, *but* this means that only two ADP molecules are needed to allow the continued metabolism from fatty substrates per oxidized fatty acid moiety. Therefore, whenever ADP availability is limited, a smaller rise in ADP is needed to stimulate oxidation with fatty acid as a fuel than with pyruvate as a fuel. This helps to explain the greater reliance on fat as a substrate for respiration at low levels of energy demands, e.g. in a fasting patient lying in bed.

Regulation of Amino Acid Metabolism

The control of flow of amino acids, either into pathways of synthesis or of amino acid catabolism, is much less well understood than for processes involving fat and carbohydrate. The transport of amino acids into tissue may, unlike the transport of glucose and fatty acids, be energy-dependent (and therefore potentially controllable) for the neutral and acidic amino acids with small side chains, and their uptake is probably stimulated by insulin. The major factor in the disposition of amino acids, however, is the extent of protein synthesis. There are large differences between the amounts of amino acids present in the free metabolic pools of the body and the amounts that have been synthesized into protein; leucine for example forms almost 10 per cent by weight of muscle protein but is one of the most scarce (~ 2 per cent) of the amino acids in the free tissue and plasma pool. This means that the concentrations of leucine and of other amino acids with a similarly high ratio between bound and free concentration are rate-limiting for protein synthesis. Under conditions in which protein synthesis is stimulated, for example by insulin, the concentration of free leucine in tissues is likely to fall as it is in-

corporated into protein. When protein synthesis is depressed, however, leucine concentrations are likely to rise. This is exactly what is seen in the muscle of patients suffering from wasting diseases of muscle, either primary diseases such as muscular dystrophy polymyositis or secondary to postoperative sepsis. The swings in the free concentrations of other amino acids which do not show such a large ratio between bound and free concentrations are likely to be less, except possibly for alanine and glutamine, which have a role as exporters of NH_2 groups from muscle. In addition, the existence of interconverting enzymes for amino acid metabolism is likely to even out the changes observed for these other amino acids, such as alanine, glutamate and aspartate.

The representation of enzymes of amino acid metabolism in muscle is much less than that in liver, but the enzymes that do occur appear to have disproportionately important roles. These roles appear to be to provide a source of amino groups for the production of alanine and glutamine by transfer of amino groups to pyruvate and glutamate, to take part in the shuttle of reducing equivalents in and out of mitochondria (by the aspartate–oxolacetate shuttle) and to transaminate the branched chain amino acids. Muscle removes their amino groups from branched chain amino acids converting them into keto acids which may then be exported for oxidation by the liver, which possesses a minor proportion of the whole body's transamination capacity. This function of muscle may be one of the most important in regulating the whole body amino acid metabolism, since it has been suggested that the branched chain amino acids have a pivotol role in control of amino acid metabolism. Increases in the supply of branched chain amino acids and keto acids to model muscle systems appear to increase protein synthesis and decrease protein degradation, and since the affinity constant of the transaminase reaction K_m for the branched chain amino acids is higher than the normal circulating concentrations, increases in the supply of the branched chain amino lead inevitably to their degradation. This factor is likely to be of some importance during conditions of decreased energy supply to the whole body when concentrations of amino acids, including the branched chain amino acids, rise in the plasma.

Fuel Metabolism

The provision of energy for any metabolic processes can be accomplished using carbohydrate, fat or amino acids derived from protein as the ultimate fuels, depending on the metabolic bank balance of the body and the capacity of the various processes involved in the breakdown of the substances. In resting post-absorptive man, energy will be initially trapped as ATP, which is later used as the ubiquitous metabolic energy currency of the cell. The measurement of blood flow across respiring tissues and organs, and the respiratory quotient (i.e. O_2/CO_2, RQ), gives valuable information about the particular sources of this metabolic energy. Thus, most of the energy in kidney and all of the energy in the brain appears to be supplied by the oxidation of blood-borne glucose, which has an RQ of 1. Since the blood flow is high and its metabolic requirements account for the largest single fraction of oxygen consumption of the total body oxygen uptake, then the brain accounts for 80 per cent of all glucose oxidized during 24 hours in the life of an average man. This amounts to some 180 g of glucose. In muscle, the situation is different. Almost all of the oxidative fuel breakdown in muscle at rest and in the heart in resting man is accounted for by the burning of fatty acids (RQ 0·7). The oxidation of glucose by heart and skeletal muscle is actually inhibited as a result of the changes (in the cellular redox state and by the production of citrate) occurring during fatty acid oxidation. Citrate feeds back to inhibit steps in glucose metabolism which control the uptake of glucose into the cell and its breakdown. Of the glucose that is taken up by skeletal muscle in post-absorptive man, about two-thirds is directed towards the storage of carbohydrate and glycogen and one-third is broken down to lactate.

The relative contributions of amino acids to the energy-supplying processes depend on whether the carbon backbones of the amino acids are of a type which predisposes them (*a*) to be directed towards the formation of intermediates which can be built up by the liver into glucose, or (*b*) of a type which may be directly oxidized within tissues to carbon dioxide and water or (*c*) may be transferred to the liver where they are converted to ketone bodies (acetoacetate and 3-hydroxybutyrate) which may act as a fuel for heart and skeletal muscle.

The relative contribution of ketone bodies in normal man to the overall fuel economy is very low, possibly because of their low circulating concentrations. However, their concentrations may increase by the largest factor of any circulating metabolite, for example, after a sustained fast or in response to trauma. In these circumstances, increases in free fatty acids may then assume a much greater importance in the provision of energy, as well as possibly acting as a metabolic signal. The ketone bodies are usually produced within the liver, not from amino acids but by a combination of 2-carbon subunits chopped-off from long fatty chains of 16–18 carbons. Ketone body production appears to be controlled by the balance of two factors—the supply of fatty acids from adipose tissue and the store of carbohydrate within the liver. The second factor appears to be of overriding significance, since in the fed state an increased supply of fat to the liver does not result in substantial increases in ketosis. However, in the fasted or stressed state, whenever carbohydrate stores are depleted, production of ketone bodies is directly related to the supply of fatty acids.

The quantitative importance of muscle to the whole body metabolic economy is shown by the fact that, although the metabolic rate of muscle is very low and its blood supply relatively limited in comparison to that of the kidney, heart and brain, nevertheless its large mass causes it to be the major consumer of metabolic fuel, and since the greatest proportion of the muscle fuel is fat, this outweighs the contribution of glucose oxidation in brain and elsewhere so that the respiratory quotient of resting post-absorptive man reflects a fat-based metabolism.

WHAT CONTROLS THE CHOICE OF FUEL BY BODY TISSUES?

Two major factors are important in the tactics of the body's fuel economy; these are (*a*) the capacity of the pathways to handle fuels, and (*b*) the size of the fuel stores.

Fuel Handling

The fastest conversion of chemical energy in nutrients to metabolic energy is achieved by the process of glycolysis and glycogenolysis (the breakdown of glucose and glucose-residues derived from the storage form of carbohydrate). The enzymatic machinery of these pathways in muscle, heart and liver has a capacity about double the metabolic capacity of pathways oxidizing pyruvate, the end product of glycolysis. When the metabolic rate of the tissue needs to be increased to supply ATP to meet its increased energy demands, for example during increased contractile activity or during metabolic stresses which would increase the ATP turnover—such as increased growth repair (i.e. protein synthesis), maintenance of ion gradients during altered acid–base status, increased cardiac work to perfuse injured tissue etc.—then pyruvate derived from glucose or glycogen will be directed at an increased rate into the oxidative processes of fuel metabolism, the Krebs cycle and electron transport chain of the mitochondrion. However, if the major regulatory step at the beginning of this metabolic sequence (the pyruvate dehydrogenase reaction) is compromised to any extent, for example by being flooded with substrate, or suffering down-regulation as a result of changes in oxidation–reduction potential of the cell secondary to the failure of oxygen supply, then pyruvate will be shunted off to form lactate. Lactate may be a major end product of carbohydrate metabolism in skeletal muscle and even in heart during respiratory failure, cardiogenic shock and fever.

The capacity for maximum flux of material through glycolysis as opposed to pyruvate oxidation is about 2:1. For fat oxidation, the maximum capacity of the oxidizing tissues is only about half as much as that for oxidizing pyruvate because of the limitations of the maximal activities of the regulatory enzymes involved. Therefore, under circumstances in which there is an increase in the metabolic load on energy-supplying mechanisms, as may occur in pre- and postoperative surgical patients with fever or in a shocked state, there will tend to be a greater reliance upon carbohydrate as a fuel than on fat, and a greater reliance on glycolysis than on glucose oxidation.

Storage

The stores of glucose and glycogen within the body are necessarily limited. Glycogen is stored within tissues in a form which binds up a large proportion of the cell's water. The maximum capacity of the muscle or liver cell for glycogen storage is therefore limited by its water content. This means that the total capacity of the body for carbohydrate storage is the equivalent of about three 1 lb loaves of bread, about half a loaf's worth in the liver and about two-and-a-half loaves' worth in the skeletal musculature. The end products of anaerobic glycolysis in muscle, lactate and pyruvate can be converted into glucose by the liver, and liver glycogen itself is broken down directly into glucose so that in theory all of the three 'loaves of bread' may be converted into glucose for the obligate glucose users of the body—the brain, white cells and the kidney medulla. Since their rate of glucose utilization is relatively large and the stores relatively limited, there is no more than $1\frac{1}{2}$–2 days' supply of carbohydrate fuel available for these tissues.

Fat may be stored within the body by a much more efficient process in terms of total energy value per unit weight than carbohydrate. Adipocytes may be 90 per cent fat by weight and the energy available from fat even in a lean 70-kg man would be enough to allow him to trot at 6 miles an hour for 4–5 days if his mechanical equipment remained usable! The upper limit of fat storage is effectively infinite, but in normal man the energy stored in fat is probably sufficient to sustain life for about 40–75 days during complete starvation.

The inability of the body to produce glucose from fat and the limited supply of carbohydrate stores means that another source of gluconeogenic carbon must be found. In the past 20 years the realization has grown that protein within the lean body mass may provide the carbon for the synthesis of new glucose from the carbon backbones of amino acids. The main source of the amino acids is in fact the depression of protein synthesis within muscle rather than an increase of protein breakdown by muscle during starvation in normal untraumatized man. (NB: Visualization of this is made easy for the reader, if he imagines what happens to the balance in his current bank account if he continues to withdraw cash but his employer ceases to pay in his salary.) As starvation continues in normal man, lipolysis becomes sufficiently accelerated to increase the circulating free fatty acid concentration to an extent where, in the absence of liver glycogen, ketogenesis by liver becomes a substantial supplier of ketones to the blood. Muscle and, more importantly, brain, are able to use ketone bodies as a fuel and therefore the need of the brain for glucose is diminished to some extent and the rate of utilization of muscle tissue falls. The increased catabolism of amino acids to provide carbon backbones for glucose and amino acid to satisfy requirements of fuel metabolism results in the production of increased amounts of end products derived from amino groups, principally urea and ammonia. Therefore there is an increase in the amount of nitrogen excretion. During the course of acute starvation, nitrogen excretion reaches a peak after about 4–7 days but thereafter the net flux of amino acids from lean tissue slowly falls. Nevertheless, the lean body mass is depleted progressively, and it would seem that the musculature as a body store is limited to the supply of about 60 days' worth of glucose carbon, this being the limiting factor for survival in starving man.

In any circumstances in which the energy needs of tissue are accelerated, for example, in response to attempted repair and mobilization of immunological defences, then the body stores will be compromised that much further unless there is additional provision of substrate (*Fig.* 16.2).

PROCESSES OF MAINTENANCE OF THE LEAN BODY MASS, GROWTH AND REPAIR OF TISSUES

Of all the processes occurring within the living cell, protein synthesis is by far the most energetically expensive except for the transduction of energy from chemical to mechanical forms. The energy cost of growth has been a major area of investigation for many years, but although it is well recognized that growth and repair of tissue is energetically expensive, reliable quantitative figures are scarce. The energy cost of maintenance of protein in the body is likely to account for something like 15–20 per cent of the total energy intake. The amount of amino acids needed for the maintenance of the normal body mass can be gauged by nitrogen balance studies when subjects are fed different amounts of protein with the same total dietary energy intake: it seems that somewhere in the region of 1 g of amino acid-derived nitrogen per

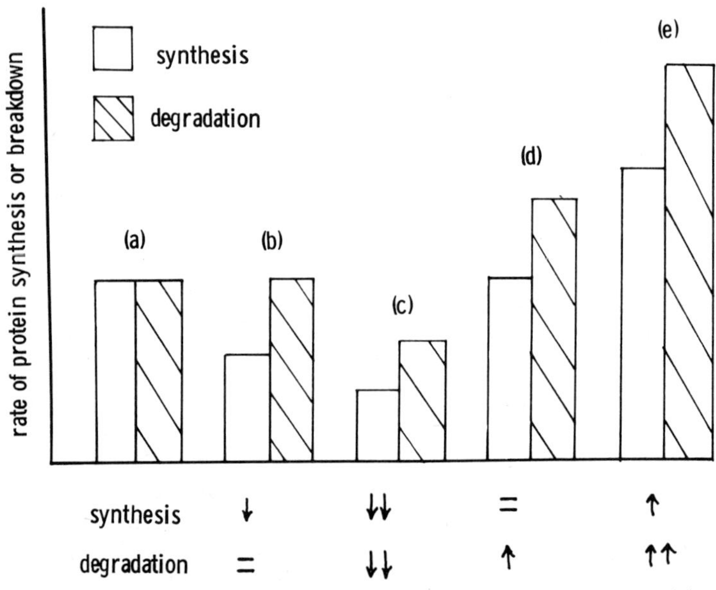

Fig. 16.2. Regulation of protein mass of the tissues. Normally synthesis and degradation are equal, i.e. there is no net loss or gain of protein—the tissue is in protein balance. (*a*) Loss of protein, i.e. wasting, can occur whenever degradation is in excess of synthesis, and in each of (*b*), (*c*), (*d*) and (*e*) this is the case, but the mechanism is different for each. In life the situations depicted occur in muscle in acute (*b*) and in chronic (*c*) starvation, in liver in acute starvation and muscle in cancer (*d*), and in muscle in inflammatory disease and some dystrophies (*e*).

kilogramme of body weight is an ample amino acid supply for the daily maintenance requirement. However, during increased protein turnover, the protein requirement is bound to go up, because whenever there is an increased flux of amino acids through the processes of biosynthesis and degradation of fixed protein in the body, the extra amino acids of the expanded metabolic pool inevitably come into contact with enzymes which cause their catabolism. Therefore, there is an inevitable obligatory wastage.

Growth and repair involve degradation as well as synthesis because these processes are remodelling processes, and therefore it is likely that proteins have to be broken down before tissues can be modified. The factors increasing synthesis and decreasing degradation have been searched for in the hope of applying them to circumstances in which encouragement of growth and repair is desirable, as in the postoperative patient, but any rationale based on the idea of depression of degradation during the simultaneous increase of growth is probably faulty, precisely because of the need for remodelling.

BIOCHEMICAL INVESTIGATION OF METABOLIC DISTURBANCES

All the metabolic systems within the body are interconnected and material is transported from one to the other constantly. It makes sense, therefore, that in order to gain some insight into these processes, measurements must, wherever possible, be designed to give information about the dynamics of the system. This does not mean that the measurements themselves must necessarily be measurements of flux of material through a pathway (although this is ideal), but the measurements should reflect the state of flux.

Dynamic Measurements

The conceptually simplest measurements of metabolic flux are those which involve measurements of input from the whole body. These include oxygen consumption and CO_2 production, food intake and urinary and faecal nitrogen production, i.e. the classical measurements. Although the information given by these measurements is extremely valuable and not directly available in any other way, their application to patients has decreased in popularity because of the difficulty in the clinical situation of arranging for adequate collection of respiratory gases, the reliable collection of urine and faeces and the difficulties of preparing and administering exact quantities of food of known composition. Nevertheless, there appears to be no absolute substitute for these methods and any derived measurements which attempt to give some of the same information must always be checked against them.

Unfortunately these classic methods do not give an insight into the components of the processes that affect the value of the net measurement made, a good example of this being the inability to determine from the size of the net negative or positive nitrogen balance the changes involved in whole-body protein synthesis and degradation. For insight into these processes recourse must ultimately be made to isotopic tracer methods which are necessarily complicated and time-consuming. They may, however, be worth the effort, since they can give information which is otherwise totally unavailable. The application of tracer methods to the study of metabolic derangement in surgical patients has grown tremendously in the past 10 years. One drawback is that most of the methods, which depend on the use of radioisotope labelled tracers, can only be applied to the measurement of turnover of substances present in the blood, and possibly to urinary and breath excretion rates because of the large radioactive doses necessary to measure incorporation into tissues. For safety reasons the methods cannot be applied to the study of young children and adults below the age of 55. The development of tracer methods depending upon the detection by mass spectrometry of heavy isotope-labelled compounds (labelled principally with ^{13}C, ^{15}N and deuterium) will inevitably extend the range of investigation possible. Even so, the methods are costly and time-consuming and the equipment needed for them only available in specialized centres, so that they are likely to remain research tools, involved in the production of definitive answers about a particular condition rather than be used in diagnosis and therapeutic guidance for particular patients.

Hydroxyproline and 3-Methylhistidine

The existence of certain 'post-translationally modified' amino acids in the urine provides the possibility of some insight into the processes involved in protein turnover. Hydroxyproline and 3-methylhistidine are two such amino acids which arise in the tissues by biochemical modification of proline and histidine of the amino acid backbones of collagen and myofibrillar protein (chiefly actin), respectively. The modifications are made *after* the processes of translation and transcription of the genetic message, i.e. protein synthesis. A knowledge of the amount of the modified amino acids in the parent protein and rate of loss from the body (assuming that the amino acids are not further metabolized) gives an estimate of the protein degradation rate.

Unfortunately the bright promise of the theory is slightly dulled in practice. Hydroxyproline is released from newly synthesized collagen only and not mature collagen, thus its urinary excretion is mainly a measure of the rapid turnover of growing connective tissue. This of course may be useful as a measure of recovery, but probably not of wasting of mature tissue. In the case of 3-methylhistidine the interpretation of the urinary excretion rate depends largely on the assumption that for practical purposes, muscle tissue contributes all of the amino acid to the urine. There seems no doubt that the greatest proportion of 3-methylhistidine in the body is bound up in muscle actin and to a lesser extent myosin, but actin is present in all tissues, some of which turn over at ten times the rate of muscle and even small pools of rapidly turning over actin (e.g. in gut or skin) could contribute markedly to the urinary excretion rate. This appears to be the case in the rat, and it is likely that in any circumstances in man in which the muscle mass is reducd (a major area of interest), the problem may become acute. It will be exacerbated if the excretion rate is based on the ratio with creatinine as a measure of muscle mass, since excretion of creatinine will fall with muscle mass, but 3-methylhistidine excretion arising from non-muscle sources will be unaffected.

A further complication of the use of hydroxyproline and 3-methylhistidine measurements is the need to modify the patient's diet to exclude collagen and all flesh. In practice this may not be a problem if enteral or parenteral feeding of synthetic nutrients is used. The doubts arising from the assumptions inherent in the theory of the use of 3-methylhistidine should not affect the interpretation of excretion rates in patients early on in the course of muscle wasting, especially if the nitrogen excretion is also known, but care should be taken in the case of data from patients of already low muscle mass.

Static Measurements

There is little point in measuring the steady-state level of a whole series of intermediates in a pathway between control points; the values will not necessarily reflect any increase or decrease in the flux through the pathway. However, if measurements are made of substrate and product on either side of a control point, then during alteration in flux through the whole pathway one would expect that the ratio between the substances would reflect the change. For example, during acceleration of glycolysis the ratio of the concentration of substrate to product for the enzyme phosphofructokinase falls; when the pathway is inhibited by control at the level of the phosphofructokinase step, the ratio rises. However, measurements of the ratio of concentrations of substrate and product for a non-regulated enzyme such as lactate dehydrogenase cannot give information about the rates of flux through glycolysis. The concentration ratio will, however, give information about the oxidation/reduction potential of the cell through the linkage between lactate and pyruvate to the reduced and oxidized forms of the nicotinamide adenine dinucleotide co-enzyme (NADH and NAD^+).

The danger of misinterpretation of the significance of single metabolite estimations becomes even more acute when the measurements are made in a compartment distinct from the actual site of interest. For example, measurements of blood glucose may or may not indicate increased glucose utilization; at the same concentration of blood glucose, glucose incorporation into glycogen and glucose oxidation may be significantly altered in, for example, normal post-absorptive man, an exercising subject, a traumatized post-operative patient with insulin resistance and a juvenile diabetic, who would all show a different pattern of the disposition of glucose at the same blood concentration. To give another example, under conditions of increased muscle wasting in postoperative patients with sepsis, and in patients suffering from muscular dystrophy, the plasma amino acid profile is not significantly altered from normal but the intramuscular profile of amino acids is fairly deranged. The normalization of the plasma amino acid profile is achieved by the action of liver in using the amino acids released from muscle during protein degradation and not used in synthesis, as gluconeogenic substrates. It is therefore important that measurement should be made, wherever possible, in the tissues.

An understanding of the constraints that affect measurement of metabolite concentrations and their interpretation should lead to a realization that similar constraints should apply in the choice of enzyme activity to be measured. There are many instances of the alteration of enzyme activities in response to alteration in metabolism, but only the alterations in rate-limiting enzymes, i.e. the control points of pathways, may be safely interpreted as reflecting changes in the capacity and possibly flux through pathways. The confidence of an investigator in interpreting the results of enzyme activities is always increased if the measurements he makes enable him to discern changes in the ratios one to another of control enzymes, since these often exist within tissues in constant proportion. It seems likely that specific changes in a particular pathway among other unaffected pathways would be easily picked up by this sort of measurement, and indeed, under circumstances of alteration of muscle metabolism in a wide variety of situations, including arterial insufficiency, muscle wasting, obesity, physical training, cancer and cardiogenic shock, there are alterations in the proportions of rate-limiting enzymes one to another.

Insufficient information has yet been collected for us to identify *in vivo* rate-limiting enzymes in the pathways of nucleic acid and protein metabolism. Thus, prediction from spot measurements of enzyme activities and metabolite concentrations of the nature of possible abnormalities is difficult. Nevertheless, there are some spot indicators that may be used and the most reliable of these are likely to be simply compositional measurements of protein RNA and DNA, and the ratios of one to another. The ratio of DNA to protein gives an indication of cell size, and measurement of the RNA/protein ratio appears both in experimental animals and in man to be directly related to the capacity for protein synthesis.

METABOLIC ABNORMALITIES AFFECTING THE FUEL AND PROTEIN METABOLISM IN THE SURGICAL PATIENT

The surgeon's main interest in nutritional metabolism inevitably stems from two main questions. First, is a particular patient sufficiently well nourished to survive surgery, and if not, can nourishment be supplied to make the outcome safe? Secondly, what is the basis of the postoperative catabolism so commonly observed in surgical patients and to what extent is it likely that nutritional intervention will prevent it. If the range of metabolic changes that are observed in a wide variety of conditions is examined from a functional viewpoint, much of the complexity of the picture disappears. The following two sections therefore describe abnormalities of metabolism commonly observed in pre- and postoperative surgical patients from a functional viewpoint, in an attempt to synthesize a coherent picture of the abnormality.

Metabolic Abnormalities in the Pre-operative Patient

Obesity

A number of metabolic abnormalities are associated with obesity and some of these will have a direct relevance to the metabolic behaviour of the patient after operation. Obese subjects have poorer glucose tolerance than normal, and this is related to peripheral insulin resistance mainly as a result of decreased insulin sensitivity of muscle tissue. The inability of muscle in obese subjects to take up glucose from the blood results in a decreased muscle glycogen content (by about 40 per cent in quadriceps of obese women compared to normal). In addition, there appear to be abnormalities of key enzymes of certain metabolic pathways which might help to explain some of the abnormality. For example, there appears to be a negative correlation between the accumulation of body fat and the enzyme activities of hexokinase, citrate synthase and the fat-metabolizing enzyme hydroxyacyl-CoA-dehydrogenase in muscle taken from obese men and women. This would partially help to explain diminished glucose uptake and low muscle glycogen content and a decreased fatty acid degradation. There is also the suggestion that the decreased physical activity associated with obesity worsens the situation by decreasing the concentration of respiratory enzymes in mitochondria, of hexokinase and of enzymes of fatty acid utilization, resulting in a vicious circle.

Little is known about protein turnover in obesity, but it has been suggested that one of the reasons for the accumulation of fat is that obese subjects have a lower rate of protein turnover associated with their lean body mass and that therefore the energy cost associated with protein synthesis is decreased, leading to a net energy surplus from dietary intake and consequently accumulation of stored energy as fat.

These metabolic alterations in the obese preoperative patient would tend to militate against a healthy metabolic response to surgery: the diminished muscle glycogen stores would result in the lean body mass being called upon for a source of gluconeogenic carbon earlier than otherwise would be the case, insulin resistance would decrease the rate of transport of glucose and amino acids into tissue for repair and, if there was a pre-existing propensity to a low protein synthetic rate, the likely rate of repair and wound healing would be lower than normal. Reduction of obesity by severe calorie restriction alone might in many ways make the circumstances worse because of further decreases of muscle glycogen content, the aerobic capacity of muscle tissue and its hexokinase activity. Exercise, however, in addition to food restriction, may mobilize fat and preserve the muscle tissue and its respiratory capacity, thus improving the metabolic responsiveness of the lean body mass.

Starvation

Severely malnourished children who have suffered the loss of a large proportion of their lean body mass show a low muscle glycogen content. Paradoxically, adolescent children suffering from anorexia nervosa may have a slightly elevated muscle glycogen content but they are also likely to show a markedly reduced RNA to protein ratio, suggesting a reduced capacity for protein synthesis. The expansion of the muscle protein stores and the body fat stores by supplementation of the diet would be of obvious benefit in these cases. A major benefit of refeeding is likely to be the normalization of deranged endocrine responses observed during protein calorie malnutrition, such as increased levels of cortisol and decreased levels of insulin and thyroxine.

Cancer

In patients suffering from cancer there may or may not be obvious gross malnutrition (i.e. more than 15 per cent weight loss). However, even in the absence of a large degree of malnutrition, it is likely that the presence of a tumour adds another factor to the derangement of the metabolic response to marginal malnutrition. A common finding in patients suffering from cancer, with or without wasting of the tissues, particularly of fat stores and muscle protein stores, is decreased insulin sensitivity, and this may be partially explained by decreases in the activities of key enzymes responsible for carbohydrate metabolism and the oxidative handling of glucose. There appear also to be abnormalities of protein metabolism: Lundholm and co-workers have shown that muscle from patients suffering from malignant tumours has a decreased rate of protein synthesis observed in muscle samples incubated *in vitro,* and that such samples of muscle tissue also contain greater than normal amounts of lysosomal enzymes. In 2 patients with oesophageal obstruction, parenteral hyperalimentation caused a substantial increase in body stores of fat and protein with concomitantly increased *in vitro* activity of protein synthesis. However, there was no effect of feeding on lysosomal enzyme activities, suggesting that the variation of nutritional status of the patient was not directly concerned in the regulation of the abnormally high catabolic apparatus of the cancer patient. The finding that RNA concentrations are largely unchanged in muscle from cancer patients suggests that the gross capacity for protein synthesis is not altered in cancer. The diminution in the protein synthetic rate observed *in vitro* may be due to dysfunctions in the aggregation of the ribosomal subunit making up the protein synthetic apparatus. Such abnormalities were suggested by Lundholm and co-workers on the basis of the ribosome sedimentation profile during centrifugation in a sucrose density gradient of ribosomal RNA from cancer patients.

A paradoxical finding in a patient suffering from cancer cachexia is the accelerated metabolic rate. It is likely that in any circumstances in which whole-body metabolism is increased that there will be a component of the increase which is due simply to the increased turnover and need for the circulation of metabolites. In addition, where protein synthesis is increased for repair and for liver export protein production, there may well be an increment due to the surgery cost of protein synthesis. However, in patients with cancer it seems that neither of these explanations will cover the relatively large increased metabolic rate. It may be that there are increases in the metabolism of other tissues than liver and muscle and the fascinating possibility exists of an abnormality existing in the metabolism of brown adipose tissue, such that its heat production becomes uncoupled from the heat requirements of the body resulting in the sucking out of substrate from the white fat and lean-body protein masses.

Whatever the basis of the acceleration in metabolic demand in surgical patients, the capacity of the heart and circulatory system to cover the additional work of servicing the increase in metabolic rate is unlikely to match the requirement; surgical patients therefore inevitably suffer a metabolic disadvantage in this respect.

THE EFFECTS OF INJURY, TRAUMA AND SEPSIS ON METABOLISM

One can differentiate between the immediate effects of physical damage to lean body tissue and the longer term effects of injury on the function of the whole body. The second category may also be divided into acute short term, and mainly hormonal, effects and longer term effects caused by alterations in the composition of the lean body mass.

Effect of Direct Trauma to Muscle

Muscle is the main component of the lean body tissue which is traumatized during surgery, and more is known about the effects of direct injury to muscle as a model system than about injury to other tissues. The common response to damage of different kinds, such as mincing, autoimplantation, administration of myotoxic drugs, burning, gross ischaemia and freezing, is initial degeneration followed by regeneration. There is disorganization and autolysis of muscle during damage and the activities of enzymes of pathways of oxidative metabolism and of glycolysis fall. Nevertheless, the fact that regeneration occurs during the diminution of the capacity of energy provision suggests that even the augmented energy needs of protein synthesis for repair are unlikely to compromise the large reserve of energy capacity in skeletal muscle.

One interesting aspect of the immediate effects of physical damage and repair to lean tissues is the observed increase in rate-limiting enzymes of one pathway of carbohydrate metabolism (the hexosemonophosphate shunt), glucose-6-phosphate dehydrogenase and 6-phosphogluconate dehydrogenase. The increase in the capacity of this pathway may be related to increased provision for nucleic acid synthesis during repair since the pathway produces ribose products which may be directly fed into nucleic acid synthesis.

Immediate Effects on Muscle of Damage to Organs other than Muscle: Shock

The well-recognized decrease in glucose tolerance associated with trauma follows early on after its occurrence. The fact that there is hyperglycaemia and decreased glucose uptake and glycolysis in the whole body, but insulin resistance of isolated muscles *in vitro* appears to be much less, points to the effects of hormonal mechanisms in mediating insulin resistance. Indeed, associated with trauma are increased cortisol, glucagon and catecholamine secretion and decreased insulin secretion. These short term responses are likely to have an immediate effect in promoting insulin resistance, partly through the metabolic effects of free fatty acids and ketone bodies (especially in the absence of glycogen stores in muscle and liver); but there also appear to be longer term effects of trauma which may significantly compromise recovery. Haemorrhagic shock induced by short term bleeding with later re-infusion of blood results in reduced cardiac and respiratory function and reduced delivery of oxygen and nutrients to skeletal muscle for the period of the bleeding. However, even this relatively mild regimen causes rapid deterioration of skeletal muscle architecture in rabbits and the pattern of disruption of myofibrils persists for up to 1 week afterwards. Possibly associated with these effects are specific defects of muscle metabolism including insulin resistance, depressed glucose oxidation and perhaps a failure of protein synthesis. Such long-lasting effects are not the consequence of trauma-induced changes in cortisol, catecholamines or insulin because manipulation of plasma hormone concentration in experimental animals to correct for the shock-induced changes fails to prevent the development of the metabolic abnormalities.

It is well known that following injury or surgery there is a period of negative nitrogen balance, the extent and duration of which is dependent upon the severity of the injury (Sir David Cuthbertson). It is likely that the loss of nitrogen can be modified by nutritional intake to some extent, possibly to the extent that protein synthesis is depressed (*Fig.* 16.3).

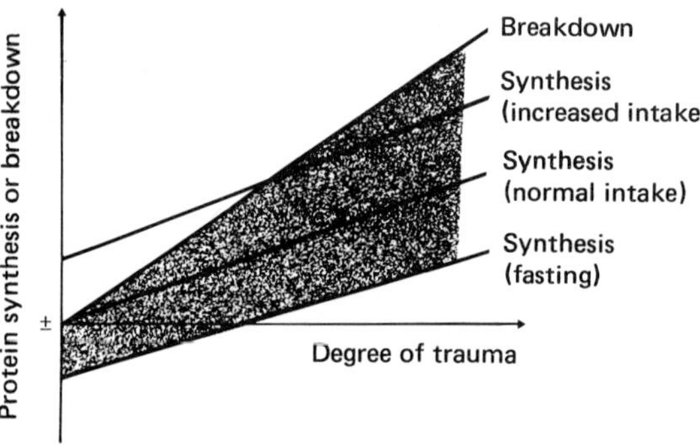

Fig. 16.3. A hypothesis concerning the regulation of whole body protein balance of lean tissue during trauma. Breakdown may increase with trauma but is not likely to be markedly affected by nutrition. On the other hand, synthesis is probably controlled by the hormonal and metabolic sequence of feeding. The shaded area represents protein imbalance (*see* Birkhaln et al., 1980).

However, if the trauma to the lean body mass, and in particular the muscle, is extended to the point that muscle protein degradation is switched on, by gross pathological changes, e.g.

in the availability of calcium causing an irreversible increase in calcium-activated proteolysis, then it is unlikely that nutritional intake will modify the response. The control of the lean body mass appears to be largely through control of the muscle mass and in normal man this appears to be affected through control of the synthesis rate of muscle protein rather than its degradation, since feeding may double the protein synthetic rate of muscle but not affect its catabolic rate. It may be that the role of nutritional support will only be of direct value when the effect of trauma on nitrogen balance is mediated via a depression of protein synthesis. Where protein degradation is accelerated by mechanisms without the normal nutritional gambit, then other methods of control may be appropriate. At present we have so little insight into the control of muscle protein degradation that this avenue of intervention is unlikely to be fruitful.

ENERGY AND PROTEIN REQUIREMENTS FOR GROWTH AND REPAIR IN THE SURGICAL PATIENT

There is no doubt that the provisions of suitable forms of energy providing substrates is central for the good management of patients recovering from operation. There is also no doubt that provision of glucose for those tissues which have an obligate need for glucose metabolism will always be necessary; however, it is also apparent that it is difficult to provide glucose in sufficient quantities at acceptable osmolality in parenteral solution to cover the often large energy needs of the postoperative catabolic patient. There is little doubt that provision of extra energy in the form of lipid emulsion, besides providing essential fatty acids etc., is able to provide energy to cover most of the needs of the patient apart from those demanding the provision of glucose. The advantages of the combination of fat and glucose are twofold. First, there is the reduction in the osmolality of the solutions being fed to the patient (there is no direct reduction in volume) so that the vessels of the peripheral circulation are occasionally suitable for parenteral infusion. There is also a second advantage, which resides in the possibility that a combination of fat and glucose is less likely to produce fatty liver than glucose alone.

Bibliography

Birkhaln R. H., Lang C. L., Fitkin D. et al.: *Surgery* 1980; **88**: 294–300.

Denton R. M., Pogson C. I.: *Metabolic Regulation*. London: Chapman & Hall, 1976.

Johnston I. D. A.: *Advances in Parenteral Nutrition*. Lancaster: MTP Press, 1978.

King R. F. G. J., MacFie J., Hill, G.: Activities of hexokinase, phosphofructokinase, fructose biphosphatase and 2-oxoglutarate dehydrogenase in muscle of normal subjects and very ill surgical patients. *Clin. Sci.* 1981; **60**: 451–6.

Lundholm K., Edström S., Ekman et al.: A comparative study of the influence of malignant tumour on host metabolism in mice and man. *Cancer (Phila.)* 1978; **42**: 453–61.

Rennie M. J., Edwards R. H. T.: Carbohydrate metabolism of skeletal muscle and its disorders. In: Randle P. J., Steiner R., Whelan W. (ed.): *Carbohydrate Metabolism and its Disorders*. London: Academic Press, 1981: **III**: 1–118.

Rennie M. J., Nathan M., Edwards R. H. T. et al.: Intracellular, plasma and urine 3-methylhistidine as an index of muscle wasting and repair. In: Rattenbury J. (ed.): *Amino Acid Analysis*. Chichester: Ellis Horwood, 1981: 210–24.

Smith R., Elia M.: The significance of urinary hydroxyproline and 3-methylhistidine changes in growth, starvation and injury. In: Rattenbury J. (ed.): *Amino Acid Analysis*. Chichester: Ellis Horwood, 1981: 225–36.

Waterlow J. C., Garlick P. J., Millward D. J.: *Protein Turnover in Mammalian Tissues and in the Whole Body*. Amsterdam: Elsevier/North Holland, 1978.

Chapter 17

Right Atrial Catheterization in Pre-term and Full-term Infants for Parenteral Nutrition

J. C. L. Shaw and J. C. St George

The technique described below was developed in the Neonatal Unit at University College Hospital, London, for parenteral nutrition in very low birth weight infants; it has, however, been used satisfactorily in full-term babies, as well as older infants and children. The procedure is performed without removing the infant from the incubator, and in skilled hands the actual catheter insertion takes less than 5 minutes and disturbs the child little more than setting up a scalp vein infusion. The resident staff in our unit feel that it takes 2 months to acquire competence in this technique, after which failure is rare.

The technique aims to place a fine silicone rubber catheter in the right atrium. When a catheter has been allowed to remain in a central vein, such as the inferior vena cava, endothelial damage has been observed. This occurs because flow in these vessels is laminar rather than turbulent, and in patients who are largely immobile and recumbent, little mixing takes place until the hypertonic solution reaches the right atrium. The heart, on the other hand, is in constant motion, and provided that the catheter is floating free in the right atrium, thrombus or epithelial damage has not been observed in those cases coming to post-mortem. The small diameter and exceptional flexibility of the catheter contribute much to its safety, and though the internal diameter is very small, volumes of 80–100 ml/h can be administered without difficulty.

Details have been included of the administration of nutrient solutions because successful use of the catheter cannot be divorced from the management of the parenteral nutrition regimen. In busy units it is essential to standardize as far as possible the solutions used for routine intravenous nutrition, and their method of administration. This relieves the medical staff of the burden of improvising a different intravenous diet for each patient, and enables each shift of nurses to quickly grasp what is happening to their patients. As a result, mistakes on the part of medical and nursing staff are largely avoided. This form of treatment, of course, requires close biochemical monitoring, and where special cases arise, such as patients with renal failure, then special solutions must obviously be devised.

PREPARATION AND STERILIZATION OF SILICONE RUBBER CATHETERS*

Materials

Medical grade Silastic tubing (No. 602–105, Dow Corning Ltd) is used for the catheters. This is supplied in 15 m coils and requires cutting, washing, packing and sterilization before use. Each catheter is cut to a length of *exactly 50 cm.* During preparation it is necessary to wear surgical gloves that have been thoroughly washed in soap and water and rinsed. Dust, lint, talc, skin oils and other surface contaminants can evoke foreign body reaction, therefore care must be taken to prevent re-contamination after cleaning and sterilization.

Cleaning

Wash the tubing thoroughly in hot soapy water to remove sodium bicarbonate (dusted on to the

*For details of equipment and manufacturers, *see* p. 230.

surface to facilitate handling) and other surface contaminants. Use a non-oily soap such as Ivory Flakes. Do not use detergents or oily-based soaps. Rinse copiously in hot water and follow through with a thorough rinse in distilled water. In rinsing, it is necessary to flush the lumen of the tubing thoroughly to ensure removal of all traces of soap.

Packaging

The catheters should be double-wrapped to reinforce protection, maintain sterility, avoid contamination on opening and facilitate handling in an aseptic manner. Peelable sterilization pouches with a transparent polyester/polypropylene front and an MG bleach kraft paper back are suitable (obtainable from DRG Hospital Supplies, Hemel Hempstead, Herts, England, or from Smiths of Whitehaven, Workington, Cumbria CA14 2DX). The catheters are first inserted in a 'U' shape into the smaller size pouch (75×240 mm). The packet is then placed inside a larger pouch (100×380 mm). At this stage it is important to ensure that the paper parts of the pouches are backing on to one another. The top of the outer pouch is then double heat-sealed at a temperature of $200\,°C$.

Sterilizing Procedure

Sterilization of the packaged catheters must only be performed in a porous load sterilizer. This type of sterilizer is designed to deal with textiles, dressing and items that are wrapped in permeable material. It is preferable to use a high vacuum machine with an efficient air removal system which incorporates either continuous steam flushing or intermittent steam pulsing. Once a pre-vacuum of -760 mmHg is attained, conditions exist for sterilizing at $130\,°C \pm 2\,°C$. The temperature-holding period is 3 minutes. After sterilization, steam is exhausted from the chamber, drying of the packets takes place and, finally, air is admitted through a 'bacterial' filter. The total cycle time should not be more than 25 minutes. Where the use of a high-vacuum machine is not possible and a gravity displacement dressing sterilizer has to be employed, which will require a longer cycle time, the following holding-time/temperature ratios must be used:

$127\,°C$ — 10 min
$121\,°C$ — 15 min
$115\,°C$ — 30 min

Sterilization by steam is the first choice for Silastic tubing as it is the most efficient method and the product does not deteriorate with repeated processes. It is strongly recommended in preference to ethylene oxide gas sterilization which calls for much higher standards in quality control.

Silastic tubing is adversely affected by ionizing radiation. Gamma-radiation is therefore unsuitable for sterilizing this material.

TECHNIQUE OF CATHETER INSERTION

Once the procedure has been observed and mastered, it usually takes between 20 and 25 minutes. If difficulty is encountered in cannulating a particular vein, it is best to have a short break before trying again. At present there is no satisfactory through-cannula technique available for the introduction of fine calibre silicone tubes. No episodes of catheter embolism have occurred. However, newcomers to the technique must perform all the following manoeuvres with care, particularly where the introducing cannula is withdrawn over the silicone and removed.

Selection of Veins

Inspect the child first and select the best vein. Shave the scalp for the superficial temporal veins, which are the easiest. The right is preferred, being usually more direct than the left. The median cubital vein at the elbow and wrist, or the basilic vein, are the best upper limb veins. The median cephalic vein can be attempted, but the catheter often sticks at the shoulder. Both long saphenous veins of the ankle may be used; once again the catheter occasionally sticks at the groin, and this is particularly so if previous femoral venepunctures have been performed.

The distance from the point of insertion to the right atrium should be measured with a tape measure, and any ECG electrodes, temperature probes and other accessory equipment should be removed from the operating area.

Sedation

In small, premature babies sedation is never necessary; in *some* older infants and young children, the use of an effective agent such as ketamine may be necessary. An anaesthetist should be consulted.

Silastic Catheter Trolley

This is prepared by the nursing staff with the following sterile equipment (*Fig.* 17.1).

Gown, towel pack and gloves
General purpose pack:
   1 pr fine scissors
   1 pr fine forceps
   1 pr artery forceps
   2 towel clips
   1 galley pot
   1 paper tape measure
   Cotton-wool balls
   Gauze swabs
   2 large green towels
19 G scalp vein needle
25 G long scalp vein needle
Silicone rubber catheter, 0·6 mm o.d. and
   exactly 50 cm long
Povidone-iodine aqueous solution 10%
No. 1 needle and 10 ml syringe
10 ml 0·9% w/v saline
1 litre sterile distilled water

Procedure

The surgeon should thoroughly scrub-up, put on a gown, mask and gloves. The gloves must then be rinsed thoroughly with distilled water to remove the adherent powder and then the pack should be opened. The catheter is unwrapped and, using forceps, coiled loosely in its wrappings ready for insertion. The 19 G needle should be prepared by trimming off the tubing close to the needle. The clinician should then draw up 10 ml of 0·9 per cent saline solution and flush the 25 G scalp vein needle, taking care to preserve the plastic sleeve.

The skin is now thoroughly cleaned with povidone-iodine solution (*Fig.* 17.2), and the infant and surrounding area are covered widely with sterile towels. If a limb is to be used, a tourniquet is next applied (*Fig.* 17.3). This may be accomplished by unwrapping a gauze swab,

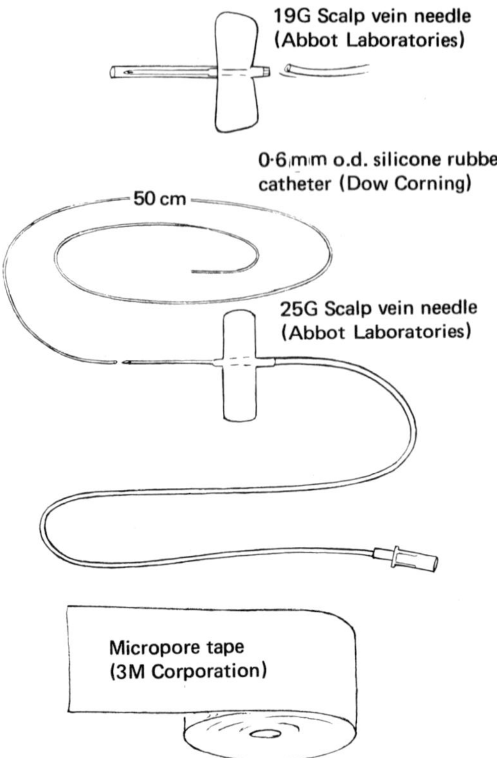

Fig. 17.1. Schematic illustration of the basic equipment required for right atrial catheterization.

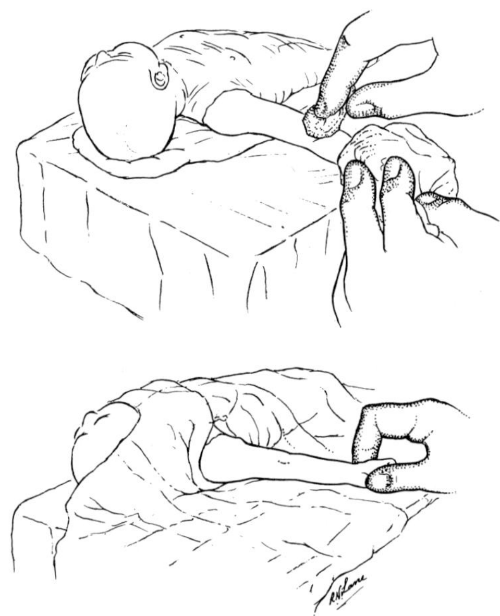

Fig. 17.2. *a*, The limb is carefully cleaned with povidone-iodine solution. *b*, The infant is carefully covered with sterile drapes. For the purposes of illustration, the incubator and other accessory tubes are not shown.

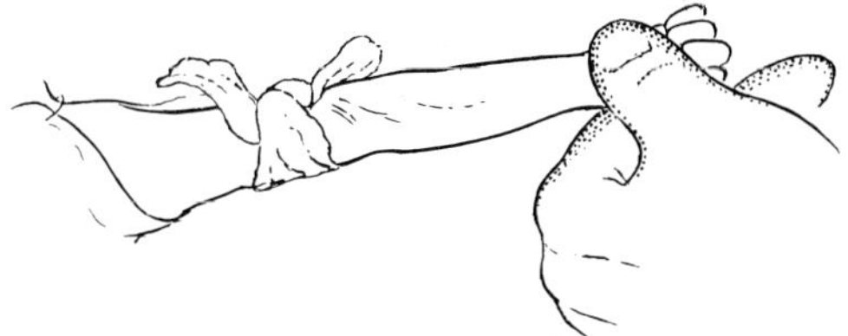

Fig. 17.3. A sterile gauze swab with a single throw (thumb) knot is used as a tourniquet.

passing it round the limb and clipping the two ends together with an artery forceps. The tension of the tourniquet may be adjusted by gently twisting; this is sterile, fine adjustment is easy and it may be readily released.

The 19 G needle is now inserted into the vein. This requires a certain degree of assurance that only comes with practice. The vein should be closely watched and the advance of the needle stopped when the vein collapses. There may not always be enough blood to run out of the needle in small infants. If blood runs out too freely, the limb can be elevated (*Figs.* 17.4, 17.5). The

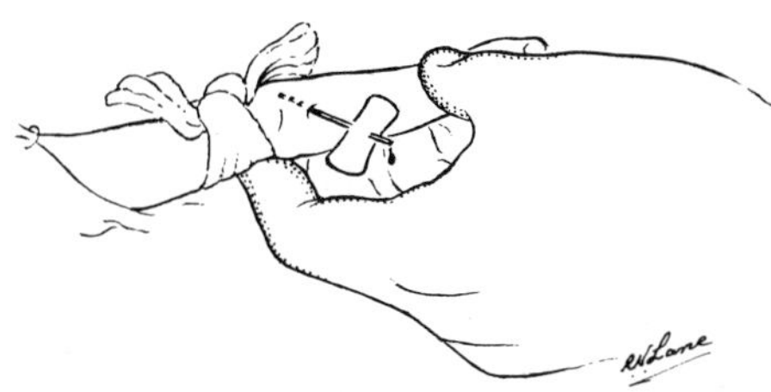

Fig. 17.4. On successful cannulation with the 19 G Butterfly scalp vein needle, blood should run back from the needle.

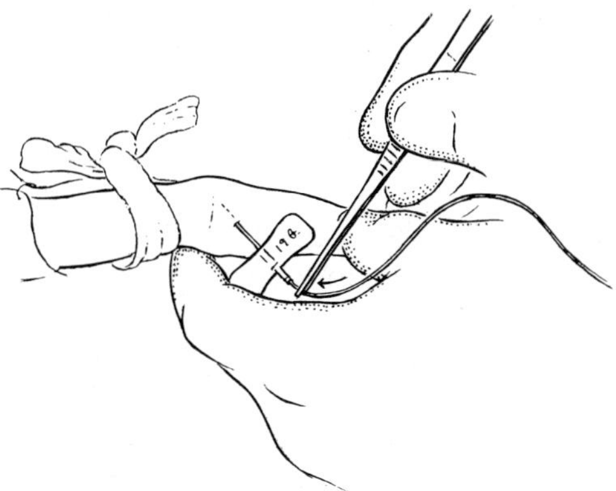

Fig. 17.5. Using a no-touch technique, the fine silicone catheter is gently threaded through the 19 G Butterfly needle into the vein, the sterile gauze thumb knot can then be gently released to facilitate passage of the catheter in 1 mm stages through the vein towards the right atrium.

catheter should next be introduced through the needle into the vein, using non-tooth forceps, and it is advanced into the heart a millimetre or so at a time. The distance inserted should be checked by measurement. When the desired length has been inserted (*Fig.* 17.6), finger pressure should be applied to the vein proximal to the needle tip. The 19 G needle is then removed and discarded and the length of catheter inserted re-measured (*Fig.* 17.7).

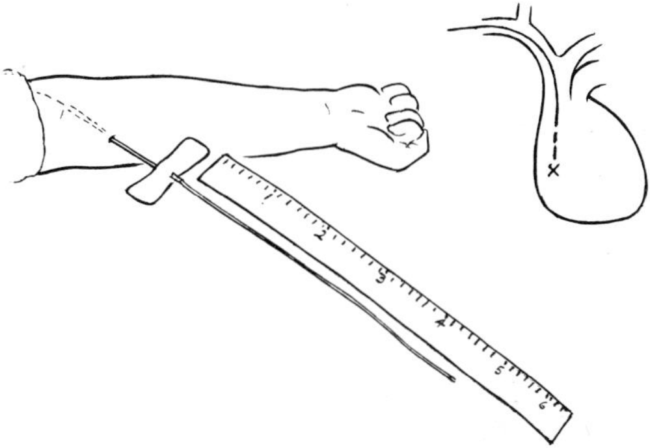

Fig. 17.6. The length of catheter inserted should be checked using a sterile tape measure so that an initial assessment of its position in the thorax can be obtained.

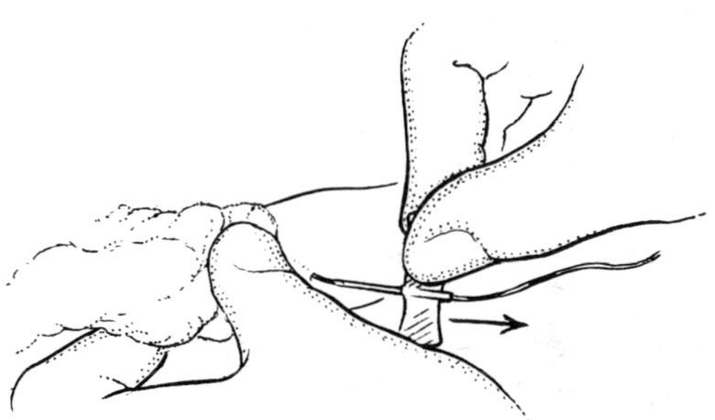

Fig. 17.7. The 19 G Butterfly needle is then carefully removed from over the silicone catheter.

The plastic sleeve of the 25 G needle, which should have been carefully preserved, is threaded on to the catheter and the 25 G needle is pushed gently about 1·5 cm into the lumen of the catheter (*Figs.* 17.8, 17.9, 17.10). This requires a little practice and is most easily learnt at leisure using unsterile components. The catheter should now be flushed through with saline. It is wise to re-measure the catheter and pull out any excess until the correctly estimated amount remains. There should be a free backflow of blood, and if this does not occur, then the catheter is probably too far in and should be withdrawn gently until

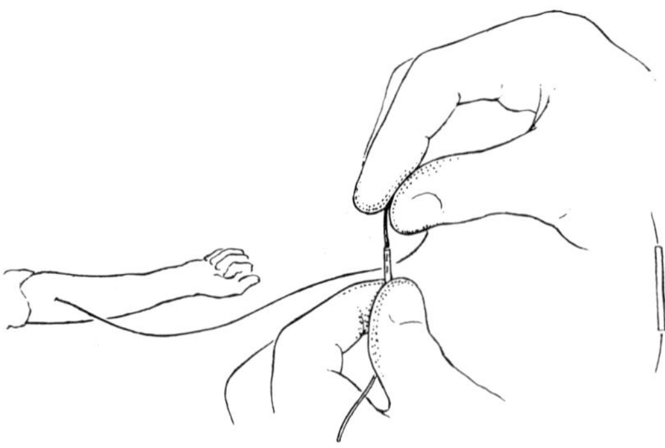

Fig. 17.8. The plastic sleeve removed from the 25 G Butterfly needle is then threaded over the silicone catheter.

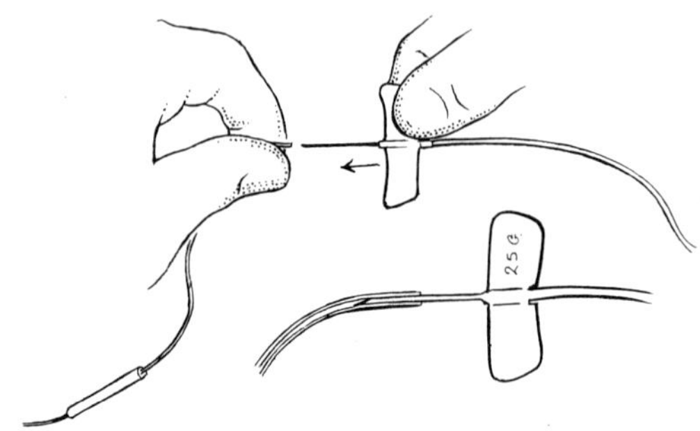

Fig. 17.9. Holding the silicone catheter very close to its end, the 25 G Butterfly needle is manoeuvred into the lumen.

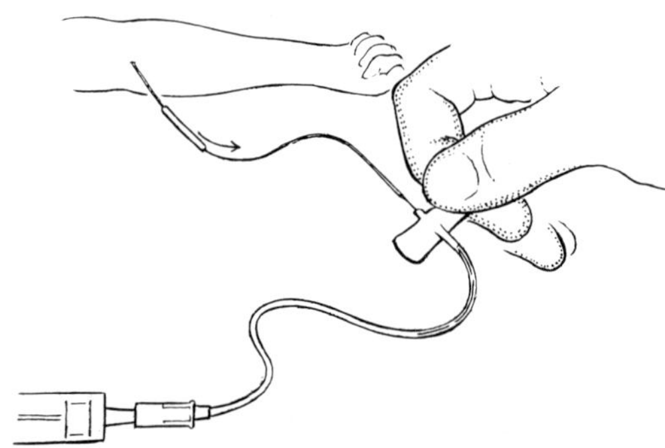

Fig. 17.10. The patency of the system is checked and the plastic sleeve moved towards the scalp vein needle/silicone catheter junction.

blood flows back on slight suction with a syringe. The skin puncture site should now be covered with a small sterile dressing and the catheter secured to the skin. The junction between the 25 G needle and the silicone tubing should be fixed by placing it, and a loop of catheter, between two pieces of Micropore tape,

i.e. sandwiched between the adhesive surfaces (*Fig.* 17.12).

The position of the catheter must next be checked radiologically after opacification with 0·6 ml meglumine iothalamate 60 per cent w/v (Conray 280) and the position adjusted (after measurement) so that the catheter tip lies freely in the centre of the right atrium (*Figs.* 17.11, 17.14). It is important to repeat the X-rays until the position is satisfactory. If the catheter is coiled or bent (*Fig.* 17.15), the tip will be jammed against the endocardium and endothelial damage with thrombus formation will result. If the catheter is not in the heart (*Figs.* 17.16, 17.17), the dangers of infusing hypertonic nutrient solutions are obvious. The catheter may now be fixed with a squirt of silicone adhesive (Dow Corning Medical Adhesive B) to the puncture site and by the application of a gauze dressing. The coils of catheter should be secured with adhesive tape or Op-Site and covered with a firm dressing held in place with tube-gauze or adhesive tape (*Fig.* 17.12). All the silicone rubber catheter must be under the dressing as well as the 25 G scalp vein connector (*Fig.* 17.13). The catheter, if exposed, will become damaged and will develop leaks. When the catheter position is satisfactory, the solutions and administration set should be set up.

ADMINISTRATION OF PARENTERAL NUTRITION SOLUTIONS

In the method below, standard solutions are used and they are administered to each patient mixed in the same fixed ratio. Only the rate of administration varies from patient to patient. As a result, the intake of any nutrient can be easily determined by reference to a single table Table 17.1). In this respect the method resembles the administration of milk, when nutrients are given in a fixed ratio to all infants. A further advantage of using standard solutions is that they are always in stock when required and can be issued with a guaranteed composition and sterility.

The solutions given here were designed specifically for the premature infant and are not necessarily suitable for older children. The composition of the solutions is undergoing constant modification in the light of ongoing research; all the allowances given below can probably be

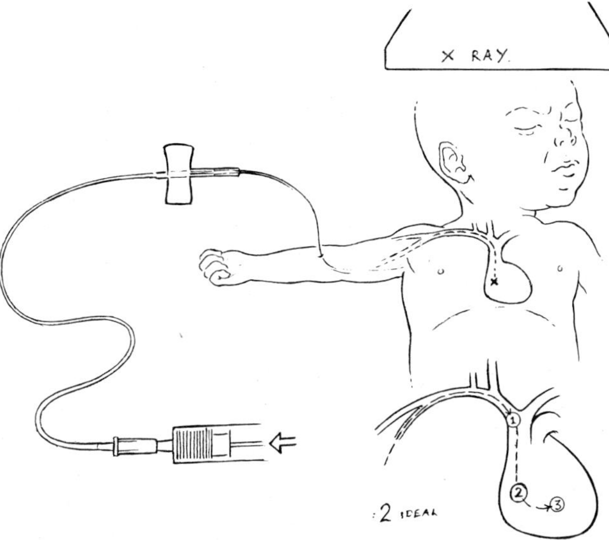

Fig. 17.11. The plastic sleeve is fixed carefully over the needle/silicone catheter junction. Correct placement in the right atrium is confirmed by performing a chest X-ray with the lumen of the catheter filled with Conray 280. The ideal final site for the catheter is at position 2 in the inset illustration.

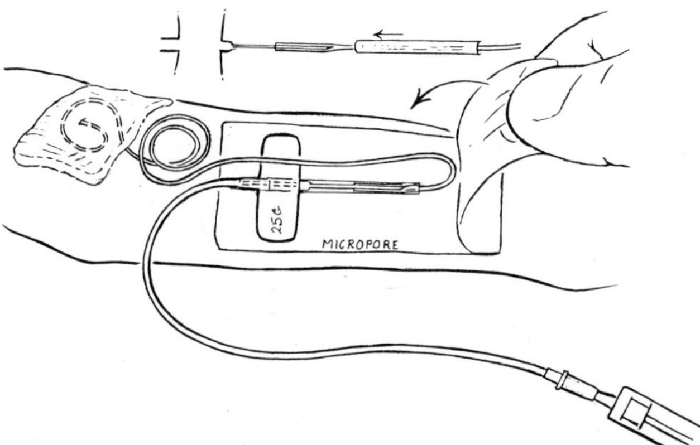

Fig. 17.12. The system must be carefully fixed to the patient with safety loops as shown. In addition, the union between the 25 G Butterfly needle and the silicone catheter must be protected in an envelope of adhesive tape. The system should be intermittently flushed with small volumes of saline during this procedure.

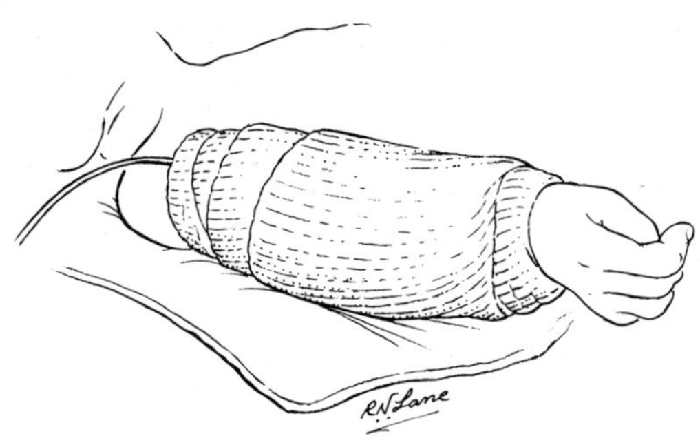

Fig. 17.13. The limb must be carefully wrapped in a sterile bandage.

improved upon. However, these solutions have been administered to numerous infants using methods outlined above. Many of these infants have been studied in detail in our long-term follow-up clinic and to date no adverse effects attributable to the use of parenteral feeding have been observed. The composition of the nutrient solutions and of the vitamin preparations are shown in Tables 17.2 and 17.3.

Administration Set

The administration set was developed in collaboration with Travenol Laboratories and is illus-

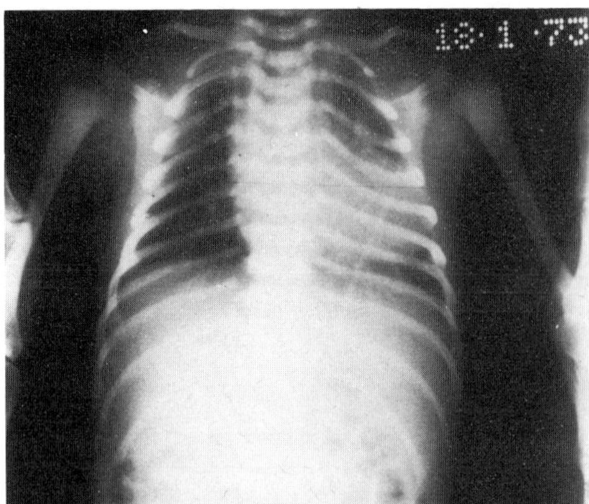

Fig. 17.14. Perfect catheter position. The catheter was inserted into the right superficial temporal vein and the tip is just below the neck of the fifth rib.

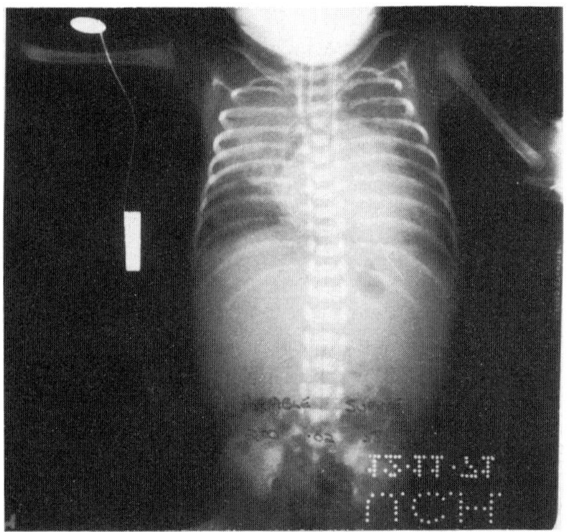

Fig. 17.15. An excess length of catheter has been inadvertently inserted forming a coil in the right atrium and ventricle. This must be corrected by withdrawal of the line and a further X-ray performed.

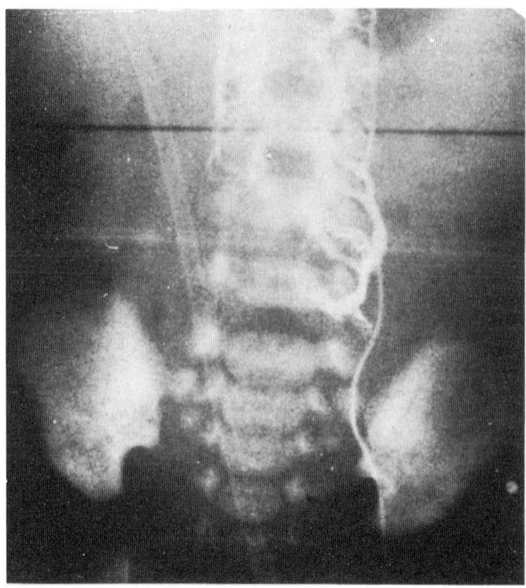

Fig. 17.16. The catheter was inserted into the long saphenous vein at the ankle and entered the pre-vertebral venous plexus. This accident is exceptionally rare. The catheter cannot be used for intravenous feeding as there is a danger of infarcting the spinal cord.

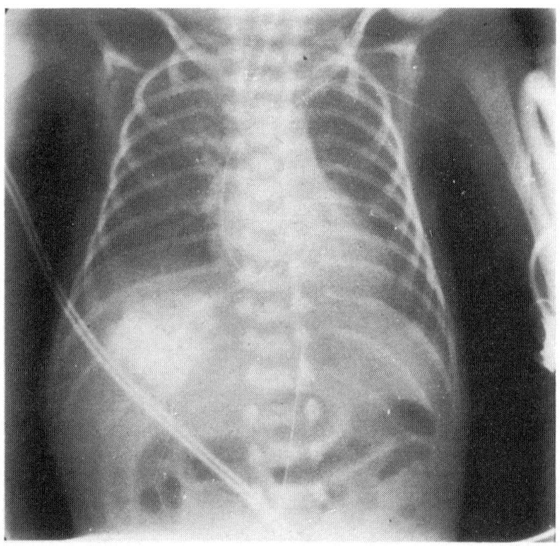

Fig. 17.17. This catheter was inserted into the left median cubital vein at the elbow. It is coiled in the right atrium and then enters the hepatic vein (possibly via the ductus venosus). If allowed to remain in this position, extensive hepatic damage will occur. *X-rays must be repeated until the catheter position is satisfactory.*

trated in *Fig.* 17.18. It comprises a 150 ml burette into which lead three lines—one from an amino acid source, one from a glucose mineral source and the third, whose use is optional. The third line may be used to give extra water to a pre-term infant under an overhead heater or to replace losses from gastric aspirate or fistulas in a surgical patient. The amino acid solution and glucose mineral solution are mixed in a fixed ratio in the burette (e.g. 25 ml + 75 ml, *see* Table 17.1) and then delivered to the patient by a peristaltic finger pump. Intralipid is given by a syringe pump through a Y-piece placed in the line close to the patient. The bottles, administra-

Table 17.1. **Composition of infusate and daily intake of different substances***

	Mol. wt.	In 25 ml Vamin Glucose +4 ml 0·5 mol K_2HPO_4/100 ml	In 75 ml glucose mineral solution	Final conc./l	Daily intake per kg body wt 150 ml $kg^{-1}d^{-1}$
Glucose (g)	180	2·5	7·5	100·0	15·0
Amino acids		1·76		17·6	2·64
Sodium (mmol)	23	1·25	1·5	27·5	4·13
Potassium (mmol)	39	1·5		15·0	2·25
Calcium (mmol)	40	0·06	0·69	7·5	1·125
Phosphorus (mmol)	31	0·48		4·8	0·73
Magnesium (mmol)	24	0·038	0·072	1·1	0·17
Chloride (mmol)	35·5	1·38	1·5	28·8	4·31
Zinc (μmol)	65		1·54	15·4	2·31
Copper (μmol)	64		0·469	4·69	0·703

Energy intake (kJ/kg day)

Glucose mineral, amino acid solution (150 ml $kg^{-1}d^{-1}$)   293

Intralipid 20% (15 ml kg^{-1} day^{-1})   126

419

*Maximum rate of administration 150 ml $kg^{-1}d^{-1}$.

Table 17.2. **Intravenous feeding: premature infant regime—composition of solutions**

Phosphate solution
0·5 M K_2HPO_4 in 10 ml ampoules. Each ampoule contains 10 mmol potassium and 4·84 mmol phosphorus. This is added to Vamin Glucose at the rate of 4·0 ml/100 ml Vamin Glucose

Vamin Glucose (Kabi-Vitrum)

Amino acids	70·2 g/l
Sodium	50·0 mmol/l
Potassium	20·0 mmol/l
Calcium	2·5 mmol/l
Magnesium	1·5 mmol/l
Chloride	55·0 mmol/l
Glucose	100·0 g/l
Energy	2717·0 kJ/l

After the addition of phosphate solution, the concentrations of potassium and phosphorus are:

Potassium	60·0 mmol/l
Phosphorus	19·4 mmol/l

Glucose mineral solution (University College Hospital)

Glucose	100·0 g/l
Sodium	20·0 mmol/l
Calcium	9·2 mmol/l
Magnesium	0·96 mmol/l
Zinc	20·50 μmol/l
Copper	6·25 μmol/l
Chloride	40·32 mmol/l

Intralipid 20%
(Kabi-Vitrum)   8400·0 kJ/l

Table 17.3. **Composition of vitamin preparations**

Vitlipid Infant (Kabi-Vitrum)

Retinol	100·0 μg (333 i.u.)/ml
Calciferol	2·5 μg (100 i.u.)/ml
Phytomenadione	50·0 μg/ml

Dosage 1·0 ml kg^{-1} d^{-1} (maximum 4·0 ml/d)
This is mixed with the Intralipid at 1·0 ml/15 ml

Solivito (Kabi-Vitrum)
Each ampoule contains:

Vitamin B1 (thiamine)	1·2 mg/ml
Vitamin B2 (riboflavin)	1·8 mg/ml
Nicotinamide	10·0 mg/ml
Vitamin B6 (pyridoxine)	2·0 mg/ml
Pantothenic acid	10·0 mg/ml
Vitamin C	30·0 mg/ml
Biotin	0·3 mg/ml
Folic acid	0·2 mg/ml
Vitamin B12	2·0 mg/ml

Dissolve ampoule in 5 ml of distilled water and give at 1·0 ml kg^{-1} d^{-1} into the burette

tion set and the Intralipid syringe are changed daily.

Bacterial Filters

The value of bacterial filters is not established. They certainly remove air bubbles and particulate matter larger than 0·22 μm diameter from the solutions, and on occasions have served to isolate infection inadvertently introduced during

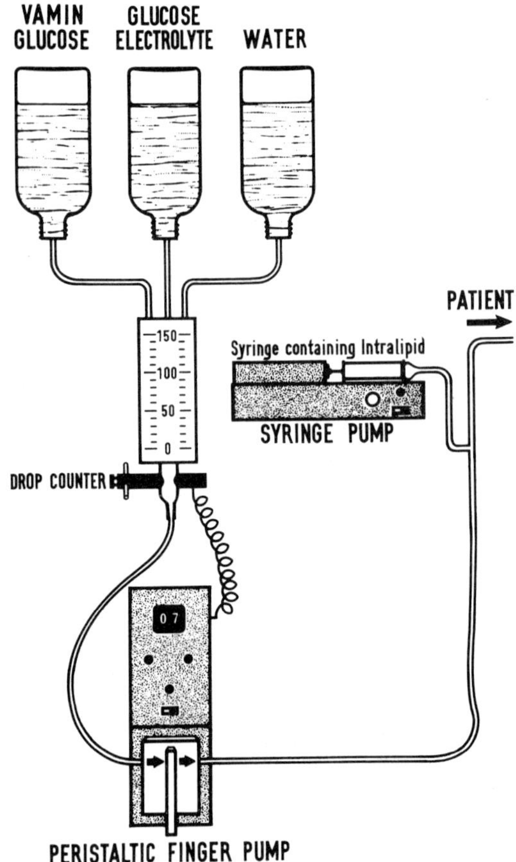

Fig. 17.18. The infusion system used, comprising a burette, peristaltic finger pump and a syringe pump.

the daily change. On the other hand, they do not remove toxins and they increase both the resistance to flow of the fluid and the number of connections in the circuit, so that leaks are more common. For these reasons we have stopped using them. Their use may be considered optional at present, until sets with integral filters become available.

Procedure for Setting up the Solutions

A detailed procedure sheet should be prepared by a senior member of the nursing staff and it should be available for reference during the procedure. All additions should be clearly charted by the medical staff and checked by two members of the nursing staff (Table 17.4).

Solutions
Amino acid solution
Glucose mineral solution
Phosphate solution
Intravenous vitamin preparations
Intravenous fat emulsion

Equipment
Paediatric drip set for total parenteral
    nutrition
Three airways
Travenol Y-type adaptor
Extension tubes × 2
Peristaltic infusion pump
Syringe pump
20 or 50 ml syringe for intravenous fat
    emulsion
10 ml syringe and needle
Medi-swabs (isopropyl alcohol 70%)
Labels

The nurse constructing the system should be thoroughly trained in the method, and the need for a fastidiously clean technique must be emphasized. The procedure should take place in a separate room and the appropriate charts and a procedure sheet should be at hand. The nurse should wash her hands thoroughly and wear a clean gown and mask. A number of technical points require emphasis:

1. After the seals of the bottles are broken, the caps should be cleaned with spirit swabs (isopropyl alcohol 70 per cent—Medi-swabs) and allowed to dry for 2 minutes.

2. The phosphate must be added to the amino acid source in order to avoid the precipitation of calcium phosphate that would occur if it were added to glucose mineral solution.

3. Before connecting the administration set to the bottles, *all clamps must be shut.* In particular, the regulating clamp below the drip chamber should be positioned as close to the drip chamber as possible before clamping. If this is not done, bubbles enter the tubing when the drip chamber is filled and these will cause an air lock in the bacterial filter, if one is used.

4. The daily dose of water soluble vitamins is added to the first burette of the day.

5. Care should be taken to prevent the accidental contamination of the junction where the daily administration set change occurs by positioning it remote from the patient, outside the incubator.

Table 17.4. **Intravenous feeding prescription: pre-term infant**

No.:   Surname:
Date of birth: First names:
Solutions to be used (infusion rate is given on chart)
1. *Glucose mineral solution* (UCH)
2. *Vamin glucose* to which has been added 4 mmol 0·5 M dipotassium
   hydrogen phosphate per 100 ml
               [or]
   20·0 ml M/2 dipotassium hydrogen phosphate per 500 ml

Mix 75 ml of (1) with 25 ml of (2) in the burette and give at the rate prescribed on the i.v. chart

3. *Intralipid 20%* (commence at $5·0$ ml kg^{-1} d^{-1} and after 24 hours give
   at 10 ml kg^{-1} d^{-1} and increase to a maximum of 15 ml kg^{-1} d^{-1})
   Rate given on i.v. chart
4. Other

VITAMINS
Vitlipid Infant   1·0 ml kg^{-1} d^{-1} (maximum 4·0 ml/d). Add
                            to Intralipid at 1·0 ml/15 ml
                            Intralipid 20%
Solivito   Dissolve ampoule in 5·0 ml distilled water
                            and give at 1·0 ml kg^{-1} d^{-1} into the burette

Date	Solutions to be given today	Any extra additives	To which solution	Signature

Table 17.5. **Routines and investigations for infants receiving parenteral nutrition**

Daily	*Once to twice per week (or as indicated)*
Weighing and measuring body weight	Length and head circumference
Fluid balance Input and output chart Urine glucose (Clinitest) 4-hourly	
Plasma chemistry Urea and electrolytes (less frequently when stable) Dextrostix (if glycosuria)	Calcium phosphorus Alkaline phosphatase Blood glucose Liver function tests Plasma proteins Ammonia Plasma copper ceruloplasmin and zinc
Bacteriology Change i.v. infusion set and filter daily Send solution for culture daily	Blood ⎫ Culture if infection CSF ⎬ suspected Urine ⎭
Haematology	Haemoglobin, haematocrit; WBC and differential; screening for disseminated intravascular coagulation if endo-toxaemia suspected

Monitoring Routines

The daily and weekly routines that should be adhered to at all times in order to anticipate serious biochemical complications are outlined in Table 17.5. In certain clinical situations it may be necessary to perform additional serum investigations at more frequent intervals.

Bacterial Contamination

Nosocomial infection is the single most important complication of intravenous nutrition. The nutrient solutions used provide an ideal culture medium for micro-organisms. The commonest contaminating bacteria is *Staphylococcus albus* arising from the hands of medical and nursing staff. The commonest fungus is *Candida albicans*. *S. albus* most commonly gains entry at the junction where the daily administration set change occurs, but may also colonize the catheter tip during a transient bacteraemia. The same is probably true for *C. albicans*, which can certainly colonize an otherwise sterile catheter system during candida septicaemia secondary to a remote infection. It is essential to take every precaution to prevent infecting the solution during the daily changeover. In view of the risk of infection, the changeover should not be left to junior or inexperienced staff.

Schedule of equipment

Betadine antiseptic solution (10% povidone-iodine
Paper tape measures (disposable)

Napp Laboratories, Watford WD2 7RA, England.

T. Lyon & Co Ltd. 142A–148 London Road, Liverpool 3, England

Silicone adhesive, Dow Corning Medical Adhesive B, Catalogue No. 895-6
Paediatric drip set for total parenteral nutrition (Code No. FKC 0788)
    Y-type adaptor, FKC 0055
Butterfly needle (19G) I/No. 4590 Luer
Butterfly needle (25G) I/No. 4506 Luer
Extension tubes 100 cm long Lectrocath (Code No. 1155-10)
Syringe pump, Sage Instruments, Model 341

Dow Corning Corporation, Medical Products, Midland, Michigan, USA.
Travenol Laboratories, Thetford, Norfolk England.

Abbot Ireland Ltd, Sligo, Republic of Ireland.

Vygon Sterile, 95440, Ecouen, France.

Arnold R. Horwell Ltd, 2 Grangeway, Kilburn High Road, London NW6 2BP, England.

Infusion pump, Ivac 231

Ivac UK, Ivac House, Bessborough Road, Harrow, Middx HA1 3DT, England.

Vamin Glucose, Intralipid 20% Vitlipid Infant, Solivito

Kabi-Vitrum Ltd, Bilton House, Uxbridge Road, London W5, England.

Chapter 18

Principles of Parenteral Nutrition in Infancy

M. Panter-Brick

Total parenteral nutrition (TPN) is now a practical alternative to enteral nutrition in paediatric patients. Most patients are infants who have either had surgery to the gastrointestinal tract or who have a malabsorption syndrome following protracted diarrhoea. The need for total parenteral nutrition in older patients is less frequent and usually follows surgery, burns, Crohn's disease or ulcerative colitis. Patients receiving cytotoxic drugs and radiotherapy may also benefit.

Because of the special difficulties associated with parenteral nutrition in childhood it is appropriate that each hospital should have a 'TPN' team to assist and advise on all aspects of parenteral nutrition for the hospital. The team should comprise a physician and a surgeon with a special interest in the subject, a senior nurse on whose ward most of the parenteral nutrition will be carried out, and the pharmacist. The actual composition of the team, however, will vary from hospital to hospital according to local expertise, and within a children's hospital the team will clearly be different from those of a district general hospital or a hospital with specialist paediatric units. It is not proposed that the TPN team should look after every patient receiving intravenous feeding on a day-to-day basis, but rather they should advise in difficult cases and should construct agreed protocols that are suitable for the conditions being treated and the ages of the patients. In this way, junior staff and nursing staff can become familiar enough with the techniques of parenteral nutrition and make it a practical and safe form of therapy in an individual hospital. Although the hospital clinical chemist should not necessarily be a primary member of the team, close consultation with his or her department will be necessary to ensure the availability of the necessary biochemical monitoring.

Many of the problems encountered with TPN stem not from the therapy but from inexperience. Similarly, the ever-present hazard of septicaemia can only be minimized by a team approach and obsessive attention to detail. Although many paediatric patients requiring prolonged intravenous feeding will receive it via a central vein catheter, many children, particularly those who are recovering from protracted diarrhoea, can be managed using peripheral veins and, as a consequence, the most important area of continuing education must be towards better care of infusions and the infusion sites by junior medical and nursing staff. An infant has a limited number of peripheral veins, and once these are used up, central venous catheterization will be necessary. In this age group, central vein catheters often have to be inserted under general anaesthesia unless a vein has been reserved for the percutaneous placement of a Silastic central venous catheter as described in the previous chapter. Thus paediatricians should be aware that parenteral nutrition may be required and be prepared to use it. It is vital to avoid serious weight loss and TPN through peripheral veins should be started early and not regarded as a last resort.

POST-SURGICAL AND OTHER INFANTS ABOVE 2500 g

Most post-surgical patients and infants with malabsorption syndromes tend to be above

2500 g, although occasionally, of course, the post-surgical infant will be smaller. Infants of less than 2500 g are best managed as described in the previous chapter. A suitable regimen for larger infants is detailed in Tables 18.1 and 18.2, and a suitable infusion system is illustrated in *Fig.* 18.1. The infusion system utilizes a triple inlet Buretrol, available from Travenol Laboratories. Great flexibility is the hallmark of the system as the glucose and nitrogen content can be altered at will and replacement of losses on an hour-to-hour basis via the same i.v. system is also possible. The two pumps permit great accuracy of delivery and avoid sudden changes in the infusion rate, thus spreading the (high) osmolar load evenly over the full 24-hour period. The simultaneous infusion of the fat emulsion reduces the likelihood of gross lipidaemia, but nevertheless, 2 hours before bloods are drawn for biochemical analysis, the lipid infusion should be discontinued to allow clearing of the plasma, otherwise spurious biochemical values will result. The use of Vamin Glucose (Kabi-Vitrum) and Ped-el (Kabi-

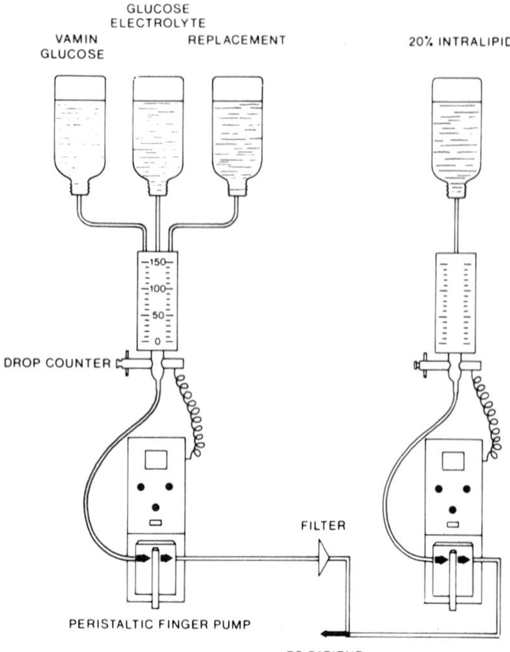

Fig. 18.1. A suitable infusion system for the supply of glucose, amino acids and Intralipid in infants.

Vitrum) is illustrated in Table 18.3 and a specimen electrolyte profile for the dextrose solutions is illustrated in Table 18.4. Vitamins are provided using the preparations Vitlipid Infant and Solivito (Kabi-Vitrum).

The regimen described (*see* Table 18.2) is suitable for most infants in the weight group 2.5–5 kg. Clearly, however, the full regimen cannot be employed immediately and about 3 days are required to achieve the volumes described. It will not be for 3 days, for example, that the maximum amount of Vamin $kg^{-1} 24 h^{-1}$ will be employed.

A child weighing 2500 g can be managed employing one 100 ml bottle of Vamin Glucose per 24-hour period. For children weighing between 2500 and 5000 g, 2 bottles of Vamin Glucose (100 ml) will be required, each with its addition of Ped-el. The 100 ml of 20% Intralipid, with its addition of 5 ml of Vitlipid Infant, will be suitable for infants up to very nearly 5 kg. When two 100 ml bottles of Vamin Glucose are used per 24 hours, one ampoule of Ped-el should be used for each addition despite the fact that there are 20 ml in the ampoule. If the pharmacist is making the additions under proper phar-

Table 18.1. **Total parenteral nutrition regimen for infants from about 2500 to 5000 g (peripheral vein)**

Vamin Glucose (100 ml) (+Ped-el 7·5 ml)	$35–40 \, ml \, kg^{-1} \, 24 \, h^{-1}$
10% glucose (+electrolytes)	$130 \, ml \, kg^{-1} \, 24 \, h^{-1}$
20% Intralipid (100 ml) (+Vitlipid Infant 5 ml +Solivito 2·5 ml)	$21 \, ml \, kg^{-1} \, 24 \, h^{-1}$
Non-protein calories approximately	$100 \, cal \, kg^{-1} \, 24 \, h^{-1}$
Nitrogen provision approximately	$350 \, mg \, kg^{-1} \, 24 \, h^{-1}$

Table 18.2. **Total parenteral nutrition regimen for infants from about 2500 to 5000 g with high calorie and nitrogen requirements (central vein)**

Vamin Glucose (100 ml) (+Ped-el 7·5 ml)	$40–45 \, ml \, kg^{-1} \, 24 \, ml^{-}$
15% glucose (+electrolytes)	$130 \, ml \, kg^{-1} \, 24 \, ml^{-1}$
20% Intrapilid (100 ml) (+Vitlipid Infant 5 ml +Solivito 2·5 ml)	$21 \, ml \, kg^{-1} \, 24 \, h^{-1}$
Non-protein calories approximately	$135 \, cal \, kg^{-1} \, 24 \, h^{-1}$
Nitrogen provision approximately	$425 \, mg \, kg^{-1} \, 24 \, h^{-1}$

Table 18.3. **Electrolytes and nitrogen provided by Vamin Glucose and Ped-el**

| Infusion rate | Vamin Glucose + Ped-el 7·5 ml/100 ml | | |
	$35\,ml\,kg^{-1}\,24\,h^{-1}$	$40\,ml\,kg^{-1}\,24\,h^{-1}$	$45\,ml\,kg^{-1}\,24\,h^{-1}$
Sodium	1·63 mmol	1·86 mmol	2·1 mmol
Potassium	0·65 mmol	0·75 mmol	0·84 mmol
Calcium	0·45 mmol	0·5 mmol	0·58 mmol
Magnesium	0·11 mmol	0·126 mmol	0·14 mmol
Phosphorus*	0·18 mmol	0·21 mmol	0·24 mmol
Nitrogen	306 mg	350 mg	394 mg

* Additional phosphorus must be provided via the glucose solutions as Na_2HPO_4 or K_2HPO_4. Ped-el also contains trace metals and iron.

Table 18.4. **Suggested electrolyte provision by total parenteral nutrition solutions for infants of between 2500 and 5000 g**

	$mmol\,kg^{-1}\,24\,h^{-1}$	$mmol\,l^{-1}\,glucose*$
Sodium	3–4	15–20
Potassium	2–3	10–15
Phosphorus	0·5	2–2·25
Calcium	0·5	In Vamin + Ped-el
Magnesium	0·125	In Vamin + Ped-el

* Average concentration which assumes a glucose infusion rate of $130\,ml\,kg^{-1}\,24\,h^{-1}$ and a Vamin Glucose Ped-el rate of $40\,ml\,kg^{-1}\,24\,h^{-1}.$
Vamin Glucose contains sodium 50 mmol/l and potassium 20 mmol/l so the actual concentration in the glucose solution must reflect this (*see* Table 18.3).

maceutical manufacturing conditions, it may be possible to use a single vial split between the two bottles of Vamin Glucose provided that the second bottle is kept refrigerated until it is used. The fat-soluble vitamins provided by Vitlipid Infant are added to the Intralipid in a ratio of 5 ml to every 100 ml of Intralipid (the maximum dose of Vitlipid Infant is 5 ml/24 h). At 21 ml/kg this will allow one bottle to be used for babies weighting up to 5 kg. Ideally, when a solution has been added to in this way it should be used within 12 hours. However, this has been found to be unnecessary in practice. Solivito can also be added to the Intralipid solution to deliver $0·5\,ml\,kg^{-1}\,24\,h^{-1}$. Alternatively, the Solvito can be added to the 500 ml of glucose solution in the correct proportions to provide $0·5\,ml^{-1}\,24\,h^{-1}$ but infused over one *12*-hour period.* Any solution containing Solivito should be protected from light.

* Solivito and Ped-el should not be added to the same solution.

Using the administration system depicted in *Fig.* 18.1, there will always be at least one bottle change every 24 hours unless the infant weighs less than 2500 g, and consequently there is both a risk of introducing infection into the solutions and also of embolization of particulate matter. In order to minimize both hazards, it is recommended that a bacterial filter should be used, as shown in *Fig.* 18.1. Ideally, the giving sets should be changed whenever a solution needs to be changed. However, this would add considerably to the cost of treatment and to its complexity and, provided that in-line bacterial filters are employed, it has been found to be unnecessary in clinical practice. In a particularly high risk situation, however, such as during parenteral nutrition in the immune-compromised patient, it is necessary to change the giving set whenever a solution container is changed.

CHILDREN FROM 6 MONTHS TO A YEAR

Up to the age of about 1 year, the infusion system described for the young infant can be employed. A regimen for such patients is detailed in Table 18.5 and examples of the glucose/electrolyte solutions needed for such patients are set out in Table 18.6. The infusion system and giving sets needed are identical to those used for younger children (*see Fig.* 18.1). The larger 500 ml bottle of Vamin Glucose will be needed and to this is added the 37·5 ml of Ped-el. The resulting mixture is delivered at 40 ml/kg at about 6 months of age, dropping to about 35 ml/kg at 12 months of age. This nitrogen provision of between 300 and 350 $mg\,kg^{-1}\,24\,h^{-1}$ is of course arbitrary and should be changed in the light of clinical needs. The risk of

Table 18.5. **Total parenteral nutrition regimen for children of 6-12 months**

Age	6 mth	12 mth
Usual weight	7·5 kg	10 kg
Fluid *	150 ml	120 ml
Glucose 15% *	90 ml	65 ml
Intralipid 20% *	20 ml	20 ml
Vamin Glucose 500 ml + Ped-el 37·5 ml *	40 ml	35 ml
Nitrogen *	350 mg	306 mg
Non-protein calories *	90	80
Calcium *	0·5	0·45
Magnesium *	0·126	0·11
Phosphorus *†	0·21	0·18

* Values are per kg per 24 h.
† Additional phosphorus is provided via the glucose solutions as Na_2HPO_4 or K_2HPO_4.

Table 18.6. **Glucose electrolyte solutions for infants from 6 to 12 months and their minimum requirements per 24 hours**

	$mmol\,kg^{-1}\,24\,h^{-1}$ (minimum)	mmol/l glucose solution (average)
Sodium	2·5	25–30 mmol/l
Potassium	2·0	20–25 mmol/l
Phosphorus *	0·50	3–3·5 mmol/l
Calcium	0·50	in Vamin + Ped-el
Magnesium	0·125	in Vamin + Ped-el

* As Na_2HPO_4 or K_2HPO_4.

hyperaminoacidaemia in this age group is negligible. The calorie provision at 80–90 calories/kg of non-protein energy is probably sufficient but under certain circumstances may need also to be increased. It is probably better to use more carbohydrate than to increase the fat beyond $20\,ml\,kg^{-1}\,24\,h^{-1}$. Vitlipid Infant and Solivito are provided in the same way as for other infants, that is 1 ml/kg of Vitlipid Infant (maximum dose 5 ml/24 h) and 0·5 ml/kg of Solivito, both added to the Intralipid.

Venous access in this age group is often particularly difficult, especially as peripheral veins may be exhausted by the time the need for parenteral nutrition is realized, and therefore central venous catheterization may be inevitable. The technique employed for neonates and older infants up to about 5000 g, as described in the previous chapter, is perfectly suitable in this age group provided a suitable vein can be found for the insertion of the catheter. If this is not possible, then recourse to placement using a

venous cut-down may well be necessary. In all such cases, the actual entry wound, be it in the neck, arm or leg, should always be completely closed and subcutaneous tunnel constructed so that the catheter exits through a separate site. This is vitally important if the long saphenous vein in the thigh has been entered; the exit wound for the catheter should be as near the knee as possible. By preference, radio-opaque Silastic catheters should be used on all occasions.

Kiely has described how fine-bore silicone catheters can be led subcutaneously from the anterior aspect of the knee to the long saphenous cut-down site in the groin, by threading the silicone cannula through the lumen of a lumbar puncture needle (*Figs.* 18.2, 18.3). He has also described an elegant technique for cannulating these fragile vessels whereby the vein is first transfixed by a small disposable hypodermic needle in order to stabilize the vessel prior to performing the venotomy and cannulation procedure (*Fig.* 18.4).

CHILDREN WEIGHING MORE THAN 15 kg.

When a child of 15 or more kilograms requires total parenteral nutrition, a central venous catheter is almost always required and needs to be placed *in situ* under general anaesthesia or ketamine sedation in the operating theatre. A suitable regimen for these patients is described in Table 18.7. The final solution containing all the nutrients, electrolytes and minerals with the exception of Intralipid, is best prepared in the pharmacy under a laminar flow hood in non-vented plastic containers which are available pre-sterilized from Travenol Laboratories. This solution is then pumped to the patient using a *volumetric* infusion pump. No airway is required and the giving set is a standard adult giving set. Intralipid is delivered via a second volumetric pump but the glass Intralipid bottle must be vented and a 0·22 µm bacterial filter should be placed on the air inlet. As before, Intralipid administration is discontinued 2 hours prior to blood being taken to check for clearing of the plasma and so that Intralipid particles do not interfere with biochemical analyses.

Using this system, it is not possible to give calcium, magnesium and phosphate on the same

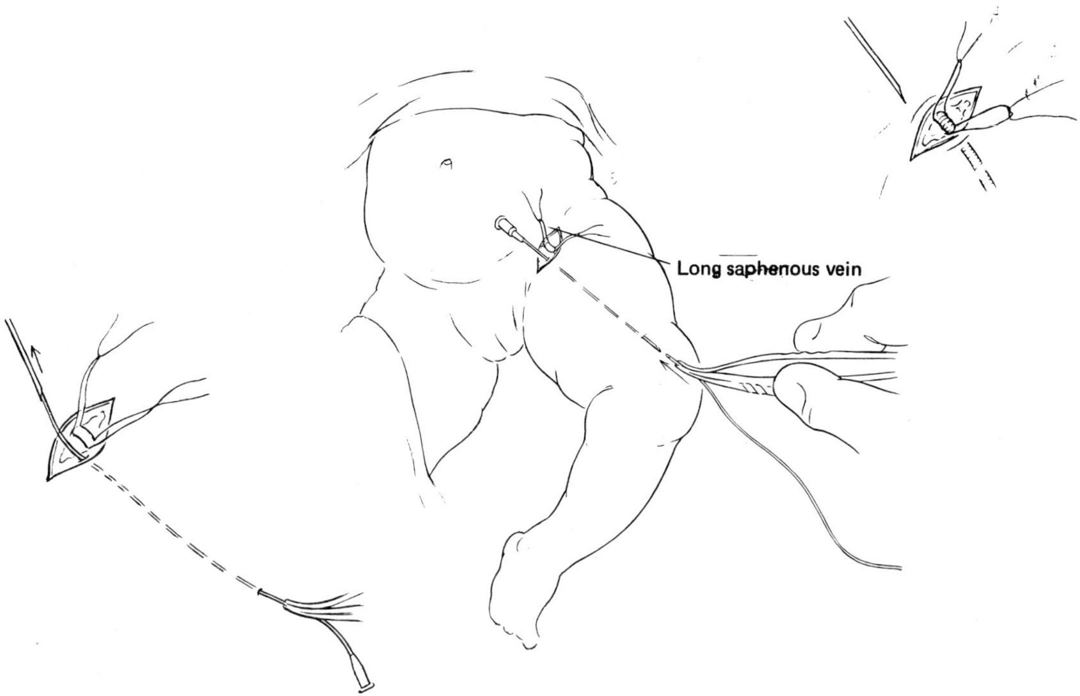

Fig. 18.2. Surgical exposure of the long saphenous vein in the groin, with retrograde passage of a fine silicone catheter through a lumbar puncture or similar needle in order to create a subcutaneous tunnel.

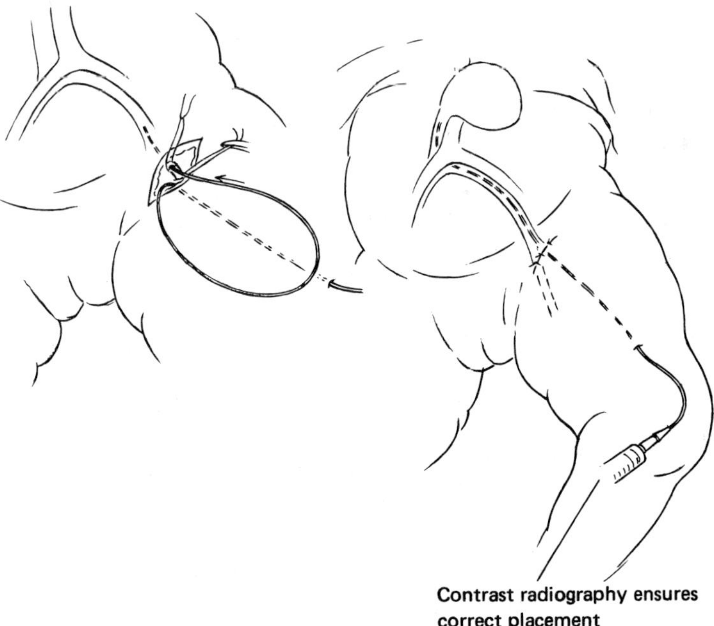

Fig. 18.3. After the passage of the catheter through the subcutaneous tunnel on the anterior aspect of the thigh, a venotomy has been performed and the catheter passed up into the inferior vena cava where its position may be confirmed radiologically with contrast medium.

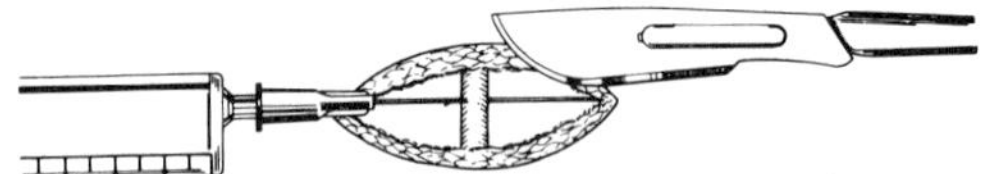

Fig. 18.4. A technique for stabilizing and opening fine veins in neonates and children. The vessel is transfixed with a very fine hypodermic needle and a scalpel blade is used to cut-down on to the needle through the vessel wall. (Reproduced by kind permission of Mr E. Kiely, FRCS and the Editor of the *British Medical Journal*.)

Table 18.7. **Total parenteral nutrition regimen for children 15–30 kg**

Age	4 yr	6 yr	10 yr
Weight	15 kg	20 kg	30 kg
Fluid *	100 ml	90 ml	70 ml
Glucose 15% *	85	75	55
Intralipid 20% *	15 ml	15 ml	15 ml
Nitrogen *†	0·3 g	0·3 g	0·2 g
Non-protein calories †	80	75	65
Calcium *	0·25	0·25	0·25
Magnesium *	0·1	0·1	0·1
Phosphorus *	0·25	0·25	0·25

* Values are per kg per 24 hours.
† The calorie and nitrogen requirements at these ages will vary enormously, and reflect the underlying condition of the patient. A clinical nitrogen balance (*see* text) is needed to evaluate the nitrogen input. Similarly, all other constituents may be significantly modified in the light of biochemical information.

day, as they would be in contact for 24 hours or longer after preparation and the risk of precipitation is marked. They are, therefore, alternated and double quantities are given on alternate days. Multivitamin infusion (USV Pharmaceutical Corp.) is a more useful preparation to provide vitamins when using the 'bag' system—2·5 ml for a 15 kg child or 5 ml when the patient is about 30 kg are given on alternate days. The vitamins are given on a day when calcium and magnesium is not present in the solution as otherwise a blackish precipitate is sometimes seen. Vitamin K, folic acid and vitamin B12 must be given each week in adequate dosage for age, as folate deficiency and a vitamin K-dependent haemorrhagic tendency can otherwise quickly occur. The adult preparation Addamel (Kabi-Vitrum) can be used to provide trace elements but is not usually necessary unless total parenteral nutrition continues beyond about 10 days. The dose is 0·14 ml kg^{-1} 24 h^{-1}. Thus a child of 15 kg will require 4 ml on every alternate day and a child of 30 kg, 8 ml on alternate days, as it should also not be mixed with the phosphate.

COMBINED ORAL AND INTRAVENOUS FEEDING

Supplemental intravenous nutrition of infants is often possible in that a certain amount of gastrointestinal function remains or becomes available as repair of the intestinal damage occurs during parenteral nutrition. Frequently, however, these infants have a secondary lactose intolerance, and may indeed have other difficulties, and so-called 'elemental' formula feed is required. A particularly suitable preparation is the new formulation of Pregestimil (Mead Johnson Ltd) or a chick diet (*see* Appendix, pp. 239–40.

During the weaning period from parenteral nutrition it is important not to reduce the calorie and nitrogen provision to the infant more than is necessary by protracted use of dilute feeds. It is far better to use a relatively concentrated feed, say half-strength, in very small quantities rather than to use larger quantities of dilute feeds. Such a trial of oral feeding can be conducted over 4–8 hours during a day and virtually full intravenous feeding continued. If the feeds then appear to be tolerated, appropriate reductions in the intravenous regimen can be made. The amount of the feeds should probably be increased at not less than 24-hour intervals. If diarrhoea occurs, then feeding should be stopped and tried again after 2–3 days. All stools passed should be tested for sugars using Clinitest tablets. If Pregestimil is being used, the sugar will be glucose, and fructose in combination with a chick diet (*see* Appendix, pp. 239–40 might then be tried. For the average infant of say 5 kg, 30 ml 3-hourly provides approximately one-third of its requirements, and at this stage Ped-el can be discontinued. A certain amount of calcium and magnesium will still be provided, however, via the nitrogen source Vamin Glucose, which is still providing two-thirds of the nitrogen intake. When about 60 ml of formula 3-hourly is being tolerated it is usually sufficient just to maintain venous access with the use of plain 10–15 per cent dextrose and gradually to increase formula feeding to provide full requirements.

In particularly difficult cases, a gastric infusion or very frequent gastric feeds may be employed and may well be successful when bottle feeding or standard tube feeding regimens fail. Sometimes oral feeding fails because of the presence of candidiasis, and this should be looked for and eradicated.

MINIMIZING COMPLICATIONS OF INTRAVENOUS FEEDING

Many adverse effects of total parenteral nutrition have been reported, but most of these can be avoided, and certainly parenteral nutrition as described is accompanied by an impressive lack of complications. In particular, infusion pumps permit flexible and reliable control and are indispensible in paediatric practice as the smooth flow of hypertonic nutrients is essential to avoid the complications of hyperglycaemia, hyperaminoacidaemia and the attendant risks of osmotic diuresis. Usually, the more problematical metabolic sequelae associated with intravenous feeding are encountered in very small infants, and using the protocols described, larger infants should tolerate parenteral nutrition very satisfactorily.

Haematological problems such as thrombocytopenia have not been seen and Intralipid has been employed when mild pre-existing thrombocytopenia has been present. However, it is wise to avoid Intralipid infusions where there is marked thrombocytopenia or during the early recovery period from septicaemia.

Satisfactory vitamin provision by the intravenous route is complicated; the range provided by Solivito and Vitlipid Infant is satisfactory provided there are no pre-existing deficiencies. If such deficiencies are suspected at the start of parenteral nutrition, it may well be appropriate to give extra folate, B12 and vitamin K, and possibly iron. In severely malnourished patients pre-treatment with frozen plasma may correct clotting deficiencies due to lack of liver-produced factors and also provide valuable plasma proteins. Trace element deficiencies are not likely to be a particular problem provided that Ped-el is used as instructed. The preparation is, however, designed for the maintenance of an otherwise satisfactory situation, and if excessive losses following surgery (such as with an intestinal fistula) occur, then measurement of trace element status and appropriate individual replacement may well be necessary. Copper and zinc are most likely to be implicated.

The most serious problem with parenteral nutrition today is the onset of cholestatic jaundice. This is only usually a problem when intravenous feeding continues beyond 2 3 weeks and the cause is unknown. Certainly, however, it is worsened by infection and every effort must be made to avoid and eradicate sepsis. The jaundice will remit when intravenous feeding is discontinued, and where the gastrointestinal tract is patent, cholestyramine administration may be of assistance. However, it is my personal view that it is in the babies whose gastrointestinal tracts are not patent that cholestatic jaundice occurs most frequently.

INFUSION PUMPS AND SKIN NECROSIS

Although infusion pumps are invaluable, they can cause skin necrosis if hypertonic fluid extravasates subcutaneously, and the necrosis is often extensive. If pumps are used when total parenteral nutrition is being given via peripheral veins, great care must be taken to avoid this serious complication. The infusate should be allowed to flow under gravity for a short period each hour. If there is any doubt thereafter, the pump should be eliminated from the system. Similarly, if there is any oedema near the drip site, pumping should be discontinued.

Butterfly needles should *never* be pumped; only when Teflon cannula are used are infusion pumps safe for peripheral veins.

CLINICAL AND BIOCHEMICAL MONITORING

Much cooperation is required from the clinical laboratory service so that the smallest amount of blood possible is used for the necessary investigations. Those investigations (together with bedside clinical assessments) are detailed in Table 18.8. Urinary electrolyte estimations can give vitally important information. If insufficient sodium or potassium is being provided in the infusate their concentrations in the urine will be extremely low and the reverse will be true if they are being provided in excess. Collecting the urine also allows a clinical nitrogen balance to be carried out; this is quite simple, and an example is given in Table 18.9.

Although metabolic acidosis was once common during total parenteral nutrition, it is now rare when the techniques described are em-

Table 18.8. **Routines and investigations for infants receiving total parenteral nutrition**

Daily	*Once to twice per week (or as indicated)*
Weighing and measuring Body weight	Length and head circumference
Fluid balance Input and output chart Urine glucose (Clinitest) 4-hourly or at least twice daily	12–24 h urine collection for clinical nitrogen balance, and sodium and potassium balance
Plasma chemistry Urea and electrolytes (less frequently when stable) Blood glucose (if glycosuria)	Calcium, phosphorus, alkaline phosphatase, blood glucose, liver function test, plasma proteins, copper* and zinc*, iron*
Bacteriology Change i.v. infusion set and filter daily Send solution for culture daily	Blood CSF } Culture if infection Urine } suspected
Haematology	Haemoglobin, haematocrit WBC and differential Prothrombin time

*Only during prolonged TPN.

Table 18.9. **Clinical nitrogen balance**

1 mmol urea = 28 mg nitrogen

A. Therefore urinary nitrogen (g) excretion is

$$\frac{\text{mmol urea}/24\,\text{h} \times 28}{1000} \times 6/5 *$$

This output can then be compared to input as 1 litre Vamin Glucose contains 9·4 g of nitrogen
NB: If there has been a change in the blood urea *upwards* then a correction as follows is added

B. $$\frac{\text{Change in urea (mmol)} \times \text{body wt kg}}{1000} \times 60/100 \times 28$$
$$= \text{gN}_2 \text{ retained as } urea$$

The two figures, A + B, added give the amount of nitrogen lost: the difference between this and input is assumed to be utilized

* 6/5 is a constant to correct for urinary nitrogen, such as uric acid etc.

ployed, and attention to hydration (usually by avoiding an osmotic diuresis) will correct any tendency in this direction. Hyperglycaemia is fairly often missed and every voided specimen of urine in a sick patient should be tested for glycosuria.

Intralipid should not be infused at a rate that will produce gross turbidity. This can be detected by the examination of the plasma after it has been centrifuged in a microhaematocrit. If Intralipid has been discontinued for 2 hours, the plasma should be clear. If it is not, the dose should be reduced.

Monitoring for sepsis during intravenous nutrition is important. Cultures must be made from any wounds or venepunctures that are red or have any discharge, and any cannula or central venous catheter must be examined routinely when removed. Febrile patients must, of course, have a blood culture, their central vein catheters removed, and the venepuncture site and catheter cultured unless there is a totally adequate explanation in another system. Prevention is all important, however, and there should be as little interference with the infusion fluids, infusion line and the sites as possible. Sampling from infusion lines is forbidden, and in any event, it is biochemically unacceptable.

THE ADMINISTRATION OF DRUGS DURING TOTAL PARENTERAL NUTRITION

It is frequently necessary to administer drugs such as antibiotics during total parenteral nutrition, and before Vitlipid, Solivito and Ped-el became available it was often necessary to give folic acid, vitamin B12, iron and vitamin K separately. This either necessitated multiple intramuscular injections or the setting up of a second infusion solely for the purpose of giving drugs. Not only did this limit the volume of fluid that could be used to deliver nutrients but also consumed precious veins. Using the modern alternatives, it is usually only necessary to give antibiotics and occasionally other drugs during parenteral nutrition, and provided a peripheral vein is being employed, it is permissible to give these through the injection port of the giving set as close to the patient as possible. However, the drug should be 'sandwiched' between 1 ml of normal saline so that there is minimal mixing with the parenteral feeding solutions. Intralipid should be switched off a few minutes prior to the administration of drugs and on again a few minute afterwards. The use of the Abbott 'T' connector (Abbott Laboratories) interposed between intravenous cannula and giving set allows the staff to give drugs directly into the intravenous cannula and therefore the mixing with parenteral nutrition solutions is truly minimal and certainly all contact with Intralipid can be avoided. When a central venous catheter is being used for intravenous feeding no additions should be made through the injection site of the giving set at any time and a second infusion or intramuscular injections may be inevitable.

Bibliography

Barness L. A.: The importance of fats and fatty acids in infant nutrition. *Curr. Med. Res. Opin*, 1976; **4** (Suppl. 1): 28–32.

Cockburn F.: The place of parenteral nutrition in the pre-term infant. *Curr. Med. Res. Opin.* 1976; **4** (Suppl.1): 90–9.

Feliciano D. V. and Telander R. L.: Total parenteral nutrition in infants and children. *Mayo Clin. Proc.* 1976; **51**: 647–54.

Hambridge K. M.: The importance of trace elements in infant nutrition. *Curr. Med. Res. Opin.* 1976; **4** (Suppl. 1): 44–53.

Heird W. C. and Winters R. W.: Total parenteral nutrition. *J. Paediatr.* 1975; **86**: 2–6.

Kiely E. M.: Placement of central feeding catheter. *Br. Med. J.* 1978; **2**: 1123.

Lee H. A. (ed.): Clinical applications in paediatric surgery and paediatrics. In: *Parenteral Nutrition in Acute Metabolic Illness.* London: Academic Press, 1974: 221–72.

Shaw J. C. L.: Parenteral nutrition in the management of sick low birth weight infants. *Pediatr. Clin. North Am.* 1973; **20**: 333–58.

APPENDIX

Comminuted chicken feed: practical details *

Comminuted chicken is purée chicken in water made by Cow & Gate, Trowbridge, Wiltshire, England. It is *not a complete feed.* Suitable carbohydrate orally or i.v. must be added; minerals including trace elements, complete vitamins and, finally, additional fat are required.

Step 1: Initially give $\frac{1}{4}$ strength Chix feed as small, frequent (e.g. hourly) feeds. If no i.v. supplement, give 200 ml volume per kg actual weight per day or build up to this volume over several days as i.v. decreases.

$\frac{1}{4}$ *strength Chix feed* is made as follows:

    12·5 g comminuted chicken (Cow & Gate)
    5 g glucose and/or fructose and/or Caloreen (Scientific Hospital Supplies, Liverpool)
    0·2 g metabolic mineral mixture (Scientific Hospital Supplies, Liverpool)
    Boiled water to 100 ml

This contains 0·94 g protein; 0·41 g fat; 5 g carbohydrate; 115 kJ or 27·5 calories; 0·46 mmol sodium; 0·55 mmol potassium; 0·44 mmol (17·5 mg) calcium

Separately give 3 Ketovite tablets, plus 5 ml Ketovite liquid per day. Check drugs are carbohydrate-free. Stop solids

Step 2: Increase *only* volume *or* strength of feed at any one time.

$\frac{1}{2}$ *strength Chix feed* is made as follows:

    25 g comminuted chicken
    5 g glucose and/or fructose and/or Caloreen
    0·4 g metabolic mineral mixture
    Boiled water to 100 ml

$\frac{3}{4}$ *strength Chix feed* is made as follows:

    37·5 g comminuted chicken
    5 g glucose and/or fructose and/or Caloreen
    0·6 g metabolic mineral mixture
    Boiled water to 100 ml

Full strength Chix feed is made as follows:

    50 g comminuted chicken
    5 g glucose and/or fructose and/or Caloreen
    0.8 g metabolic mineral mixture †
    Boiled water to 100 ml

* *From* Larcher V. F., Sheppard R., Francis D. E. M. et al.: Protracted diarrhoea in infancy: An analysis of 82 cases with particular reference to diagnosis and management. *Arch. Dis. Child.* 1977; **52**: 597–605.

† The full dose of minerals is 1·5 g per kg actual weight per day to a maximum of 8 g daily but never add more than 1 g to each 100 ml feed volume or osmolarity of feed is too high. Added calcium gluconate should be given if less then 6 g of minerals is given per day on a long term basis.

Do not exceed 10 g protein per kg actual weight per day
This full strength feed contains in 100 ml

Protein (contained in comminuted chicken)	3·75 g
Fat (contained in chicken)	1·65 g
Caloreen	5·0 g
Sodium	1·85 mmol
Potassium	2·32 mmol
Calcium	1·75 mmol

Total energy provided: approximately 211 kJ

Step 3: Build up feed carbohydrate to 10 per cent by approximate daily increments, i.e., 50 mg comminuted chicken 1·5 metabolic mineral mixture per kg actual weight per day.

Start with 5 g glucose and/or fructose and/or Caloreen

then 6 g	,,	,,	,,
then 7 g	,,	,,	,,
then 8 g	,,	,,	,,
then 9 g	,,	,,	,,
then 10 g	,,	,,	,,

Boiled water to 100 ml

Step 4: Slowly build up fat in feed by adding Prosparol (Duncan Flockhart) 1 per cent per day (Prosparol is a 50 per cent arachis oil emulsion of long-chain triglycerides, i.e. peanut oil) (*or* MCT oil where MCT is clinically indicated)

This can be done either after carbohydrate is at 10 per cent or alternatively added to the carbohydrate increases of Step 3.

Basic feed = 50 g comminuted chicken
          1·5 g metabolic mineral mixture per kg actual weight per day
          10 g glucose and/or fructose and/or Caloreen
          Boiled water to 100 ml

Add 2–5 ml Prosparol (1 to 2·5 ml MCT oil) to full volume of day's feed in daily increments as tolerated until total fat = 4 g/100 ml from chicken fat plus Prosparol (or MCT oil), i.e. a total of 5 ml Prosparol (or 2·5 ml MCT oil) to each 100 ml feed.

The final feed details:
Constituents
Comminuted chicken
  Not more than 10 g protein $kg^{-1} d^{-1}$
Caloreen
  10 g/100 ml of feed
Fat (from Prosparol and comminuted chicken)
  4 g/100 ml of feed
Metabolic mineral mixture
  1·5 $kg^{-1} d^{-1}$ (provided quantities do not exceed 1 g/100 ml of feed, or a total of 8 g/d)

Calcium (from comminuted chicken, metabolic mineral mixture and added calcium gluconate)
  At least 1·25 mmol/100 ml of feed of a minimum of 12·5 mmol/d
Feed volume
  200 ml $kg^{-1} d^{-1}$
Total energy provided
  750 or more kJ/$kg^{-1} d^{-1}$

Step 5: Increase volume to achieve weight gain but do not exceed the 10 g protein per kg actual weight per day and the 1·5 g minerals per kg actual weight per day (or 8 g maximum). Change to less frequent feeds 2-hourly, 3-hourly, then 4-hourly.

Step 6: Introduce suitable solids, e.g.:
1. Rice cereal (Robinson's Baby Rice; Milupa Rice mixed with 5 per cent dextrose
2. Milk-free mashed potato and gluten-free gravy
3. Purée meat
4. Egg yolk

Commercial baby foods may be suitable but must be milk-free, sucrose-free, lactose-free and gluten-free. *Drugs should be carbohydrate-free.*

Step 7: Continue the final feeding regimen and Ketovite until weight gain is satisfactory and/or reintroduction of disaccharides and milk is planned.

Home-made alternatives

Instead of 50 g comminuted chicken, 11·5 g of chicken meat (boiled, drained, cooked weight, preferably chicken breast) can be used and puréed aseptically in a liquidizer.* All weight should be chicken meat and not meat juices.

The disadvantages of home-prepared chicken are:
1. Salmonella contamination.
2. Aseptic preparation of freshly cooked chicken daily.
3. Difficulty in getting the fibres fine enough to go through an infant's feeding bottle teat. If all the meat is not puréed sufficiently the protein calorie content of the feed is lowered as the infant does not consume the calculated feed.

Rabbit fibre is finer than chicken and has been used (same weight as chicken meat) *or* egg 25 g instead of 50 g comminuted chicken. The latter must be cooked and does *not* require additional fat,† (Eggs can cause allergy or intolerance.)

* *See* Francis D. E. M.: *Diets for Sick Children,* 3rd ed. Oxford: Blackwell Scientific, 1974: 265–7.
† *See ibid*: Table 86: 267.

Chapter 19

Principles of Parenteral Nutrition in the Adult

P. D. Wright

An essential pre-requisite to the survival of the human organism, both in health and disease, is an adequate supply of nutrition sufficient to meet the prevailing physiological and environmental demands being faced by the individual. This can only be achieved by supplying appropriate quantities of water, electrolytes, vitamins, trace elements, calories as either carbohydrate or fat, and protein as a source of nitrogen. Long term existence without even one of these nutrients is not possible. Normal nutrition is dependent upon satisfactory oral assimilation of the food and adequate absorption from the gut. Even during illness, it is frequently possible for adequate nutrition to be maintained by the oral route, and there is little doubt that, wherever possible, nutrition during an illness should be encouraged by this natural route. This may entail the encouragement by the nursing staff of oral sip-feeding or the insertion of fine bore naso-enteral tubes to carry appropriate mixtures which, by virtue of their viscosity, may require propulsion by a pump. However, circumstances do occur after sickness and injury where the gut is no longer able to transport or absorb adequate quantities of food, either as a result of absolute deficiency of the gut, as in a short bowel syndrome, or as in a malfunction of the gut, such as might occur in inflammatory bowel disease or malabsorption syndrome (*Fig.* 19.1). In these circumstances, the body's demand for nutrition persists and can only be supplied by the intravenous route.

PATIENT SELECTION

The admission to hospital of a patient who is clearly underweight is a common occurrence, and it is important to identify such individuals by taking a careful history and performing a comprehensive physical examination. A firm diagnosis should be reached as to why the patient is underweight. Protein-energy malnutrition, both overt and subclinical, is common in hospital patients. Unfortunately, it is often unrecognized and hence goes untreated (1). A study in the United States concluded that nearly 50 per cent of surgical patients in a large city hospital had some evidence of protein-energy malnutrition (2).

In addition to a careful assessment of the patient's weight loss, other parameters have been used to try to determine the degree of protein-energy malnutrition. Anthropometric measurements, involving the mid-arm circumference and axillary and triceps skinfold thickness, have been used as a correlation with reserves of fatty tissue and lean body mass. These measurements have also been estimated recently using the Dopler ultrasound probe in an effort to improve accuracy (3). For many years, an estimation of the serum protein levels has been used as a guide to the patient's nutritional status. A serum albumin level of $3.5\,g/100\,ml$ is considered to be normal; a concentration of between 2.8 and $3.5\,g/100\,ml$ is indicative of mild visceral protein depletion; $2.1–2.7\,g$ denotes moderate depletion; less than $2.1\,g/100\,ml$ is evidence of severe depletion. Other groups of workers have utilized delayed cutaneous hypersensitivity reactions to several antigens (e.g. PPD, streptokinase, streptodornase, candida and mumps), and a battery of laboratory tests in an effort to quantify the individual patient's

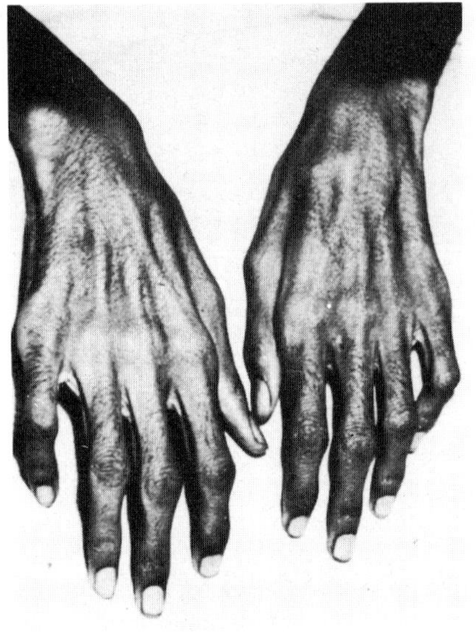

a

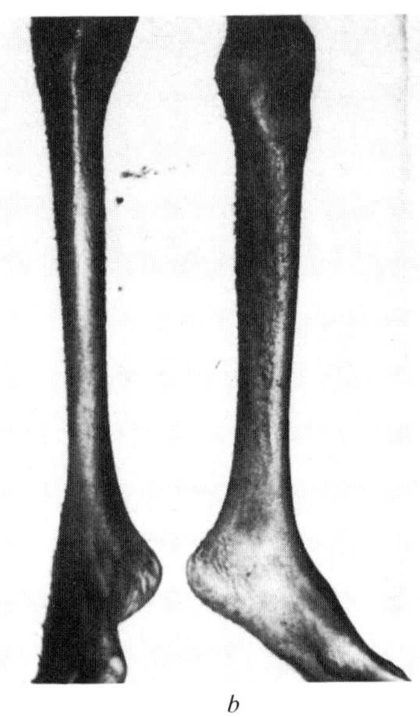

b

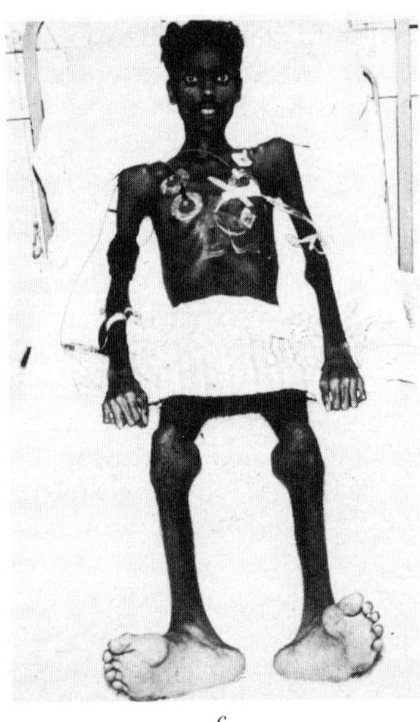

c

Fig. 19.1. An extreme case of protein-energy malnutrition arising with a severe malabsorption state and complicated by profound hypokalaemia and a peripheral neuropathy (*a, b*). This patient was 6 feet 2 inches tall and weighed only 29 kg. In addition to an oral diet, he was resuscitated with supplementary intravenous parenteral nutrition via a tunnelled catheter inserted through the right infraclavicular subclavian route (*c*). Subsequent investigations and a laparotomy unfortunately revealed the presence of intestinal lymphoma. (Reproduced by kind permission of Dr G. M. Stern, FRCP, Dr M. Sarner, FRCP and Prof. C. G. Clark.)

circulating humoral and cellular immune deficit. Some success has been claimed in identifying those at greatest risk prior to major surgical procedures (4). Skin testing for anergy can be affected by other factors in addition to impairment of immune defence mechanism induced by protein-energy malnutrition, e.g. fever, steroid therapy, tumours, shock and anaesthetic agents (5, 6). Recently, the value of the total white cell and absolute lymphocyte count has been realized as an indicator of immune paresis. Total lymphocyte counts of below $1·5 \times 10^9/l$ are seen with moderate depletion and counts of less than $0·8 \times 10^9/l$ indicate a severe depletion. The search for a suitable *in vitro* test of leucocyte function is progressing and both lymphocyte transformation assays and macrophage inhibition factor testing have recently showed promise (6).

Other traditional indices of a satisfactory protein-calorie status have included a satisfactory red blood cell count, haemoglobin, haematocrit, serum albumin and serum transferrin levels. These latter visceral protein levels may not fall until quite late in the process of malnutrition. The relative stability of albumin levels can be explained by the relatively long half-life (19 days) (7), the large total albumin mass, by mobilization of albumin from the extravascular pool to the intravascular pool and also by the capacity to maintain a high level of albumin synthesis as a result of diverting amino-acids from muscle to liver. The normal levels of transferrin (half-life, 8 days) also vary widely. More accurate indicators of subclinical protein malnutrition are the plasma levels of thyroxine-binding prealbumin (half-life, 2 days) and retinol-binding protein (half-life, 12 hours) (7). Thus, the problem of assessing the overall extent of protein-calorie malnutrition and the degree of tissue catabolism has stimulated many lines for research beyond the standard daily urinary nitrogen excretion and balance studies. Such interesting lines of inquiry have included the role of scalp hair root morphology and the suggestion has emerged that the growth of hair roots can act as a sensitive indicator of the recovery of protein synthesizing capacity (8, 9). Continuing research into this sphere of nutritional assessment is of great importance, so that a cost-effective screening profile can be achieved and implemented by clinical chemical pathologists.

Whilst the value of intravenous feeding in the management of prolonged postoperative complications is undeniable, there is an element of controversy surrounding the effectiveness of preoperative parenteral nutrition and peroperative support in reducing the incidence of morbidity and mortality. Despite the extensive use of preoperative parenteral nutrition and a strong clinical impression that it is a valuable therapeutic aid, conclusive documentation of its efficacy in reducing operative complications is still awaited (10, 11). A recent study in the United States has indicated that 'eye-ball' evaluation of nutritional status cannot identify high-risk individuals, and this series did suggest that significant reductions in the operative morbidity and mortality could be achieved by combined pre- and postoperative nutritional support (12). Other groups have also correlated the improved outcome after surgery with the provision of intravenous hyperalimentation (13, 14). The hypothesis appears to be sound, namely that protein-calorie malnutrition leads to immunosuppression which in turn increases the susceptibility to both sepsis (which naturally includes infection of the respiratory and urinary tracts in addition to the surgical wound) and failure of anastomotic and wound healing.

Undernutrition itself is frequently a manifestation of diseases such as cancer or inflammatory bowel disease. It is important to determine accurately the absolute weight loss and to detect whether or not the weight loss is progressive or static. If the patient's weight has reached a plateau, it is frequently possible to maintain adequate nutrition by continued oral feeding. However, if the patient continues to lose weight despite intensive efforts at oral feeding, then total parenteral nutrition has to be considered. It is important that weight loss should not be considered out of context with the disease process as a whole, and similarly, any decision to undertake total parenteral nutrition cannot be taken without careful consideration of the ultimate prognosis, so that treatment is undertaken with some idea of what is to be achieved by intravenous feeding. For example, it is probably not justifiable to nourish a patient who is suffering from severe advanced malignant disease when one does not propose to use nutritional treatment in relation to any other form of therapy, but is merely using it to prolong life for a short while in a patient who has a fatal disease.

The most important features in the assessment of patients who are underweight are to make a diagnosis, establish the extent of their protein-calorie malnutrition and then provide adequate treatment with total parenteral nutrition in association with the management of their particular disease process. However, circumstances do occur when a patient is so ill that total parenteral nutrition becomes necessary to buy time in order that the patient may be investigated without further deterioration. When deciding to undertake parenteral nutrition in a patient with a severe weight-losing disease, one has to be very clear of what one is trying to achieve.

Inflammatory Bowel Disease

Patients with severe diarrhoea, associated with weight loss, are a common clinical problem. Disease such as malabsorption and inflammatory bowel disease often present with severe diarrhoea, weight loss and anaemia. Where possible, it is, of course, desirable to treat the underlying disease. For example, coeliac disease is better managed with a gluten-free diet than with parenteral nutrition. However, severe and extensive Crohn's disease causing diarrhoea and weight loss has few primary treatments and some form of parenteral nutrition may become essential.

An important feature of many of the inflammatory diseases of the bowel is that they do not only cause the patient to lose weight, by virtue of their tendency to inhibit malabsorption of the bowel contents, but also, because of their inflammatory nature, they tend to cause a protein-losing enteropathy. There is an increasing body of evidence that multifocal inflammatory bowel disorders, such as Crohn's disease, can be managed satisfactorily by total parenteral nutrition as a form of primary therapy. Evidence has been obtained in the United States of America and the United Kingdom that by instituting a full regimen of total parenteral nutrition, and allowing the bowel complete rest, a significant degree of clinical improvement can take place and has been associated with quite marked radiological improvement in the disease process (15, 16). Any form of malabsorption syndrome which does not respond well to a primary form of treatment also represents a situation in which parenteral nutrition must be considered to maintain the patient through a period of treatment so that further nutritional deterioration may be kept to a minimum—'Holding the line'. This is particularly important where major surgery may have to be contemplated.

Gastrointestinal Fistulas

The management of small bowel fistulas frequently requires therapy with total parenteral nutrition (17–19). This is particularly the case in a situation where a high small bowel fistula occurs, the losses being particularly large and the amounts absorbed by the bowel low. Whilst it is important to know the pathophysiological cause of the fistula and to determine the presence or absence of distal obstruction in the bowel, an important feature of the treatment of such problems is first to assess the level at which a fistula has occurred, and then, by careful measurements of the amount of fistula output together with quantitation of the contents of the fistula fluid, to make a fairly accurate estimate of the total losses. It is only by accurate replacement of the losses, together with a proper supply of nutritional requirements, that a successful outcome will be achieved in these patients. Satisfactory control of the patient's metabolism must be re-established and simultaneously the bowel rested, adjacent abscesses drained and the site of the fistula (or fistulas) controlled by an appropriate drainage or suction system. Fistulas between loops of bowel may give rise to blind loop syndromes which themselves cause a significant degree of malnutrition. This can be brought under control by total parenteral nutrition, and the cause of the problem may then be corrected by surgical intervention at the most appropriate opportunity.

Surgery

The role of parenteral nutrition in the surgical patient is quite clear. There is little evidence to suggest that well-nourished patients undergoing routine elective surgery represent a nutritional problem of sufficient severity to require parenteral nutrition. The importance of correcting preoperative anaemia, hypoproteinaemia and water and electrolyte disturbances by the infusion of the appropriate fluids has been appreciated for many years. This aspect of patient care should not be neglected because of the current availability of suitable sources of parenteral nutrition. However, if a surgical patient undergoes a procedure, or develops a complication, that means that he is to be maintained without adequate oral nutrition for more than 3–5 days, then the patient has to be carefully assessed and some prediction made as whether this situation is likely to continue. If the patient is going to remain without adequate oral nutrition for more than 5 days, then the institution of perioperative total parenteral nutrition must be seriously considered. The form of treatment must depend very much on the type of surgery that the patient has undergone, and the extent of any pre-existing nutritional deficit. For example, if a patient is unable to swallow after head and neck or oesophageal surgery and the rest of the bowel is functioning fairly normally, then it is reasonable to feed such a patient through a fine bore nasogastric or naso-enteral tube. Occasionally, a gastrostomy or fine bore feeding tube jejunostomy may be created to carry the patient through this critical period. If the surgery has resulted in a significant degree of paralytic ileus, rendering most of the bowel non-functional, then total parenteral nutrition becomes a necessity. The provision of supplementary intravenous nutrition will also provide cancer patients with a useful adjunctive energy source enabling them to withstand palliative resections, radiotherapy and chemotherapy with fewer associated complications (19, 20).

Burns and Severe Sepsis

Patients with burns and severe sepsis represent a special group on their own, in whom the demands for nutrition may be extremely high. The energy demands in a patient who has undergone a significant degree of burn injury may be enormous and it is almost impossible immediately following a burn to supply these requirements adequately by mouth. In these circumstances, intravenous replacement has to be seriously considered. It is not unusual for a period of ileus to follow a severe burn and then, if adequate calorie replacement is to be provided, parenteral nutrition is mandatory. As improvement occurs, as much of this as possible should be transferred to the gut as soon as the bowel function returns to normal, so that the central venous catheters, with their inherent risks of thrombosis and infection, can be used for the shortest possible period of time.

In the patient with severe sepsis, as a complication following surgery for example, similar considerations apply, but these patients are almost invariably unable to undertake any form of oral nutrition. In these circumstances, adequate replacement by total parenteral nutrition, making allowance for the high demands of a septic patient, must be arranged without delay. In patients with a continuing fever, in addition to providing extra water for metabolism, as much as a 12 per cent increase has to be made in the calorific supply per 1 °C rise in the temperature (*Fig.* 19.2).

All the categories of patient discussed serve to highlight the major groups who, in recent years, have required total parenteral nutrition. There are many other sub-sets of patients who may be suffering from chronic obstructive airways disease, cardiac cachexia or moderate to severe degrees of hepatic or renal failure, in addition to patients with severe musculoskeletal trauma, who might benefit from intravenous nutrition. Each patient must be considered as an individual, and in simple terms, what makes us decide in any of these categories whether a patient needs total parenteral nutrition or not, is whether the total available oral intake of fluid and food, taking account of such problems as the degree of absorption, exceeds the demands or not. If the demands of energy are exceeded by the protein-calorie supply, then total parenteral nutrition or supplementary intravenous nutrition is not necessary. However, if the supply via the enteral route is less, and likely to be less on a continuing basis than the demands of energy and repair, then total parenteral nutrition must be seriously considered as a form of treatment for such a patient. It is essential that the decision to start treatment is made without undue delay.

PLANNING A REGIMEN FOR TOTAL PARENTERAL NUTRITION

To provide adequate nutritional support, a regimen must contain energy sources such as carbohydrate or fat, amino acids, water, electrolytes, trace elements and vitamins. In order to get this combination of substrates into a patient within 24 hours in a reasonable volume, the solution must be almost certainly hypertonic and this means that, for most circumstances, some form of central venous catheterization is essential.

What is the Role of the Various Substrates that are Available?

Carbohydrates

Glucose (Dextrose)

Glucose is by far the most satisfactory calorie source available, being both physiological, cheap and easily obtained. It has the complications of any hypertonic solution, in that if it is infused through a peripheral vein, it will cause phlebothrombosis. Also, careful attention must be paid to the monitoring of such a patient to make sure that the glucose concentration in the serum does not become excessively high, or that hyperosmolar situations do not occur. In any patient receiving intravenous glucose as a nutritional support, the prime consideration is the amount of energy that the patient requires as carbohydrate. This amount of carbohydrate is then given as a continuous infusion. If the patient becomes hyperglycaemic as a result of such an infusion, then insulin will need to be given in adequate dosage. Insulin may be added directly to the infusion of glucose or be given separately by an infusion at a rate appro-

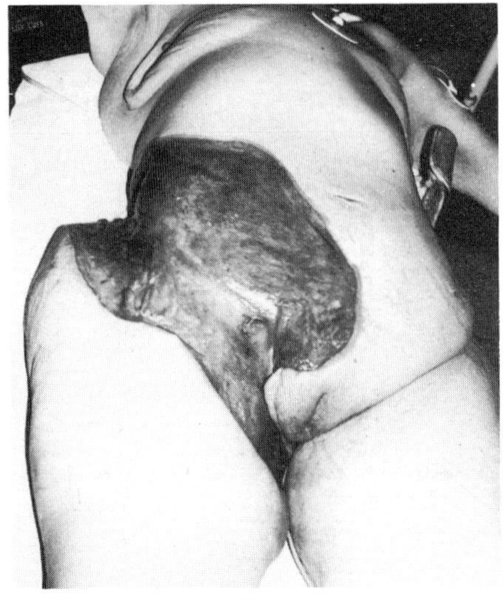

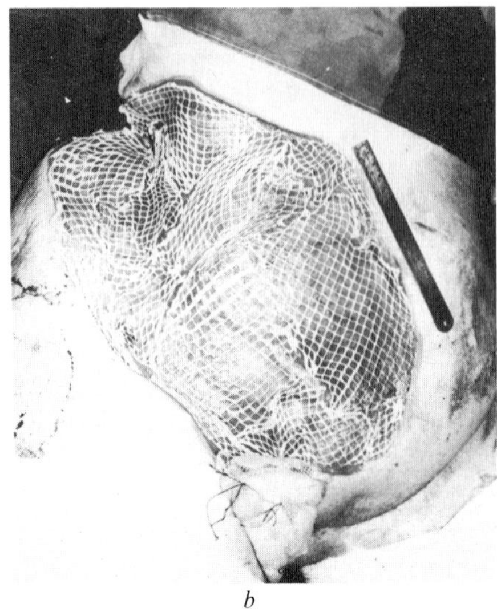

a

b

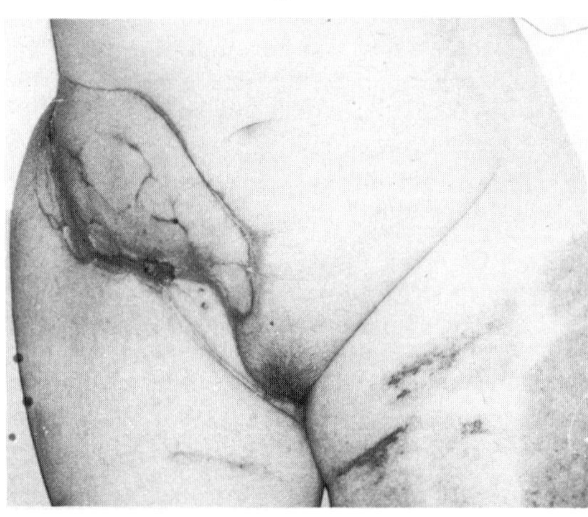

c

Fig. 19.2. This shows the consequences of fulminant synergistic necrotizing fasciitis which followed an emergency femoral hernia repair and bowel resection in a 75-year-old lady. After extensive debridement and resuscitation, this lady received supplementary parenteral nutrition via a tunnelled central catheter until satisfactory granulation tissue formed (*a*). A mesh of split skin was applied (*b*) and the successful healing outcome is shown in (*c*), just prior to her discharge.

priate to maintain a relatively normal glucose concentration. The molecule is adsorbed both to glass and plastic and, therefore, if insulin is added to the infusate an allowance may have to be made for this loss. The presence of diabetes mellitus in the patient requiring treatment with intravenous glucose does not preclude the use of adequate quantities of glucose for maintaining normal nutrition. Additional care must be taken with the glucose concentration in the serum and the amount of insulin that must be added in order to maintain normoglycaemia. It is important that the amount of infused glucose should be limited to less than $60\,\mathrm{kcal\,kg^{-1}\,d^{-1}}$ since it is known that excessive glucose loads have been incriminated in the development of fatty liver—likened to a form of human glucose-induced 'pâté de foie gras' (21).

Fructose

Fructose has been used in many intravenous solutions, and it does have the advantage that in patients who become hyperglycaemic following injury, there is some evidence that fructose bypasses the point at which the patient's inhibition of glucose metabolism occurs and is potentially used more satisfactorily. However, it does have a significant risk in that it can be associated with the development of lactic acidosis in certain situations, particularly when used in neonates. In general terms, the advantages of fructose are really outweighed by their disadvantages and it is more satisfactory to use glucose, which is a more physiological substrate. In the rare circumstance that this is the only energy source available for intravenous feeding, it is important not to infuse more than $0\cdot5\,\mathrm{g\,kg^{-1}\,h^{-1}}$

Sorbitol

Sorbitol is a relatively unphysiological substrate to be used in large quantities, and has no advantages over glucose. A 30 per cent solution of Sorbitol contains some 1250 kcal/l.

Ethanol

Ethanol has a relatively high calorie value (7·1 kcal/g) and has been used in a number of commercially available parenteral nutrition solutions. However, it really ought not to be recommended for general use in parenteral nutrition regimens as many of the patients who require intravenous feeding suffer from some form of intra-abdominal sepsis or general sepsis resulting potentially in a degree of portal pyaemia, when it might be expected that any ethanol-containing substrate should be contra-indicated. Similarly, many underweight patients who require parenteral nutrition are extremely sensitive to the cerebral effects of alcohol, and this can confuse the clinical assessment of any patient who is liable to develop clinical changes as a result of their primary disease. In general terms, alcohol should not be recommended for regular use. It does, however, have a role in the management of the patient with severe alcoholism who requires surgery and it can be very effective in the treatment of delirium tremens when provided under controlled conditions.

Fat

The only satisfactory commercially available fat solution at the present time in the United Kingdom is Intralipid, which is a soya bean emulsion. This is a very satisfactory form of calories and has been used extensively with very few side-effects (1 litre of 10% provides 1100 kcal; 1 litre of 20% provides 2000 kcal). It has the advantage that it contains the essential fatty acids that are so important in the patient receiving long-term parenteral nutrition. Furthermore, 30 i.u. of vitamin E are provided per 500 ml of Intralipid 20%. Although very valuable, many consider that it should not need to be given in quantities any greater than 500 ml of 20% Intralipid each day and would probably be more satisfactory given at a level 500 ml of 20% Intralipid every 3 days, which maintains essential fatty stores at a satisfactory level throughout a long period. There is some evidence emerging that septic and injured man prefers to utilize endogenous fat as an energy source and that the body cannot tolerate large glucose loads as the principal source of calories. Indeed, in patients with pulmonary dysfunction receiving high glucose loads, elevated levels of CO_2 production have been recorded sufficient to cause respiratory distress, and this has been reversed by switching to fat as the source of intravenous calories (22–24).

Amino Acids

In recent years there have become available a large number of commercially prepared amino acid solutions suitable for parenteral nutrition. In spite of the wide claims that may be made by the manufacturers for these various solutions, there is little evidence that any one of these amino acid solutions confers any specific clinical benefit, and one might just as well choose the cheapest solution containing the most satisfactory quantity of nitrogen for each individual's needs. All now contain the essential L-amino acids—isoleucine; leucine; lysine; methionine; valine; phenylalanine; threonine; tryptophan.

Branch Chain Amino Acids

Extensive research work has been performed on the role of branch chain amino acids in the management of patients requiring total parenteral nutrition. There are two particular groups of patients who might benefit from this type of solution. First, there is some evidence that the encephalopathy in patients with severe liver disease is related to high levels of phenylalanine, tyrosine and methionine in the serum. By providing branch chain amino acid solutions, one can obtain a significant lowering in the serum concentrations of these amino acids and there is some experimental evidence to suggest that they may well be of benefit in patients with incipient hepatic encephalopathy. However, they are not at present commercially available in the United Kingdom and, depending on the results of further studies, their availability may increase over the next few years. Secondly, in renal failure there is some evidence that the use of branch chain amino acids can reduce the rate of ureagenesis and can therefore potentially increase the time interval between haemodialysis sessions.

Isotonic Amino Acids

There has been extensive study of the value of isotonic amino acids in the management of patients who require parenteral nutrition after surgery. The advantage of these is that they do not need to be given through a central vein catheter. However, the evidence suggesting their usefulness is somewhat doubtful, and their particular limitation is that if adequate quantities of nitrogen or calories are to be given in the postoperative situation to restore nitrogen balance, they have to be accompanied by an almost unacceptable volume of water to maintain isotonicity, with the consequent danger of overhydration.

An excellent and comprehensive review of the role of amino acids in parenteral nutrition and the prospects for the future have recently been provided by Okada et al. (25).

Vitamins

In any patient undergoing long term parenteral nutrition, the addition of vitamins, both water-soluble and fat-soluble, is essential (26, 27). These may be given as daily injections, separate from the intravenous feeding regimen, or incorporated into the regimen. If they are placed within the hyperalimentation fluid containers, there can be rapid decay and only a small proportion of that which is injected into the containers eventually reaches the patient in an active form. The only way of preventing this is to wrap the containers in aluminium foil or other screening film to minimize light penetration. This must be seriously considered in certain wards depending upon the local climatic conditions. Furthermore, vitamins given intravenously tend to be more rapidly excreted by the kidneys, so that the daily intravenous requirements may be greater than the oral dose. It must also be remembered that although the oral daily dose of water-soluble vitamins can be doubled without evidence of toxic effects, this is not the case for fat-soluble vitamins. Hypervitaminosis A can cause exfoliative dermatitis and hypervitaminosis D may cause hypercalcaemia. There are special fat-soluble vitamin preparations which can be added to Intralipid solutions which are highly satisfactory (e.g. Vitlipid, Kabi-Vitrum). With water-soluble solutions, it is essential to make sure that you are giving the full spectrum of vitamins, as many commercial preparations are highly selective in the compounds which they contain (Table 19.1). At present Solivito (Kabi-Vitrum) contains the most appropriate combination of water-soluble vitamins.

It is particularly important to provide folic acid in parenteral nutrition regimens as many serious defects may occur as a result of deficiency. Acute pancytopenia can arise with disas-

Table 19.1. **Vitamin preparations for intravenous infusion**

Vitamin	Units	Recommended daily intake	Solivito (Kabi-Vitrum)	Vitlipid (Kabi-Vitrum)	Multibionta (BDH)	Parenterovite (Bencard) Ampoule 1	Ampoule 2
Thiamine B1	mg	1·4	1·2	—	50	250	—
Riboflavin B2	mg	2·1	1·8	—	7·29	4·0	—
Pyridoxine B6	mg	2·1	2·0	—	15	50	—
Cyanocobalamin B12	μg	2·0	2·0	—	—	—	—
Nicotinamide	mg	14	10	—	100	—	160
Biotin	mg	0·35	0·3	—	—	—	—
Pantothenic acid	mg	14	10	—	25	—	—
Folic acid	mg	2	0·2	—	—	—	—
Ascorbic acid C	mg	35	30	—	500	—	500
Calciferol D	i.u.	100	—	120	—	—	—
Phytylmenaquinone K	μg	140	—	150	—	—	—
Retinol A	i.u.	700	—	2500	10 000	—	—
Tocopheryl acetate E	i.u.	30	—	—	5	—	—

trous consequences and falls in the serum folate concentration have been noted within 24 hours of starting intravenous nutrition (28). This was initially ascribed to ethanol in the infusate, but other reports have appeared in which this factor could not be incriminated (29, 30). This haemotological syndrome was traced back and the first description credited to Harvier and Mallarme (31). Intravenous methionine can lower the serum folic acid level and supplementation with 15 mg/week should stop this problem arising (32).

It is important to observe patients closely for the development of vitamin dificiency when parenteral nutrition is prolonged. Bozetti has noted a case of development of a sensorimotor peripheral neuropathy, particularly involving the peroneal nerves, due to a relative thiamine deficiency (33). The patient was receiving high doses of glucose and Bozetti postulated that, because thiamine is an important co-factor in carbohydrate metabolism (participating in the oxidative decarboxylation of pyruvate and alpha-ketoglutarate, and also in the trans-ketolase reaction of the pentose shunt), the patient was in fact relatively deficient of this vitamin. Although the normal daily requirements are only in the range of 1·5 mg, and this had been adequately covered in the feeding regimen, the addition of 100 mg of thiamine per day resulted in a resolution of the patient's leg pains and sensory symptoms. Thus, the development of a beri-beri-like syndrome related to parenteral nutrition should be considered. On the basis of red-cell transketolase levels, the thiamine requirement for patients receiving prolonged parenteral nutrition should be $0.3 \, \mathrm{mg \, kg^{-1} \, d^{-1}}$ (34). Bozetti also mentioned the potential for these patients to develop cerebral manifestations of thiamine deficiency in the form of Wernicke's encephalopathy; any derangement of the patient's level of consciousness, understanding, or the development of nystagmus and ophthalmoplegia, especially involving the sixth cranial nerve, should arouse the clinician's suspicions concerning the possibility of thiamine deficiency.

Vitamin C or ascorbic acid is intimately concerned with the healing of wounds by virtue of its role in the formation of collagen and intercellular cement substance. The normal body pool amounts to 1500 mg, and in the absence of any vitamin C, this is depleted at the rate of 3 per cent per day, so that the clinical manifestations of scurvy appear after 84–97 days, when the total body reserves have fallen below 300 mg (35). Even before the overt and classic signs of scurvy appear, personality changes occur with depression, hypochondriasis, reduced arousal and loss of motivation. Once such a deficiency is established, the patients present a picture of fatigue, petcchial haemorrhages, follicular hyperkeratosis, swollen and bleeding gums and joint effusions. Anaemia occurs and may be normocytic or macrocytic and true megaloblastic anaemia also occurs. The factors responsible for the anaemia are haemolysis, bleeding and a dietary iron deficiency. Vitamin C deficiency also impairs folate metabolism and it plays an important role in maintaining a pool of folate.

There is evidence accumulating that the requirements of the body for vitamin C are increased by surgery and that supplements may be of benefit in augmenting wound healing.

A regular review of the vitamin status of patients who are receiving prolonged intravenous feeding should always be maintained. Vitamin K should be added by intermittent intramuscular or intravenous injections. Satisfactory amounts of vitamin E are provided in Intralipid (Kabi-Vitrum). The development of bizarre nutritional deficiency syndromes, such as the diarrhoea, dementia and dermatitis of pellagra, are best prevented by regular replacement therapy. Even in the midst of plenty and despite the assistance of the DHSS, lonely individuals unwittingly neglect themselves, especially in inner-city areas where neighbours fail to notice or care about the patient's declining health until hospital admission is precipitated by some medical or surgical catastrophe. Such patients are not always elderly, and a careful dietary history is invaluable as it usually reveals why they are harbouring significant vitamin deficiencies.

Electrolytes

It is important before any parenteral hyperalimentation regimen is commenced to ensure that, first, the serum electrolytes are stabilized and abnormalities corrected to as near normal as possible within the constraints of the patient's renal, cardiac and hepatic problems, should they exist. Subsequently, adequate quantities of all the routine electrolytes, such as sodium, potassium, chloride, magnesium and phosphate, must be added in appropriate quantities to maintain normal serum concentrations (Table 19.2) (36).

Table 19.2. **Recommended adult daily allowances per kg body weight in intravenous nutrition (36)**

Substance	Unit	Basal	Increased losses or depleted status	Severe catabolism
Water	ml	30	50	100–150
Energy	kcal	30	35–40	50–50
	MJ	0·13	0·15–0·17	0·21–0·25
Sodium	mmol	1–1·4	2·3	3·4
Potassium	mmol	0·7–0·9	2	3–4
Calcium	mmol	0·11	0·15	0·2
Magnesium	mmol	0·04	0·15–0·20	0·3–0·4
Phosphorus	mmol	0·15	0·4	0·6–1·0

Phosphate is particularly important, as are calcium and magnesium, for maintaining homeostasis and must not be left out of any regimen, particularly those containing hypertonic glucose, as this solution on its own can cause significant depression of the serum phosphate concentration. Hypophosphataemia interferes with the oxygen dissociation curve by increasing the red cell affinity for oxygen, and this is of importance where good tissue oxygenation is required. An adequate supply of phosphate is invariably provided when Intralipid is included in the regimen.

Trace Elements

An adequate provision of trace elements must also be considered, particularly in those patients undergoing long term parenteral nutrition. These can be obtained as commercially available trace element solutions for addition to intravenous feeding fluids. The most widely used mixture at the present time in the United Kingdom is Addamel (Kabi-Vitrum), which contains the following amounts of elements in each ampoule: magnesium, 1·5 mmol; calcium, 5 mmol; zinc, 20 µmol; manganese, 4·0 µmol; iron, 50 µmol; copper, 5 µmol; chloride ion, 13 mmol; fluorine, 50 µmol; and iodine, 1 µmol.

Many commerically available amino acid and dextrose solutions now contain significant quantities of both electrolytes and trace elements, making administration of these substances significantly easier. It must, of course, be remembered that the provision of the basic requirements may not be sufficient to correct a longstanding deficiency. As in the case of potassium, care must naturally be exercised when replacing elements such as magnesium and zinc via the intravenous route, particularly when there is impaired renal function. The recommended daily adult allowances are illustrated in Table 19.3 (36).

The possibility of deficiency states with these elements usually only arises after very prolonged total intravenous feeding, in the presence of excessive gastrointestinal, fistula or urinary losses. It has been realized for some time that magnesium and zinc are particularly important to replace in surgical patients. Zinc has an important role to play in protein synthesis, wound healing and growth. Replacement

Table 19.3. **Recommended daily adult allowances per kg body weight of trace elements in intravenous nutrition**

Substance	Unit	Basal requirements	Increased losses or depleted status	Severe catabolism
Iron	µmol	0·25–1	1·0	1·0
Zinc	µmol	0·7	0·7–1·5	1·5–3·0
Manganese	µmol	0·1	0·3	0·6
Copper	µmol	0·07	0·3–0·4	0·4–1
Chromium	µmol	0·015	—	—
Iodine	µmol	0·015	—	—
Fluorine	µmol	0·7	0·7–1·5	—
Molybdenum	µmol	0·003	—	—
Selenium	µmol	0·006	—	—

therapy with this element should not be performed too rapidly and extreme care should be taken when supplementing the feeding regimen since episodes of toxicity have been reported causing nausea, gastric erosions, renal failure and death (37). Serum zinc levels may not be a satisfactory index of total zinc depletion. Wolman et al. have developed a formula for replacement in order to achieve a balance in the face of the gastrointestinal disease frequently found in surgical practice (38).

Zinc replacement (mg/d)
$$= 2 \cdot 0 + 17 \cdot 1a + 12 \cdot 2b$$

$2 \cdot 0$ = replacement for urinary losses

a = mass (kg) of stool or ileostomy output

b = mass (kg) of small bowel fluid lost via a fistula or stoma.

Agget has provided a comprehensive review of the current understanding of trace elements (39), and suggests that they can be envisaged as having a spectrum of biological effects. Sub-optimal concentrations of an essential element cause a deficiency state and there is no doubt that they have an important role to play incorporated in metalloenzymes. At higher concentrations, normal physiological effects are apparent until the homeostatic capacity is exceeded with pharmacological and toxic effects appearing.

Recently it has been suggested that selenium is essential in the human diet (40). Deficiency of this element is known to cause a form of muscular dystrophy in sheep and cattle, pancreatic degeneration in poultry and liver necrosis in rats. There is a selenium-dependent glutathione peroxidase in human erythrocytes and this strongly suggests that selenium is an important trace element. Furthermore, Keshan disease, a cardiomyopathy, occurs in children from a region of China where selenium levels are low in staple foods. Recently, a possible case following prolonged parenteral nutrition has been reported from New Zealand by Johnston et al. (41). This highlights the need for vigilant surveillance of the status of micro-nutrient supply when total parenteral nutrition is carried on for months and years. Further guidance in this area has been provided by the American Medical Association's Department of Foods and Nutrition (42).

SELECTION OF A PARENTERAL NUTRITION REGIMEN

The first step in selecting a parenteral nutrition regimen is to make an accurate assessment of the patient's day-to-day requirements, taking into account all fluid and electrolyte losses. The patient's calorie requirements must be calculated with care, depending on the patient's body weight and also the severity of disease. If a patient is particularly hypercatabolic, for instance in association with sepsis or burns, then the calorie requirement may have to be increased by up to 50 or 100 per cent, depending on the severity of the illness. The estimation of urinary nitrogen will allow adequate replacement of nitrogen losses with amino acids. For the calculation of how much nitrogen to give a patient suffering from under-nutrition or injury, nitrogen should be given at the rate of $0 \cdot 2 \, \text{g kg}^{-1} \text{d}^{-1}$, for most circumstances; thus, for a 70-kg man, approximately 14 g of nitrogen should be given each day. An extra provision of nitrogen should be made whenever there are severe purulent wounds. For such patients it is wise for an accurate assessment of the discharge losses to be made since significant amounts of protein can be shed from the patient's body via this route.

It is important to obtain a satisfactory ratio of calories to nitrogen, and for most circumstances, the ratio of 200 calories to 1 g of nitrogen is adequate. The energy and nitrogen supply required to achieve a balance situation obviously varies with the metabolic state of the patient, and the proposals of Woolfson are considered satisfactory for most situations (Table 19.4) (43).

In general terms, all the calories may be given as carbohydrate for a considerable time without the patient suffering deleterious effects. However, it is generally recommended that fat should

Table 19.4. **Energy and nitrogen requirements**

	Fasting	Intermediate	Catabolic
Nitrogen (g/24 h) for equilibrium	7·5	14	25
Kcal (including protein)	2000	3000	4000
Non-protein calorie:nitrogen ratio	250	200	135

be given as a source of calories so that the patient receives at least 1000 calories as a fat solution at least twice a week. Vitamins and trace elements need to be provided as previously indicated.

PRESENTATION OF THE REGIMEN

The presentation of the regimen to the bedside depends very much on the facilities available in the individual hospital. Most hospitals do not have the benefit of laminar flow facilities and are forced to present their intravenous regimens in fluid bottles. In these circumstances, the most satisfactory way of administering an intravenous feeding regimen is by means of a Y, V or W tube arrangement whereby bottles of calories and amino acids run into the patient simultaneously through a manifold type of connection into a central vein. Because of the importance of ensuring adequate quantities of added electrolytes and trace elements, it is most satisfactory to use fluids which already contain a number of these substances. However, when selecting an amino acid solution for use in parenteral nutrition, it is best to select one which contains just amino acids and very few additional calories as this simplifies the calorie calculation significantly. When selecting a calorie source, particularly glucose, there are a number of available solutions on the market which contain either 20 per cent or 40 per cent glucose and also adequate amounts of electrolytes, particularly calcium, magnesium, phosphate, zinc, sodium and potassium. By judicious selection of these bottles, an adequate regimen can be formulated without difficulty for most patients.

Preparation in the Pharmacy

For those hospitals who are fortunate enough to have laminar flow facilities, the optimum way of presenting an intravenous feeding regimen is to have it prepared under laminar flow conditions in bags tailored to the individual patient, whereby calories and amino acids can be added at source, together with the appropriate electrolyte additives. This minimizes the risk of infection caused by changing bottles and adding various substances at the bedside. The one limiting factor to this is that it is only now becoming

possible to add Intralipid to a bag containing carbohydrate or amino acid, because it does have the significant disadvantage, being a lipid compound, of floating and it is not possible to maintain an adequate mixture of the fluid throughout the time of administration. In view of this, most centres administer Intralipid separately as an individual bolus of 500 ml daily, twice a week or once a week as appropriate for the individual patient's requirements.

Administration

Normally, it is possible to administer the fluid into a central vein by the simple expedient of gravity drip infusion. However, the success of this method depends very much on the motivation and skill of the nursing staff in maintaining an adequate flow rate to ensure that fluids enter the patient at an appropriate rate. If this is not possible, an intravenous fluid pump may be added to the administration system so that more accurate metering of fluids can be achieved. This is particularly satisfactory when dealing with fluids that have been added to a single bag in the dispensary. However, problems can arise when a pump is added to a V or Y tube arrangement where the fluids are mixed before entering the pump. In these circumstances, the differential viscosities of the glucose and amino acid solutions can allow the less viscous amino acid solution to run in disproportionately fast, unless very careful adjustment of the metering valves is made.

Mobilization and Morale

In the management of long term parenteral nutrition patients, one of the most important aspects is the maintenance of adequate morale through what is usually a serious illness. There is little doubt that if optimum protein utilization and synthesis is to be obtained, then the patient's muscles must be used as much as possible. It is our practice that wherever possible the patient should be fully mobilized. If this is impracticable, then he should be given full and vigorous physiotherapy to maintain adequate muscle activity. Those patients who are able to walk are encouraged, to have their infusion fluids attached to a highly portable drip stand so that they can move around the ward freely. We also encourage a parenteral nutrition regimen designed for 24 hours to be given over a period of 18–20 hours, thus allowing the patient to be disconnected from the intravenous catheter which can be filled with a heparin lock for the remaining 4–6 hours under full· sterile precautions. This allows the patient to walk normally and allows him to leave hospital and go for a walk outside, which has significant effects on maintaining the morale.

METABOLIC COMPLICATIONS

Overhydration

The commonest complication that is seen in intravenous feeding is overhydration, and this is frequently missed because it is easy for the inexperienced clinician to mistake weight gain due to excessive water with the weight gain from the build-up of tissue mass. Wherever possible, the volume of administered solution and the volume of sensible and insensible fluid loss must be carefully monitored to exclude a persistently positive water balance. This surveillance is particularly important in the elderly, and regular examination of the ankles, pre-tibial tissue, the posterior aspect of the calves and thighs, in addition to the sacral area, should be performed. Pulmonary and cerebral oedema can easily occur when intravenous feeding regimens are prolonged.

Hyperosmolar syndrome

The normal serum osmolality is 290 mosmol/kg of water. Normal saline has an osmolality of 285 mosmol and 5 per cent glucose, an osmolality of 278 mosmol. The osmolality of some feeding solutions are listed below:

10% Intralipid	280 mosmol/kg of water
20% Intralipid	330 mosmol/kg of water
10% glucose	523 mosmol/kg of water
20% glucose	1250 mosmol/kg of water
30% glucose	2100 mosmol/kg of water
50% glucose	3800 mosmol/kg of water

The osmolality of many of the amino acid solutions is also more than 1000 mosmol/kg of water. Since the movement of water between the different compartments of the body is determined by the concentration of dissolved par-

ticles, it is extremely important not to change the osmotic pressure of the blood too rapidly during an intravenous infusion. Thus, it is vital that the nursing and clinical staff do not try to 'catch up' with concentrated solutions. This can precipitate acute intracerebral dehydration with resultant convulsions, coma and severe neurological deficit. It is not unknown for the controlling clamps of infusion sets to fail, and the sudden surge of 500 ml of 50 per cent glucose into the circulation would be an extremely serious event. Similarly, such solutions when contained in a 3-litre bag compound this potential danger, and therefore every precaution must be taken to eliminate this risk by using an appropriate pump or more than one control device. The administration of hypertonic glucose can cause hyperglycaemia. A regular examination of the urine for glycosuria should be carried out each day on all patients receiving total parenteral nutrition.

It is a wise precaution to commence intravenous feeding slowly in the elderly, with reduced concentrations of glucose for the first 2–3 days, and similarly, at the end of the intravenous feeding programme, the concentrations should be scaled down so that rebound hypoglycaemia does not occur. Hyperglycaemia will occur when glucose is supplied faster than it can enter cells; this may precipitate an osmotic diuresis with the development of dehydration. An osmotic diuresis will also occur if the osmotic load of other nutrient solutions is too great. This problem can easily be detected by regular surveillance of the serum electrolytes and osmolality. The osmotic load can be scaled down and extra water for metabolism supplied in the regimen. Hyperglycaemia can naturally be controlled by appropriate doses of insulin; however, if more glucose enters into the cells than can be catabolized, intracellular accumulation can lead to a state of intracellular overhydration clinically resembling dehydration. Intracellular overhydration therefore requires a restriction in the calorie load of the regimen. Calorie requirements can easily be overestimated, particularly in seriously ill patients.

Metabolic Acidosis

The titratable acidity of amino acid solutions is relatively high, and it is possible when giving large quantities of these solutions, to generate a metabolic acidosis. Also, patients suffering from liver disease may be unable to tolerate the high concentration of aromatic amino acids and may develop hepatic encephalopathy. Another factor in the creation of a metabolic acidosis is that some amino acid solutions contain an excess of cationic amino acids such as lysine, arginine and histidine; this problem is further accentuated when some solutions have been formulated with deficiencies of anionic amino acid, e.g. glutamic acid and aspartic acid.

Essential Fatty Acid Deficiency

This has only been described following prolonged intravenous nutrition in which intravenous fat emulsions have not been used. The fatty acids which cannot be produced in the body are linoleic acid and linolenic acid, with 2 and 3 double bonds respectively. Arachidonic acid with 4 double bonds, which is also necessary for normal metabolism, can be produced in the body from linoleic acid. When deficiency of these fatty acids does occur, a characteristic dermatitis develops with scaly skin lesions, sparse hair growth and a degree of thrombocytopenia. Essential fatty acids are also required to maintain a normal lipid composition in other tissues, e.g. the brain. Fat infusions also prevent the development of fatty liver when patients receive prolonged parenteral nutrition.

Complications with the administration of Intralipid are relatively uncommon. Febrile reactions have been recorded, together with occasional blood dyscrasias and coagulation defects. Jaundice has also been noted in patients receiving Intralipid which spontaneously resolves on cessation of the therapy. The administration of Intralipid is contraindicated in patients with severe disturbances of fat metabolism. A severe degree of hyperlipidaemia can develop in such individuals. In order to control the supply of fat to a patient unable to eliminate fat from the bloodstream adequately, on the morning following the first day's infusion of fat emulsion, a citrated blood sample should be centrifuged at 1200–1500 rev/min. If the plasma is strongly opalescent or milky, further infusion should be postponed or smaller doses of fat administered. In most patients the plasma should be completely cleared 12 hours after the conclusion of an infusion of fat. This point is important since the apparatus of the biochemical laboratory can be contaminated and subsequent electrolyte estimations be spurious and inaccurate. Therefore, the regimen should be so designed that fat has cleared from the circulation well before venesection is carried out on the following morning.

Many of the deficiency syndromes, e.g. hypophosphataemia, hypomagnesaemia, have already been mentioned and these should no longer arise. The key to successful management of patients receiving total parenteral nutrition is the application of sound measurement in the formulation of the individual patient's protein and energy requirements; vigilance and care during the infusion; regular biochemical monitoring, and a lively awareness of the rare syndromes that can arise from the relative excess or deficiency of particular nutrients essential for life. A great deal of skill is required to artificially maintain serum and cellular homeostasis, particularly in the presence of disordered cardiac, renal or hepatic function. In patients suffering from such conditions, constraints may well have to be applied to the volume of fluid infused per day, and the amount of amino acid supplied. Hyperammonaemia and abnormally elevated levels of amino acids can rapidly precipitate the onset of confusion, drowsiness and then coma. More sophisticated biochemical surveillance involving serum aminograms may be required in addition to the following measurements recommended as a routine, whilst the patient's metabolism is being stabilized:

Daily
    Haemoglobin
    White cell count
    Urea and electrolytes
    Blood sugar
Twice weekly
    Liver function tests
    Serum proteins
    Calcium and phosphate
    Platelets
    Prothrombin time
    Urinary electrolyte analysis
    Nasogastric and fistula fluid
        analysis (where applicable)
    Body weight
    Osmolality

Every 2 weeks
Serum cholesterol and
triglyceride levels
Serum iron and TIBC
Magnesium
Zinc
Creatinine
Serum B12
Red cell folate levels
Urinary calcium, phosphate
and urate

Naturally, the interval between such investigations can be extended once control has been achieved.

PROSPECTS FOR THE FUTURE

The continuing development of various amino acid and calorie solutions, together with methods of administration, will almost certainly make the application of total parenteral nutrition safer and more available in a wider variety of clinical situations. However, the one limitation in the field is the tendency to generalize over the appropriate fluids for certain circumstances together with the various forms of administration. The reason for this is the intrinsic heterogeneity of the population that is to be treated. In the ideal world, an intravenous feeding regimen would be tailored to the individual patient. However, logistically, this is just not possible for the majority of circumstances and a number of compromises have to be made. Perhaps with the advent of computers and microprocessors it is going to become increasingly easy to calculate an accurate regimen for a patient on the ward in a minimum of time, and transfer this to the pharmacy to allow a regimen to be prepared for each patient each day. Although this may take some time to come about, it is clearly the most satisfactory approach in the long term for the patient who requires parenteral nutrition.

References

1. Randell H. T.: Diet and nutrition in the care of the surgical patient. In: Goodhart R. S., Shils M. E. (ed.): *Modern Nutrition in Health and Disease*. Philadelphia: Lea & Febiger, 1973; 961–5.
2. Bistrian R. B., Blackburn G. L., Halowell H. et al.: Protein status of general surgical patients. *JAMA* 1974; **230**: 858–60.
3. Balta P. J., Ward M. W. M., Tomkins A. M.: Ultrasound for measurement of subcutaneous fat. *Lancet* 1981; **2**: 504–5.
4. Blackburn G. L., Bistrian B. R., Maini B. S. et al.: Nutritional and metabolic assessment of the hospitalised patient. *J. Parent. Enteral. Nutr.* 1977; **1**: 11–22.
5. Michel L., Serrano A., Malt R. A.: Nutritional support of hospitalised patients. *N. Engl. J. Med.* 1981; **304**: 1147–52.
6. Ota D. M., Copeland E. M., Corriere J. N. et al.: The effects of nutrition and treatment of cancer on host immunocompetence. *Surg. Gynecol. Obstet.* 1979; **148**: 104–10.
7. Shetty P. S., Jung R. T., Watrasiewicz K. E. et al.: Rapid-turnover transport proteins: an index of subclinical protein-energy malnutrition. *Lancet* 1979; **2**: 230–2.
8. Bradfield R. B.: A rapid tissue technique for the field assessment of protein calorie malnutrition. *Am. J. Clin. Nutr.* 1972; **25**: 720–9.
9. Jourdan M. H.: Some aspects of protein metabolism in postoperative surgical patients requiring intravenous nutrition. In: Baxter D. H., Jackson G. M. (ed.): *Clinical Parenteral Nutrition*. Chester: Geistlich Education, 1977: 158–68.
10. Editorial: Parenteral nutrition before surgery? *Br. Med. J.* 1979; **2**: 1529–30.
11. Heatley R. V., Williams R. H. P., Lewis M. H.: Preoperative intravenous feeding—a controlled trial. *Postgrad. Med. J.* 1979; **55**: 541–5.
12. Mullen J. L., Buzby G. P., Matthews D. C. et al.: Reduction of operative morbidity and mortality by combined pre-operative and post-operative nutritional support. *Ann. Surg.* 1980; **192**: 604–13.
13. Daly J. M., Dudrick S. J., Copeland E. M.: Intravenous hyperalimentation. Effect on delayed cutanous hypersensitivity in cancer patients. *Ann. Surg.* 1980; **192**: 587–92.
14. Copeland E. M., Dudrick S. J.: Nutritional complications in post-surgical patients. *Am. Surg.* 1981; **47**: 67–71.
15. Fischer J. E., Foster G. S., Abel R. M.: Hyperalimentation as primary therapy for inflammatory bowel disease. *Surgery* 1973; **125**: 165–75.
16. Mullen J. L., Hargrove W. C., Dudrick S. J.: Ten years' experience with hyperalimentation and inflammatory bowel disease. *Ann. Surg.* 1978; **187**: 523–9.
17. Thomas R. J. S., Rosalion A.: The use of parenteral nutrition in the management of external gastrointestinal fistulae. *Aust. NZ J. Surg.* 1978; **48**: 535–9.
18. Soeters P. B., Ebeid A. M., Fischer J. E.: Review of 404 patients with gastrointestinal fistulae: impact of parenteral nutrition. *Ann. Surg.* 1979; **190**: 189–202.
19. Johnston I. D. A.: Parenteral nutrition in the cancer patie t. *J. Human Nutr.* 1979; **33**: 189–96.
20. Copeland E. M., Dudrick S. J.: In: *Current Problems in Cancer*, vol. I. Chicago: Year Book, 1976.
21. Missing B., Bitoun A., Galian A.: Fatty liver during parenteral nutrition. Does it depend upon the amount of calories given as glucose? *Gastroenterol. Clin. Biol.* 1977; **1**: 1015–25.

22. Ashkanazi J., Elwyn D. H., Silverberg P. A. et al.: Respiratory distress secondary to a high carbohydrate load. *Surgery* 1980; **87**: 596–8.
23. Ashkanazi J., Carpentier Y. A., Elwyn D. H. et al.: Influence of total parenteral nutrition on fuel utilization in injury and sepsis. *Ann. Surg.* 1980; **191**: 40–6.
24. Stoner H. B., Little R. A., Gross E. et al.: Metabolic complications of parenteral nutrition. *Acta Chir. Belg.* (In press.) Quoted by Bancewicz J.: Intravenous feeding: Complications, their prevention and management. 2nd European Congress on Parenteral and Enteral Nutrition. *Acta Chir. Scand.* 1981; Suppl. 507: 200–7.
25. Okada A., Itakura T., Kim C. W. et al.: The prospects for amino acid infusion. *Jpn. J. Surg.* 1980; **10**: 353–63.
26. Editorial: Deficiencies in parenteral nutrition. *Br. Med. J.* 1978; **2**: 913–14.
27. Anon: Adult parenteral nutrition: which preparations? *Drug Ther. Bull.* 1980; **18**: 85–8.
28. Wardrop C. A. J., Heatley R. W., Tennant G. P. et al.: Acute folate deficiency in surgical patients on amino acid ethanol intravenous nutrition. *Lancet* 1975; **2**: 640.
29. Ibbotson R. M., Colvin B. T., Colvin M. P.: Folic acid deficiency during intensive therapy. *Br. Med. J.* 1975; **4**: 145–6.
30. Saary M., Hoffbrand A. V.: Folic acid deficiency during intensive therapy. *Br. Med. J.* 1976; **1**: 461.
31. Harvier P., Mallarme J.: Maladie de Biermier à formé hepatomégalique avec pigmentation simulant une cirrhose pigmentaire. *Sang* 1938; **12**: 883–90.
32. Connor H., Preston F. E., Newton D. J. et al.: Oral methionine loading as a cause of acute serum folate deficiency: its relevance to parenteral nutrition. *Postgrad. Med. J.* 1978; **54**: 318–20.
33. Bozetti F.: Long term parenteral nutrition. *Br. Med. J.* 1979; **1**: 487–8.
34. Wretlind A.: Parenteral nutrition. *Surg. Clin. North Am.* 1978; **58**: 1055–70.
35. Editorial: Vitamin C, disease and surgical trauma. *Br. Med. J.* 1979; **1**: 437.
36. Shenkin A., Wretlind A.: Parenteral nutrition. *World Rev. Nutr. Dietet.* 1978; **28**: 1–111.
37. Brocks A., Reid H., Glazer G.: Acute intravenous zinc poisoning. *Br. Med. J.* 1977; **1**: 1390–1.
38. Wolman S. L., Anderson H., Merliss E. B. et al.: Zinc in total parenteral nutrition. Requirements and metabolic effects. *Gastroenterology* 1979; **76**: 458–9.
39. Aggett P. J.: Trace elements in medicine. *Hospital Update* 1979; November: 981–9.
40. Young V. R.: Selenium: a case for its essentiality in man. *N. Engl. J. Med.* 1981; **304**: 1228–30.
41. Johnson R. A., Baker S. S., Fellon J. T. et al.: An occidental case of cardiomyopathy and Selenium deficiency. *N. Engl. J. Med.* 1981; **304**: 1210–12.
42. Special Communication: Guidelines for essential trace element preparations for parenteral use. A statement by an Expert Panel. *JAMA* 1979; **241**: 2051–3.
43. Woolfson A. M. J.: Metabolic considerations in nutritional support. *Res. Clin. Forum* 1979; **1**: 35–7.

Further Recommended Reading

Brennan M. F.: Total parenteral nutrition in the cancer patient. *N. Engl. J. Med.* 1981; **305**: 372–82.
Fischer J. E. (ed.): *Total Parenteral Nutrition.* Boston, Mass.: Little, Brown & Co., 1976.
Grant J. P.: *Handbook of Total Parenteral Nutrition.* Philadelphia: Saunders, 1980.
Johnston I. D. A. (ed.): *Advances in Parenteral Nutrition.* Lancaster: MTP Press, 1978.
Lee H. A. (ed.): *Parenteral Nutrition in Acute Metabolic Illness.* London: Academic Press, 1974.
Moore F. D.: *Metabolic Care of the Surgical Patient.* Philadelphia: Saunders, 1959.
Wretlind A.: Complete intravenous nutrition. *Nutr. Metab.* 1972; **14**: 1–170.
Wright P. D. (ed.): Parenteral and Enteral Nutrition: Proceedings of the symposium for the 2nd European Congress. *Acta Chir. Scand.* 1980; Suppl. 507.

Chapter 20

Techniques for Parenteral Nutrition in the Ambulatory Patient

A. J. Macnab

In the past 12 years, technical improvements and increasing clinical experience have enabled total parenteral nutrition (TPN) to become a reality for the ambulant patient and even to be feasible in a home base setting (1–5). TPN is assuming an increasing clinical relevance in conditions other than chronic gastrointestinal disease— noticeably as an adjunct to cancer therapy (6–8) and in the management of cystic fibrosis (9). Renal dialysis at home has become an established concept, and home-based parenteral nutrition can prove less complex and more immediately attractive (10–12). Some patients have a definite potential for recovery, so that TPN may be dispensed with ultimately after months or years (9, 12, 13).

The potential benefits for the ambulant patient are considerable and the physician must not allow the possible problems to outweigh these advantages. However, the logistics of ambulatory TPN require careful attention in order to balance the benefit/problem ratio adequately (3, 6, 14–16). Centres in Europe and North America have almost 10 years' experience with ambulatory TPN (4, 8–10, 12, 13, 17). The techniques used vary, as does the choice of indwelling catheter, nutrient solutions used and the exact programme of infusion. However, their success depends upon three concepts crucial to ambulatory nutritional care. These are:

1. Careful attention to patient selection.
2. The use of a parenteral nutrition team made up of hospital and family physician, pharmacist, social worker and parenteral nutrition nurse.
3. A portable infusion system.

PATIENT SELECTION

Consider both medical and psychosocial factors. The disease process must warrant the extreme measures of TPN and be unremediable by other treatment entities. The management of patients in the terminal stages of disease is not warranted (16). The patient must be physically and mentally able to participate fully. Motivation is usually high in view of the lack of other treatment alternatives, but encouragement is necessary, although the advantages must always be explained in context with the inconveniences and potential problems entailed. The family must be prepared to become actively involved and take on TPN as a round-the-clock priority (3, 8, 18). The stress for both patient and family cannot be underestimated, and a level of manual dexterity and technical ability are essential if the system is to be maintained adequately. Previous psychiatric disorders may well be enhanced (13, 14). Age need not be a limiting factor—patients from 6 weeks to 66 years have been managed (9, 10).

Hospitalization for TPN is costly in terms of actual expense and psychological disability for the patient. Attempts to cost home TPN involve complex calculations, and figures vary from £40 to £125 per day (10, 13–15). These costs are less when infusion can be intermittent (i.e. 12–14 hours per day). The major justification for this expense is the impressive improvement in well-being reported in the majority of patients, and the definite positive impact of TPN on their management and rehabilitation. The majority of children from active home nutrition programmes attend normal school and take part in recreational activities (9). Many adults contribute actively within the home environment and some have even returned to work (3, 10, 13, 14).

THE AMBULATORY TPN SERVICE TEAM

The function of this team is to select, train, supply and support the ambulant patient around the clock. The activities of the hospital physician, family physician, pharmacist, social worker and TPN nurse are best coordinated by a team nurse. TPN nurses should be ward-based. They must be experienced in the logistics and management of the catheter and delivery system, (3, 6, 16) and will have the closest regular contact with the patients.

The team trains all selected patients at the hospital and supports them in the home (8, 13, 14). This continuity is critical. It is also imperative that there is no deviation from the established protocols by the staff, as this can be both confusing and potentially dangerous to the patient (6). Training must cover every aspect of the TPN system, the daily routine and potential problems. The use of display units to demonstrate the delivery system is helpful (8). A clear step-by-step protocol must be evolved, and discussion with other home-based patients aids the individual and the family during their orientation. Comprehensive written instructions reduce the incidence of complications (9, 12). Training has to be thorough and a mean of 3 weeks should be planned, although some patients have required more than 2 months to become competent (3, 10, 11).

Support services include supplies, technical assistance and psychosocial input (6, 13). In the latter context, the family must be viewed as a whole. A social worker can act effectively as a neutral third party and monitor of morale. The lack of direct technical involvement makes a remarkably frank rapport possible.

Domiciliary nursing care must be on a daily basis to start with (8). The nurse should work through the protocol with the patient to reinforce good habits and supervise dressings and catheter care. Nobody has a keener interest in the asepsis of their system than the patients themselves. Once involved and correctly trained, their motivation is enormous.

An on-call system must be available to allow immediate access to the team. Often, this is best based on the hospital ward. TPN nurses can be scheduled to be on duty and available throughout the day and night to answer questions, check the system and organize any necessary emergency investigation or treatment.

This team concept is vital. As with any form of intensive care, the quality of the personnel involved ultimately dictates the degree of success achieved by the programme.

THE INFUSION SYSTEM

Central venous catheters are now preferred to arteriovenous shunts as a means of circulatory access (3, 8–10). The choice, availability and insertion of these catheters are dealt with in other chapters. The basic components of a portable infusion system are shown in *Fig.* 20.1. Highly individual variations on this design have been described. Advice should be sought from a local biomedical engineering department, as current technical advances mean that modified systems, more sophisticated pumps, newer alarm and monitoring mechanisms and lighter-weight power sources are becoming available.

Infusion may be continuous or intermittent depending upon the needs of the patient. With intermittent infusion the catheters can be flushed after use with a heparinized solution to maintain their patency, and capped with a spigot using a strict sterile technique (8, 11, 13, 15, 18). An impressive range of home-based activity is reported with cyclic infusions. The patient is relatively free of worry and equipment between infusions and there is a low incidence of metabolic reactions. Some patients, however, cannot be maintained on 12–14 hours of infusion per day. A continuous infusion can combine a light-weight, battery-powered infusion system by day, with the convenience and alarm system of a bedside alternating-current-powered unit by night. (19).

Infusion can be achieved by gravity drip or by forced flow. The simplest and cheapest systems use gravity flow and are sometimes satisfactory (15, 18), but pumps are necessary for most ambulant patients, particularly with:

1. The paediatric age group—due to the range of activity and lack of appropriate awareness.

2. Complex programmes where a variety of

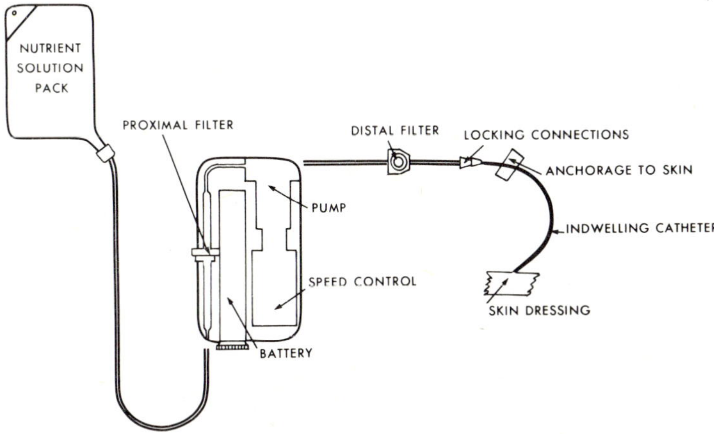

Fig. 20.1. The basic components of a portable infusion system.

fluids is required or intricacies of rate control develop.

Infusion fluid may be propelled either by using external compression of the nutrient pack or by a delivery pump within the system. Scribner and Broviac combined a Holter pump and counterbalanced scale which incorporated an alarm (10). Although portable and operable in the home, this system does not allow the patient to be fully ambulant, and battery life is only a matter of hours. Jeejeebhoy's pneumatic cuff infusion system is relatively bulky, but has advantages of simplicity and a low incidence of problems (13). The 1-litre plastic packs of nutrient solution are placed inside the cuff of the pressure infusor (Fenwall pressure infusor, Baxter; or PAC:300, Cutter). When inflated, this cuff compresses the nutrient pack and the pressure generated within the system infuses fluid via the patient's central vein catheter. A sudden massive infusion is avoided by a screw clamp between the nutrient reservoir and the catheter. The pressure maintained prevents blood flowing back into the catheter even if a delivery tube becomes kinked. Another major advantage is that air cannot enter the system when the infusate is exhausted. The incidence of metabolic sequelae appears less than with intermittent infusions in the 46 patients treated to date (20). Strobel uses an IMED volumetric pump (9). A built-in alarm will stop the infusion if air enters the system, the delivery tube becomes occluded, or the nutrient solution is exhausted. Fleming reports experience with the EPIC pump, which also has alarm facilities (14).

The choice of pump is important. It must be reliable and able to supply fluids accurately over the required range (0·5–12 l/24 h) and incapable of infusing air (11). The pressure generated by the pump must not be so high that it causes leakage from the catheter or connections if flow is obstructed; nor must it be so low that back flow of blood into the catheter is possible. Because pumps are relatively inexpensive patients can be given a spare unit. This allows the unit to be changed immediately in the event of failure and also permits routine servicing (19). The first small pumps were custom-made (21) (*Fig.* 20.2). Many compact units are now commercially available. Flow rates depend upon gearbox ratios, pump chamber diameter and flow resistance. Within the chosen range, flow can be altered by including an adjustable potentiometer within the circuit. Constant motor speed can be maintained at any given setting, and in spite of variation in load or battery voltage, by delivering a higher current in response to an increase on motor load (21).

If the delivery system and nutrient solution are sufficiently compact, they can be carried in pouches on a waist-coat back-pack. The author first designed and used this concept for paediatric work at University College Hospital, London, in conjunction with workers from the Hammersmith Hospital (19) (*Fig.* 20.3), and Dudrick modified it successfully for adults (17).

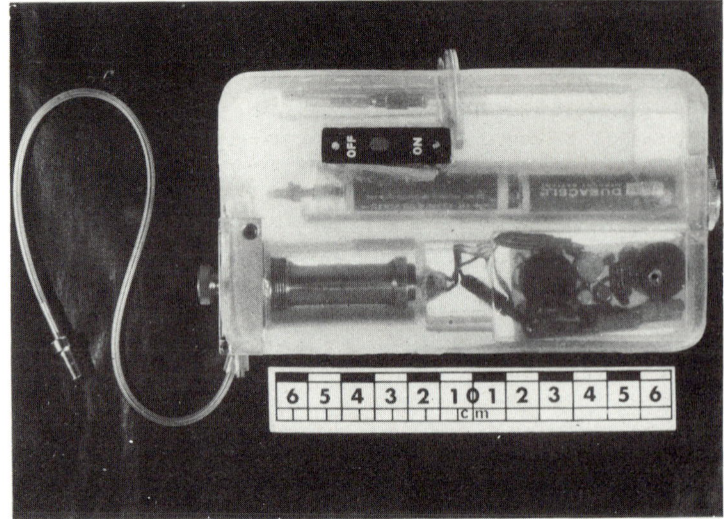

Fig. 20.2. The earliest custom-made portable infusion pump.

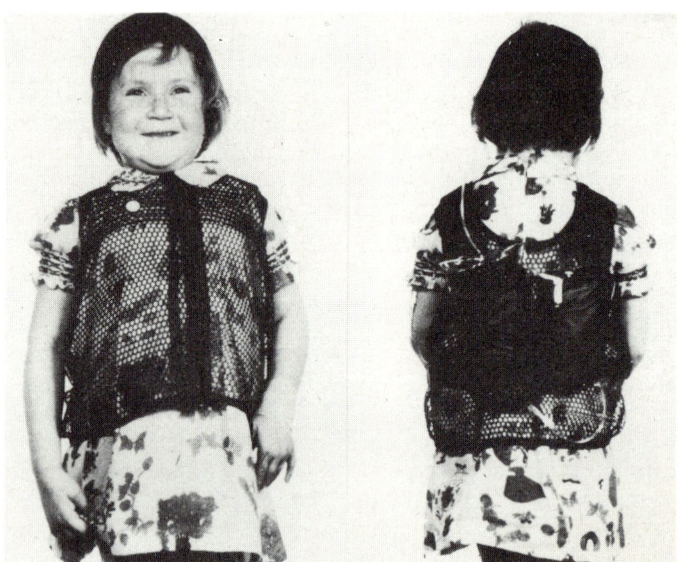

Fig. 20.3. The first vest for use with a portable infusion system.

This has given TPN a genuinely ambulant potential; Dudrick's current pump weighs 13 oz (370 g) and can run for 24 hours on battery power. Rates are set and periodically checked against a detachable meter, which saves weight. The unit is light, custom-fitted to the patient, inexpensive and can be worn over or under conventional clothing.

With gravity drip and pressure infusion systems, regular giving sets can be used (3, 9, 15) provided that locking connectors are chosen (11). Non-kinking tubing should be used whenever possible. Silicone rubber pump chambers and additional connections are necessary with rotary pumps. Some are available commercially; others must be made individually. Connections should be cleansed with a povidone-iodine solution (Betadine) prior to disconnection (3, 18) and should not be taped. Epidemiologic evaluation has implicated use of Elastoplast as a possible cause of bacteraemia related to TPN lines (22).

The nutrient solutions can be packed in 1–3 litre plastic bags (e.g. Fenwall arterio-pak, Baxter). These and similar units are readily available commercially for filling by pharmacy. More specialized bags are used by other centres. Solassol has extended the concept of the artificial gut (8) and uses a Scurasil bag of 3-litre capacity which can be washed, sterilized and refilled (16). A three-speed pump allows a choice of flow rates from a nomogram which plots pump speed against blood pressure (1). Mixed nutrients are infused; this reduces the number of disconnections necessary in the feed-line, and daily infusions run over 8–12 hours. Infusion may thus be diurnal or nocturnal depending upon the wishes of the patient.

Modern alarms can detect air or drained reservoirs in systems infusing clear fluids. More complex devices utilizing ultrasound or thermistor technology are necessary for tinted or opaque solutions. Drop counters detect occluded flow but necessitate an air space within the system. A compact experimental pressure infusor which uses a cartridge of compressed carbon dioxide has been designed. The size and low weight make this attractive and worthy of further development.

It can be seen that various techniques and apparatus have evolved which permit patients to receive TPN without restricting them either to bed or to hospital. The degree of ambulatory potential varies, and equipment of the genuinely ambulant patient is still limited. The ultimate objectives are still to provide independence and comfort for the patients, allow them continuation of their family life and perhaps permit them to resume some form of recreation and occupational activity.

COMPLICATIONS

The problems of ambulatory TPN are similar in range to those seen with the hospitalized patient, but can vary in degree if there is a delay before they receive attention. Problem-solving protocols can prompt appropriate action and minimize the chance of metabolic difficulties (9, 12). An emergency pack enables the catheter to be preserved by means of a flush of heparinized solution under appropriate conditions (8). The ward and TPN nurse provide the necessary advice and treatment back-up. Problems include sepsis, thromboembolism, nutrient deficiency and metabolic disturbance.

The incidence of sepsis need be no higher during home TPN. Infection control can be as thorough, and lack of contact with hospital pathogenic flora is probably a positive advantage. Several years of therapy without catheter-related sepsis have been achieved in home-based groups (14, 20). Thromboembolism occurs less often with modern silicone rubber catheters, but patients with malignant disease appear to have a higher incidence (6). The risk of acute metabolic disturbance is reduced by alarm systems that warn if flow is interrupted and in programmes that reduce infusion rate towards the end of cyclic therapy (3, 9, 14). However, acute glucose intoxication with high infusion rates and endogenous insulin reactions during rapid withdrawal are regularly reported (3, 10, 12). Particulate matter within the solutions can make in-line filters difficult to manage (9, 19).

No TPN system is problem-free, and deaths have occurred during home TPN (15). Some centres have found it difficult to maintain a standardized infusion programme. However, with thorough training, strict surveillance and team support, the domiciliary patient need have no higher incidence of complication than his hospital counterpart.

CONCLUSION

There is no doubt that total parenteral nutrition is an essential component of some medical treatments and can prolong useful life. As Dudrick has recognized, we have been guilty of encouraging some patients to eat, knowing that they probably have neither the appetite nor the digestive capacity (15). Nowadays, with prudent application of parenteral nutrition techniques, we can abandon these meaningless requests and initiate a therapeutic process capable of real physical and mental benefit to the patient. Recent technical advances have added a new dimension to the quality of life for these patients. The ability to be ambulant within the hospital, and even on occasion to be based at home, can enhance patient morale enormously. With a good programme, less then 10 per cent of the ambulant TPN patient's time need be spent in hospital. The freezing of hospital beds and direct involvement of the patient's family are very relevant (12, 14). However, the major incentive should be the opportunity to offer the patient a realistic alternative to chronic malnutrition on the one hand, or permanent hospitalization on the other.

In the United Kingdom, experience of home parenteral nutrition has been limited to a few centres with encouraging early results reported (23). Although the cost of this form of treatment per patient is high, it will have to be provided for only a few patients by the National Health Service. Furthermore, the majority of patients treated in this way have been found to be able to resume feeding by mouth (24).

References

1. Dudrick S. J., MacFadyen B. V., Copeland E. M. et al.: Manni C., Magalini S. I., Scrascia E. (ed.) Experimental aspects of total parenteral nutrition. In: *Total Parenteral Alimentation.* Amsterdam: Excerpta Medica 1976: 3.
2. Scribner B. H. Cole J. J., Christopher T. G.: Long-term total parenteral nutritions: the concept of the artificial gut. *JAMA* 1970; **212**: 457.
3. Shils M. E.: A program for total parenteral nutrition at home. *Am. J. Clin. Nutr.* 1975; **28**: 1429.
4. Miller D. G., Ivey M., Ivey T., et al.: Experience with an indwelling right atrial catheter for home parenteral nutrition. *Surg. Gynecol. Obstet.* 1980; **151**: 108–10.
5. Byrne W. J., Ament M. E., Burke M., et al.: Home parenteral nutrition. *Surg. Gynecol Obstet.* 1979; **149**: 593–9.
6. Dudrick S. J., MacFadyen B. V., Souchon E. A., et al.: Parenteral nutrition techniques in cancer patients. *Cancer Res.* 1977; **37**: 2440.
7. Editorial: Nutrition and the patient with cancer. *Br. Med. J.* 1978; **2**: 846.
8. Solassol C., Joyeux H.: Ambulatory parenteral nutrition. In: Manni C., Magalini S. I., Scrascia E. (ed.) *Total Parenteral Alimentation.* Amsterdam: Excerpta Medica, 1976: 138.
9. Strobel C. T., Byrne W. J., Fonkalsrud E. W. et al.: Home parenteral nutrition: results in 34 pediatric patients. *Ann-Surg.* 1978; **188**: 394.
10. Broviac J. W., Scribner B. H.: Prolonged parenteral nutrition in the home. *Surg. Gynecol. Obstet.* 1974; **139**: 24.
11. Powell-Tuck J., Farwell J. A., Nielsen T. et al.: Team approach to long-term intravenous feeding in patients with gastro-intestinal disorders. *Lancet* 1978; **2**: 825.
12. Rault R. M. J., Scribner B. H.: Treatment of Crohn's disease with home parenteral nutrition. *Gastroenterology* 1977; **72**: 1249.
13. Jeejeebhoy K. N., Langer B., Tsallas G., et al.: Total parenteral nutrition at home: studies in patients surviving 4 months to 5 years. *Gastroenterology* 1976; **71**: 943.
14. Fleming C. R., McGill D. B., Berkner S.: Home parenteral nutrition as primary therapy in patients with extensive Crohn's disease of the small bowel and malnutrition. *Gastroenterology* 1977; **73**: 1077.
15. Ladefoged K., Jarnum S.: Long-term parenteral nutrition. *Br. Med. J.* 1978; **2**: 262.
16. Solassol C., Joyeux H.: Logistic problems of artificial nutrition. *Biomedicine* 1978; **28**: 85.
17. Dudrick S. J., Englert D. M., MacFadyen B. V. et al.: A vest for ambulatory patients receiving hyperalimentation. *Surg. Gynecol. Obstet.* 1979; **148**: 587.
18. Bordos D. C., Cameron J. L.: Successful long-term intravenous hyperalimentation in the hospital and at home. *Arch. Surg.* 1975; **110**: 439.
19. Macnab A. J.: A portable infusion system for the ambulant child. *Paediatr.* 1976; **88**: 654.
20. Jeejeebhoy K. N.: Personal communication. 1979.
21. Ball G., Chenery L., Hemsley, D. et al.: A miniature peristaltic pump with electronic rate control: technical adaptation to a clinical need. *Biomed. Eng. J.* 1974; **9**: 565.
22. Bauer E., Denson P. Infections from contaminated Elastoplast. *N. Engl. J. Med.* 1979; **300**: 370.
23. Milewski R. J., Gross E., Holbrook I. et al.: Parenteral nutrition at home in the management of intestinal failure. *Br. Med. J.* 1980; **281**: 1356–7.
24. Bambach C. P., Lennard–Jones J. et al.: Occasional review—home parenteral nutrition in England and Wales. *Br. Med. J.* 1980; **281**: 1407–9.

Appendix

The following is a list of manufacturers of equipment and products that are mentioned throughout the text. Complementary to it is the list of equipment and manufacturers on p. 00 which relates specifically to the technique of right atrial catheterization described in Chapter 17.

Abbott Laboratories Ltd, Queenborough, Kent ME11 5EL.

B. Braun Melsungen A.G., Carl-Braun Strasse 1, 3508 Melsungen, West Germany.

BDH Chemicals Ltd, Poole, Dorset BH12 4NN.

Baxter and Cutler, England.

Becton, Dickinson UK Ltd, York House, Empire Way, Wembley, Middlesex HA9 0PS.

Bencard, Great West Road, Brentford, Middx TW8 9BD.

C. R. Bard International Ltd, Pennywell Industrial Estate, Sunderland SR4 9EW.

Cambridge Instruments, Melbourn, Royston, Herts SG8 6EJ.

DRG Hospital Supplies, Brislington, Bristol.

Deseret–Messrs Warner-Lambert, University Precinct, Oxford Road, Manchester M13 9QB.

Dow Corning Ltd, Reading Bridge House, Reading RG1 8PW.

Duncan Flockhart & Co. Ltd, Birbeck Street, London E2 6LA.

Edwards Laboratories, AHS (UK) Ltd, Station Road, Didcot, Oxfordshire OX11 7NP.

Evermed, PO Box 296, Medina, Washington 98039, USA.

H. G. Wallace & Co. Ltd, Chandlers Row, Port Lane, Colchester, Essex CO1 2JP.

ICI, Medical Aids Department, Pharmaceutical Division, Alderley Park, Macclesfield, Cheshire.

IVAC Ltd, Ivac House, Bessborough Road, Harrow, Middlesex HA1 3DT.

J. M. Loveridge Ltd, Manufacturing Chemist, Southampton, Hants.

Kabi-Vitrum Ltd, Bilton House, Uxbridge Road, London W5 2TH.

Kifa, Stockholm, Sweden.

May & Baker Ltd, Dagenham, Essex RM10 7XS.

Mead Johnson Ltd, Bristol Labs, Stamford House, Langley, Berks SL3 6EB.

Medishield BOC, Priestley House, Priestley Way, London NW2 7AG.

Portex Ltd, Hythe, Kent CT21 6JL.

Pye Dynamics Ltd, Park Avenue, Bushey, Herts WD2 2BW.

Sage Instruments, 380 Putnam Avenue, Cambridge, Massachusetts 02139, USA.

Sherwood Medical Industries Ltd, Sherwood House, London Road, Crawley RH10 2TA.

Smiths, Workington, Cumbria.

Sonicaid Ltd, Bognor Regis, Sussex.

Sorensen Research Co., 4387 Atherton Drive, Salt Lake City, Utah 84115, USA.

Steriseal Ltd, Redditch, Worcestershire.

Stille-Werner (UK) Ltd, 24 York Road, Maidenhead, Berkshire SL6 1SF.

Stuart Pharmaceuticals Ltd, Carr House, Carrs Road, Cheadle, Cheshire SK8 2EG.

T. J. Smith & Nephew Ltd, Bessemer Road, Welwyn Garden City, Herts AL7 1HF.

Tekmar Medical Ltd, 57A Milton Trading Estate, Nr Abingdon, Oxon OX14 4RX.

Travenol Laboratories Ltd, Caxton Way, Thetford, Norfolk IP24 3SE.

USV Pharmaceutical Corp., 1 Scarsdale Road, Tuckahoe, New York 10707, USA.

Van Leer Verpackungen, 784 Mullheim/Baden, POB 84, West Germany.

Vickers Ltd, Medical Engineering, Priestley Road, Basingstoke, Hants RG24 9NP.

Viggo, Isis Trading Estate, Stratton Road, Swindon SN1 2PT.

Vygon (UK) Ltd, Eskdale Road, Uxbridge, Middlesex UB8 2RT.

Watson-Marlow Ltd, Falmouth, Cornwall TR11 4RU.

Weddell Pharmaceuticals Ltd, Salisbury House, London Wall, London WC2M 5XD.

Index